T0383308

ANXIETY IN CHILDREN AND ADOLESCENTS WITH AUTISM SPECTRUM DISORDER

ANXIETY IN CHILDREN AND ADOLESCENTS WITH AUTISM SPECTRUM DISORDER

Evidence-Based Assessment and Treatment

Edited by

CONNOR M. KERNS
Drexel University, Philadelphia, PA, United States

PATRICIA RENNO
University of California, Los Angeles, CA, United States

ERIC A. STORCH
University of South Florida, Tampa, FL, United States

PHILIP C. KENDALL
Temple University, Philadelphia, PA, United States

JEFFREY J. WOOD
University of California, Los Angeles, CA, United States

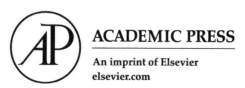

ACADEMIC PRESS

An imprint of Elsevier
elsevier.com

ELSEVIER

Academic Press is an imprint of Elsevier
125 London Wall, London EC2Y 5AS, United Kingdom
525 B Street, Suite 1800, San Diego, CA 92101-4495, United States
50 Hampshire Street, 5th Floor, Cambridge, MA 02139, United States
The Boulevard, Langford Lane, Kidlington, Oxford OX5 1GB, United Kingdom

Copyright © 2017 Elsevier Inc. All rights reserved.

No part of this publication may be reproduced or transmitted in any form or by any means, electronic or
mechanical, including photocopying, recording, or any information storage and retrieval system, without
permission in writing from the publisher. Details on how to seek permission, further information about the
Publisher's permissions policies and our arrangements with organizations such as the Copyright Clearance
Center and the Copyright Licensing Agency, can be found at our website: www.elsevier.com/permissions.

This book and the individual contributions contained in it are protected under copyright by the Publisher
(other than as may be noted herein).

Notices
Knowledge and best practice in this field are constantly changing. As new research and experience broaden
our understanding, changes in research methods, professional practices, or medical treatment may become
necessary.

Practitioners and researchers must always rely on their own experience and knowledge in evaluating and
using any information, methods, compounds, or experiments described herein. In using such information or
methods they should be mindful of their own safety and the safety of others, including parties for whom they
have a professional responsibility.

To the fullest extent of the law, neither the Publisher nor the authors, contributors, or editors, assume any
liability for any injury and/or damage to persons or property as a matter of products liability, negligence or
otherwise, or from any use or operation of any methods, products, instructions, or ideas contained in the
material herein.

British Library Cataloguing-in-Publication Data
A catalogue record for this book is available from the British Library

Library of Congress Cataloging-in-Publication Data
A catalog record for this book is available from the Library of Congress

ISBN: 978-0-12-805122-1

For Information on all Academic Press publications
visit our website at https://www.elsevier.com

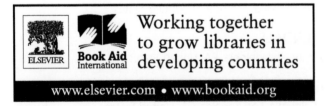

Working together
to grow libraries in
developing countries

www.elsevier.com • www.bookaid.org

Publisher: Nikki Levy
Acquisition Editor: Emily Ekle
Editorial Project Manager: Barbara Makinster
Production Project Manager: Nicky Carter
Designer: Matthew Limbert

To Mike, Finn, Rebecca and Graham
Connor M. Kerns

To Sue and Paul Renno
Patricia Renno

With love to Maya, Noah, Ellie, and Jill
Eric A. Storch

For all of the youth and their families who have
contributed to our knowledge and our ability to
provide improved services through their
participation in research
Philip C. Kendall

This book is dedicated to my two sons,
Jonah and Elliott, the two sweetest boys
I could ever have imagined
Jeffrey J. Wood

CONTENTS

Future Directions and Applications   117
References   118

7. **Individual CBT for Anxiety and Related Symptoms
    in Children With Autism Spectrum Disorders   123**
    Jeffrey J. Wood, Sami Klebanoff, Patricia Renno, Cori Fujii
    and John Danial

    Use of Unproven Treatments by Parents and Professionals   125
    Summary of EBT Classification System   126
    Method   126
    Results   127
    Discussion   136
    References   138

8. **Group Cognitive Behavior Therapy for Children
    and Adolescents With Anxiety and
    Autism Spectrum Disorders   143**
    Judy Reaven and Kirsten Willar

    Introduction   143
    Group Treatment for Youth With ASD—Initial Focus   145
    Determining Treatment Focus—Social Skills or Anxiety-Based Interventions?   146
    Group Therapy for Anxiety in Youth With ASD   147
    Challenges/Recommendations for Conducting Group Therapy With Youth
    With ASD and Anxiety   150
    Summary   164
    Future Directions   164
    Acknowledgments   165
    References   165

9. **Behavioral Treatments for Anxiety in Adults With Autism
    Spectrum Disorder   171**
    Susan W. White, Caitlin M. Conner and Brenna B. Maddox

    Introduction   171
    Prevalence and Clinical Presentation   171
    Evidence-Informed Assessment of Anxiety in Adults With ASD   174
    Targeting Key Mechanisms   177
    Basic Processes Underlying Anxiety in ASD   177

LIST OF CONTRIBUTORS

Mary Baker-Ericzén
Child & Adolescent Services Research Center, San Diego, CA, United States;
Rady Children's Hospital, San Diego, CA, United States

Lauren Brookman-Frazee
Child & Adolescent Services Research Center, San Diego, CA, United States;
University of California, San Diego, CA, United States

Colby Chlebowski
Child & Adolescent Services Research Center, San Diego, CA, United States;
University of California, San Diego, CA, United States

Caitlin M. Conner
University of Colorado School of Medicine, Aurora, CO, United States

John Danial
University of California, Los Angeles, CA, United States

Thompson E. Davis
Louisiana State University, Baton Rouge, LA, United States

James P. Donnelly
Institute for Autism Research, Canisius College, Buffalo, NY, United States

Amy Drahota
Michigan State University, East Lansing, MI, United States; Child & Adolescent
Services Research Center, San Diego, CA, United States

Cori Fujii
University of California, Los Angeles, CA, United States

Louis P. Hagopian
Kennedy Krieger Institute, Baltimore, MD, United States; Johns Hopkins
University School of Medicine, Baltimore, MD, United States

John D. Herrington
The Children's Hospital of Philadelphia, Philadelphia, PA, United States;
University of Pennsylvania, Philadelphia, PA, United States

Maysa M. Kaskas
Louisiana State University, Baton Rouge, LA, United States

Philip C. Kendall
Temple University, Philadelphia, PA, United States

Rachel Kent
Institute of Psychiatry, Psychology & Neuroscience, London, United Kingdom

Connor M. Kerns
Drexel University, Philadelphia, PA, United States

Sami Klebanoff
University of California, Los Angeles, CA, United States

Matthew D. Lerner
Stony Brook University, Stony Brook, NY, United States

Karen Levine
Harvard Medical School, Lexington, MA, United States

Megan Lilly
Louisiana State University, Baton Rouge, LA, United States

Christopher Lopata
Institute for Autism Research, Canisius College, Buffalo, NY, United States

Brenna B. Maddox
The Children's Hospital of Philadelphia, Philadelphia, PA, United States

Iliana Magiati
National University of Singapore, Singapore

Judith S. Miller
The Children's Hospital of Philadelphia, Philadelphia, PA, United States;
University of Pennsylvania, Philadelphia, PA, United States

Lauren J. Moskowitz
St. John's University, Queens, NY, United States

Ann Ozsivadjian
Guy's and St. Thomas Foundation Trust, London, United Kingdom

Valentina Parma
Scuola Internazionale Superiore di Studi Avanzati, Trieste, Italy

Judy Reaven
University of Colorado Anschutz Medical Campus School of Medicine, Aurora,
CO, United States; Children's Hospital Colorado, Aurora, CO, United States

Patricia Renno
University of California, Los Angeles, CA, United States

Tamara Rosen
Stony Brook University, Stony Brook, NY, United States

Paige M. Ryan
Louisiana State University, Baton Rouge, LA, United States

Emily Simonoff
Institute of Psychiatry, Psychology & Neuroscience, London, United Kingdom

Nicole Stadnick
Child & Adolescent Services Research Center, San Diego, CA, United States;
University of California, San Diego, CA, United States

Eric A. Storch
University of South Florida, Tampa, FL, United States

Marcus L. Thomeer
Institute for Autism Research, Canisius College, Buffalo, NY, United States

Susan W. White
Virginia Tech, Blacksburg, VA, United States

Kirsten Willar
University of Colorado Anschutz Medical Campus School of Medicine, Aurora, CO, United States; Children's Hospital Colorado, Aurora, CO, United States

Jeffrey J. Wood
University of California, Los Angeles, CA, United States

CHAPTER 1

Introduction

Connor M. Kerns[1], Patricia Renno[2], Eric A. Storch[3],
Philip C. Kendall[4] and Jeffrey J. Wood[2]
[1]Drexel University, Philadelphia, PA, United States
[2]University of California, Los Angeles, CA, United States
[3]University of South Florida, Tampa, FL, United States
[4]Temple University, Philadelphia, PA, United States

Anxiety has been discussed within the context of autism spectrum disorder (ASD) since Kanner and Asperger's initial accounts of autism, in the
descriptions of ASD in the Diagnostic and Statistical Manual (DSM), and
in the burgeoning research on the prevalence, presentation, and treatment
of ASD that has emerged over the last decade. Kanner (1943) noted high
levels of anxiety in several of his case studies. For example, he described
one child as being "very timid, fearful of various and changing things,
wind, large animals, etc." (p. 228). Another child displayed "...a good
deal of 'worrying.' He frets when the bread is put in the oven to be made
into toast, and is afraid it will get burned and be hurt..." (p. 233).
Criteria for ASD in the DSM over the last several editions have included
symptoms that often overlap with anxiety (e.g., adherence to rituals, difficulties with minor changes in routine). Recent research provides evidence
that anxiety disorders affect approximately 40–50% of children with ASD
(van Steensel et al., 2011) and cause substantial distress and impairment
over and above that caused by ASD alone (Bellini, 2004; Chang et al.,
2012; Sukhodolsky et al., 2008).

Although anxiety has been consistently noted in ASD, efforts to
understand and explain the role and significance of this cooccurrence are
more recent. Cooccurrence of psychological disorders is common and yet
there is something particular about the relationship of anxiety in ASD.
Anxiety is more prevalent in ASD than other developmental and learning
disorders. Further, anxiety is both independent and distinguishable from
core ASD deficits and also influenced by and influential to them (Kerns
and Kendall, 2012). The relationship of ASD and anxiety may thus teach
us much about the underlying etiology and maintenance of these psychological conditions and the increased functional impairments related to

Anxiety in Children and Adolescents with Autism Spectrum Disorder.
DOI: http://dx.doi.org/10.1016/B978-0-12-805122-1.00001-6
© 2017 Elsevier Inc.
All rights reserved.
1

their cooccurence. The study of anxiety in ASD may demonstrate neurobiological and behavioral patterns associated with comorbidity generally but also elucidate patterns specific to the cooccurrence of these particular symptoms. Further, recent research has indicated that anxiety is a valid treatment target among children with ASD based on emerging genetic, psychophysiological, and psychometric evidence. As a result of the increased awareness of the prevalence and impact of anxiety on individuals with ASD, several interventions have been developed and tested and found to be efficacious in treating anxiety in ASD.

This book begins with chapters focusing on the nature of ASD and anxiety cooccurrence. Authors delve into the current literature on the prevalence, presentation, and underlying mechanisms of anxiety in ASD. These chapters highlight classical presentations of anxiety in youth with ASD, as well as, more ambiguous presentations, the correct diagnostic classification of which is unclear. Additional chapters discuss recent research findings on neurobiological mechanisms underlying anxiety in ASD.

Chapters are then devoted to discussion of assessment and treatment of anxiety in ASD, with several chapters on evidence-based practices. Basic cognitive behavioral therapy principles are introduced as well as how this treatment approach can be applied to children and youth with ASD. Authors review the existing literature on the efficacy of individual and group CBT therapies for anxiety in ASD. Further, authors describe individual and group CBT approaches that have been employed in successful treatment programs and provide case studies to exemplify how these types of interventions can be implemented by clinicians to treat anxiety in youth with ASD. Chapters detailing psychosocial treatment have a pragmatic flavor to them allowing the reader to apply skills and techniques immediately. Particular attention is also given to treatment considerations for symptoms related to anxiety in ASD that can complicate case conceptualization, treatment planning, and implementation.

Further chapters include preliminary findings and future research directions related to the treatment of anxiety in individuals with ASD. These sections are devoted to the assessment and treatment of anxiety in adults and minimally verbal children. There is also a chapter on school-related issues that are relevant for youth with anxiety and ASD. Topics include how anxiety can manifest and interfere in the school setting and discussion of accommodations and supports that can be employed in the school for anxious children on the spectrum. Lastly, there is a chapter on the use of evidence-based psychosocial treatments for anxiety in youth with ASD in the community. It discusses current efforts to disseminate psychosocial approaches and future directions for implementing psychosocial treatments to treat anxiety and related conditions in children and youth with ASD in the community.

This edited book covers broad ground and targets the scientist, the clinician, and those who combine these disciplines in their daily work. It provides reviews of literature, covering topics such as the prevalence, etiology, presentation, and assessment of anxiety in ASD with chapters submitted from leaders in the field. This compilation combines scientific richness and evidence with clinical "how to's" and practical illustrations and suggestions. The chapters cover newly developing areas and areas of important future research and clinical practice. There should be something in this book for all those who support individuals with ASD in their lives and careers and who wonder about the essential nature of social development and cognition and its connectedness with mental health, quality of life and well-being. Further, we see this book as a medium to deliver the scientific literature to those outside of academia who nonetheless want to know as much as they can know, know what has been tested, and offer treatments and approaches that can be expected to have an impact on the lives of individuals with ASD.

This edited book provides the current state of knowledge of the presentation, assessment, and treatment of anxiety in ASD, but there are future research directions that the authors note in their chapters. Of considerable importance is the need for further research in the assessment and treatment of anxiety in under-represented subpopulations on the autism spectrum, including individuals who are minimally verbal, individuals with intellectual disability and adults. The majority of the current assessment and treatment research has been conducted in school-age children with average intellectual abilities. Additionally, with research demonstrating the efficacy of individual and group treatment approaches for anxiety in ASD, further research on how these treatments can be successfully disseminated and implemented in the community is needed.

Anxiety disorders in children and adolescents with ASD have been rigorously studied over the last decade and continue to receive considerable attention. Explicit studies of anxiety in ASD have increased our knowledge of the prevalence, presentation, assessment and treatment of these constructs and their connectedness. Further, this research suggests that regardless of how it is conceptualized or what it is called, anxiety plays a role in the long-term development, functioning and well-being of individuals with ASD and their families. Moreover, it may provide a gateway to global improvements for individuals and their families.

REFERENCES

Bellini, S., 2004. Social skill deficits and anxiety in high-functioning adolescents with autism spectrum disorders. Focus Autism Other Dev. Disabil. 19, 78–86. Available from: http://dx.doi.org/10.1177/10883576040190020201.

Chang, Y., Quan, J., Wood, J.J., 2012. Effects of anxiety disorder severity on social functioning in children with autism spectrum disorders. J. Dev. Phys. Disabil. 24, 235–245. Available from: http://dx.doi.org/10.1007/s10882-012-9268-2.

Kanner, L., 1943. Autistic disturbances of affective contact. Pathology217–250.

Kerns, C.M., Kendall, P.C., 2012. The presentation and classification of anxiety in autism spectrum disorder. Clin. Psychol. 19 (4), 323–347. Available from: http://dx.doi.org/10.1111/cpsp.12009.

Sukhodolsky, D.G., Scahill, L., Gadow, K.D., Arnold, L.E., Aman, M.G., McDougle, C.J., et al., 2008. Parent-rated anxiety symptoms in children with pervasive developmental disorders: frequency and association with core autism symptoms and cognitive functioning. J. Abnorm. Child Psychol. 36, 117, 117. doi:10.1007/s10802-007-9165-9.

van Steensel, F.J., Bögels, S.M., Perrin, S., 2011. Anxiety disorders in children and adolescents with autistic spectrum disorders: a meta-analysis. Clin. Child Fam. Psychol. Rev. 14, 302–317. Available from: http://dx.doi.org/10.1007/s10567-011-0097-0.

CHAPTER 2

Prevalence of Anxiety in Autism Spectrum Disorders

Rachel Kent and Emily Simonoff
Institute of Psychiatry, Psychology & Neuroscience, London, United Kingdom

AUTISM SPECTRUM DISORDER

Autism spectrum disorder (ASD) is a developmental disorder characterized by qualitative impairments in social interaction and social communication such as difficulties in engaging in normal reciprocal conversation and difficulties understanding relationships in addition to a pattern of restricted interests and repetitive or stereotyped behavior such as an insistence on sameness. Recent estimates of the prevalence of ASD from the Centers for Disease Control and Prevention indicate that ASD occurs in as many as one in 68 people and is about 4.5 times more common among boys than girls (Christensen et al., 2016).

The most recent revision of the classification of psychiatric disorders, the Diagnostic and Statistical Manual, Fifth Edition (DSM-5; American Psychological Association, 2013) collapsed under the single term "autism spectrum disorder" a number of diagnostic entities that had been differentiated in the previous classifications (the Diagnostic and Statistical Manual, Fourth Edition (DSM-IV) and the International Classification of Disease, 10th Edition (ICD-10)). These included: autistic disorder, Asperger's disorder (also known as Asperger syndrome), pervasive developmental disorder not otherwise specified (PDD-NOS), and atypical autism. Research involving any of these categorical disorders will be covered in this chapter and referred to as ASD unless results specifically address differences between previous diagnostic subgroups.

Individuals with ASD vary widely in their presentation of autistic symptoms, cognitive and language abilities, and the additional co-occurring disorders they experience. Other neurodevelopmental disorders including intellectual disability (e.g., Dykens and Lense, 2011), dyspraxia (e.g., Dziuk et al., 2007), and language impairment (e.g., Loucas et al., 2008) are increased in ASD, as is epilepsy. People with ASD also have

Anxiety in Children and Adolescents with Autism Spectrum Disorder.
DOI: http://dx.doi.org/10.1016/B978-0-12-805122-1.00002-8
© 2017 Elsevier Inc.
All rights reserved.
5

elevated rates of a range of psychiatric disorders compared to the general population (de Bruin et al., 2007; Mukaddes and Fateh, 2010; Simonoff et al., 2008). One of these frequently co-occurring psychiatric disorders with ASD is anxiety.

ANXIETY

Anxiety disorders embrace a constellation of conditions marked by subjective experiences of worry or fear. Such symptoms are part of normal experience and should only be considered indicative of an anxiety disorder when they are sufficiently frequent or severe to cause sustained and high levels of distress and/or impairment in everyday functioning. Classification systems subsume under anxiety a number of different disorders and, in general, the same criteria are used to classify anxiety disorders among people with ASD as in the general population. In this chapter, we will largely refer to disorders as described under DSM-IV, as much of the relevant research uses this system. This review summarizes the prevalence of anxiety disorders in aggregate and provides an overview of the prevalence rates for individual disorders.

The main changes between DSM-IV and DSM-5 are that obsessive compulsive disorder (OCD) and posttraumatic stress disorder (PTSD) are now included in domains other than anxiety. In addition, for agoraphobia, specific phobia, and social anxiety disorder (used interchangeably with social phobia) it is no longer necessary for the individual to recognize their anxiety as being excessive or unreasonable. Agoraphobia can also now be diagnosed as a distinct disorder without panic disorder. Finally, the diagnostic criteria for separation anxiety disorder no longer require an onset before 18 years of age.

PREVALENCE OF ANXIETY DISORDERS IN THE GENERAL POPULATION

Children and adolescents. A review of general population prevalence studies found rates in children and adolescents to vary widely depending on methodological differences, including the assessment period; prevalence rates for any anxiety disorder ranged from 2.2–8.6% in studies measuring the prevalence over three month periods, to 5.5–7.7% over a six-month period, 8.6–20.9% over a 12-month period, and 8.3–27% for lifetime prevalence (Costello et al., 2005). A systematic review (1980–2004) also found lifetime prevalence (16.6%) of any anxiety disorder to be higher than the 12-month prevalence (10.6%); in this review social anxiety disorder (4.5%), specific phobia (3%), and generalized anxiety disorder (GAD; 2.6%) were the most common anxiety disorders and OCD (0.54%), panic disorder (0.99%), and agoraphobia (1.6%) were less common (Somers et al., 2006).

Adults. In a U.S. population-representative study of adults the 12-month prevalence rate of DSM-IV anxiety disorders was 18.1% and the lifetime prevalence was 28.8% (Kessler et al., 2005; Kessler et al., 2005). In contrast, a population study in Europe found a 12-month prevalence of 6.4% and lifetime prevalence of 13.6% (Alonso et al., 2004). For the 12-month prevalence, across both samples of adults, specific phobia (8.7%; 3.5%) was the most prevalent, followed by social anxiety disorder (6.8%; 1.2%). GAD (3.1%; 1.0%) and panic disorder (2.7%) were also common whereas separation anxiety (0.9%), OCD (1.0%), and agoraphobia (0.8%; 0.4%) were the least frequent (Alonso et al., 2004; Kessler et al., 2005). A general finding, for both youth and adult populations, is the higher rate of anxiety disorders in females with a ratio of around 1.5:1 (Alonso et al., 2004; Costello et al., 2005).

Prevalence in individuals with intellectual disability (ID). In considering the rates of anxiety disorders in people with ASD, it is helpful to contrast these with rates reported for those with ID. About half the ASD population also have ID (Charman et al., 2011). ID may both constitute a risk factor for anxiety disorders and also a barrier to its detection as people with ID may have more difficulty communicating the subjective experiences and cognitions that underpin diagnosis.

Children and adolescents. In a UK national sample, Emerson and Hatton (2007) defined ID by parent- and teacher-reported significant learning problems and found a point prevalence of any impairing anxiety disorder was 11.4% compared to 3.2% in those without ID. Consistent with this, Dekker and Koot (2003) assessed Dutch children attending schools for individuals with ID and reported that for 12-month prevalence rates 21.9% of the children met the criteria for an anxiety disorder with 10.5% having a significant level of impairment. Across studies, specific phobia (2.0%; 6.8%), separation anxiety (2.7%; 1.9%), GAD (1.6%), and social anxiety disorder (1.9%) were the most common (Dekker and Koot, 2003; Emerson and Hatton, 2007).

Adults. In a population sample of adults with ID, the point prevalence of any DSM-IV anxiety disorder was 2.4% (Reid et al., 2011); GAD was the most common (1.3%), and other disorders had very low rates (agoraphobia, 0.2%; panic disorder, 0.2%; social anxiety disorder, 0.1%). In a randomly selected sample of adults with moderate to profound ID the DSM-IV prevalence of any anxiety disorder was similar at 3.3%; 2.5% met criteria for specific phobia, and 0.8% for agoraphobia without panic (Bailey, 2007).

ANXIETY IN ASD

The co-occurrence of anxiety symptoms in ASD has been noted since the first descriptions of the condition by Leo Kanner (1943) and Hans Asperger (see Frith, 1991), both of whom observed that the children they described were fearful of both common and unusual or novel situations and objects as well as presenting with high levels of generalized worry, fear of social encounters, and obsessionality. Despite these early observations, there still remain a number of challenges, both conceptual and methodological, to the accurate diagnosis of anxiety disorders in people with ASD.

Conceptual considerations. First, there is a lack of consensus on what constitutes gold standard measures of anxiety in ASD and whether these measures should take account possible differences in the manifestation of symptoms in the ASD population. While there is general agreement that assessments need to distinguish the superficial similarities of core ASD symptoms where they overlap, e.g., social avoidance versus social anxiety, repetitive, stereotyped language versus reassurance-seeking, there is presently no agreement whether anxiety symptom definitions and/or criteria should be modified in ASD. Second, many people with ASD experience difficulties with emotional literacy and may find it difficult to express emotions. In assessing internal experiences, this leads to using informants, rather than self-reports, who are often inferring internal states based on contextual cues and other suppositions. Third, among those with more significant levels of ID, it is uncertain how to conceptualize the cognitive components of anxiety, including worry and anticipatory fear. Currently, as there are no reliable and valid biomarkers for anxiety, these issues remain unresolved.

Methodological considerations. A number of methodological considerations may influence the findings, and the most important ones are considered below.

Implementing diagnostic criteria and clinical thresholds. Diagnostic classification systems are designed primarily to assist clinicians in determining which condition(s) apply to patients presenting with psychiatric disorder. While these systems indicate which symptoms are subsumed under different disorders, they give much less guidance with respect to the operationalization into research criteria and how these should be applied in epidemiological studies. Diagnostic assessments ordinarily require the use of a psychiatric interview but these vary in mode administration (structured/semi-structured), the definitions of individual symptoms, and the application of diagnostic algorithms. Diagnostic assessments vary in whether they include a measure of functional impairment, and whether this is applied implicitly or later, more explicitly, in the diagnostic process. These methodological problems are pervasive in psychiatry research and not limited to studies in people with ASD but are likely an important contributor to variability across studies.

Sample ascertainment. The most accurate prevalence estimates will be obtained from studies that use epidemiological methods to derive samples that either include the entire population of interest (target population) or are randomly selected from this population. These methods of complete ascertainment require that the target population can be accurately identified and, for selected groups, this can be a time-consuming aspect of research. Many studies in ASD use other methods to identify the population of interest, leading to incomplete ascertainment. These may involve health registers, clinic or special school populations, and volunteer samples. All have the potential to deliver biased findings and it is often difficult to judge the degree of inaccuracy. As a general principle, ascertainment from more selected samples, particularly where the selection is associated with the area of interest, is more likely to be biased.

Control groups. Control or comparison groups refer to an additional sample of participants that may help to contextualize the findings reported for the target population. However the selection of control groups raises questions about whether to match or control for certain features when drawing comparisons. In ASD, such features might include the high proportion of affected males and the relatively lower IQ. There is no clear scientific consensus on how best to select control groups or account for sample differences in analysis, although "matching" eliminates the possibility of exploring in analysis the effect of that characteristic. Comparison groups should be assessed in a manner that is similar, if not identical, to the target population. Sometimes, comparisons are made with published normative data; in such cases, the applicability of these norms to the population from which ASD participants were drawn should be carefully considered.

Informants. In assessing psychiatric status among adults, self-reports are the most common source of information. Among youth and people with ASD and/or ID, however, a variety of different informants may be used, including self, parent/carer, and teacher. The agreement among these different informants is limited, however, with a meta-analysis reporting only a modest correlation between self-report and other informants (0.22 and 0.28) on questionnaire measures of behavioral and emotional problems (Achenbach et al., 1987; Rey et al., 1992).

Comer and Kendall (2004) found parent–child agreement for symptoms was better than agreement at the diagnostic level for three anxiety disorders measured using a diagnostic interview. Agreement between parent and child has also been found to be higher on reports of conduct or behavioral problems (0.51) than anxiety, fear, and obsessions (0.17; Edelbrock et al., 1986).

Inconsistency across informants may reflect actual variation in psychopathology across situations, failure of an informant to detect or endorse psychopathology, or other factors that affect the ability to respond accurately (Grills and Ollendick, 2003). Younger children are known to have comprehension difficulties with questions about psychopathology (Breton et al., 1995) and these may apply to older children and adults with ASD. The gold standard for research-level diagnoses is to use multiple informant data but it is not always possible in ASD as youth populations may not be able to complete a psychiatric interview.

Period of assessment. Prevalence estimates refer to the presence of a disorder during a particular time period, typically either "current" or lifetime. The duration of the current period may vary, usually between the last month and the last year, but this variation can have a considerable impact on prevalence rates especially for disorders that remit and recur.

Methods of assessment. Structured or semi-structured interviews, which vary in the degree of structure applied and extent to which the interviewer probes and makes judgments, are the gold standard for psychiatric diagnoses. Interviews allow clinicians or researchers to request additional information when symptoms are unclear. While questionnaire measures have been used to report psychopathology, even when validated cut-offs are available, these are considered inferior to interview measures and ordinarily would be used for screening rather than diagnostic purposes, especially when applied at the individual clinical level. In population studies, they have the advantage of ease of administration and may be useful in providing indicative prevalence rates, although these should always be viewed with caution.

PREVALENCE RATES OF ANXIETY IN ASD

In order to review the most reliable and valid data on the prevalence of anxiety disorders in ASD, only studies using diagnostic interviews that apply specific DSM or ICD criteria will be used. The studies' methodological characteristics are summarized in Table 2.1 and the prevalence rates of both aggregate and specific anxiety disorders are shown in Table 2.2. In total 17 studies used clinical interviews to assess anxiety disorders in ASD. The majority ($N = 12$) focused on children and adolescents and only four studies examined prevalence in adults. Maddox and White (2015) looked only at social anxiety in a sample of adolescents and adults.

Prevalence of any anxiety disorder. In a population cohort of children with PDD or a statement of special educational needs, Simonoff et al. (2008) found a 3-month prevalence of 42% for any anxiety disorder. In contrast, the community sample used by Salazar et al. (2015) reported a 3-month prevalence of 78.9%; however, the interview used in this study is known to produce relatively high rates of disorders (see Egger and Angold, 2006). Mattila et al. (2010) directly compared recruitment strategies and period prevalence; using a sample of children with Asperger Syndrome (AS) or high-functioning autism (HFA), they found rates of 45% and 58%, respectively for current and lifetime prevalence among those who were clinically referred compared to rates of 39% and 50% among those recruited from the community.

There is consensus among the 12 studies that the proportion of children and adolescents with ASD and one or more anxiety disorders is high. The majority of studies report a prevalence rate of around 50%, although some, such as Mukaddes et al. (2010) and Salazar et al. (2015), report levels as high as 78% and 79%, respectively. The variability in rates is likely due to the methodological differences highlighted. Overall prevalence estimates range from 42% to 79%, which is considerably higher than rates reported in the general or ID population of children and adolescents (e.g., Costello et al., 2005; Dekker and Koot, 2003).

Tables 2.1 and 2.2 categorize the reviewed studies into child/adolescent and adult samples, although some overlap does occur in the younger samples extending up to 20 years old (Green et al., 2000; Mukaddes and Fateh, 2010) whereas the adult sample used by Hofvander et al. (2009) included participants from 16 years old. The lifetime prevalence rates of any anxiety disorder among adults with ASD who had been recruited from clinical samples ranged from 50% to 59%. These rates are substantially

Table 2.1 Table presenting the sample characteristics and measurement instruments used for studies assessing the prevalence of anxiety in ASD using diagnostic interviews

Study	# ASD	Control group	Age	Ability level[a]	Gender; % males	Diagnosis of ASD	Sampling technique (ASD)	Anxiety measure
Children and adolescents								
Population studies								
Simonoff et al. (2008)	112	–	M = 11.5 R = 10–13.9	M = 72.7 SD = 21.6 R = 19–124	88%	Clinical consensus diagnosis (ICD-10 criteria) informed by ADOS & ADI-R	Population cohort (56,946) of children with PDD diagnosis or Statement of Special Educational Needs	CAPA; Parent report
Community samples								
Matrila et al. (2010)	50	–	M = 12.7 SD = 1.5 R = 9.8–16.3	FSIQ > 75	76%	ADI-R, ADOS & ASSQ	Combination of community sample (n = 18) and a clinic study (n = 32)	K-SADS; Parent and self-report
Leyfer et al. (2006)	109	–	M = 9.2 SD = 2.7 R = 5.1–17	M = 82.6 SD = 23.4 R = 42–141	94%	ADI-R, ADOS & DSM-IV-TR criteria	Two previous samples. Not clinically referred.	ACI; Parent report
Salazar et al. (2015)	101	–	M = 6.7 SD = 1.1 R = 4.5–9.3	M = 66.4 SD = 28 R = 19–120	56%	ADI-R, 3di, DISCO, ADOS	Population sample living in either of two London boroughs with an ASD diagnosis	PAPA; Parent report
Clinic samples								
de Bruin et al. (2007)	94	–	M = 8.5 SD = 1.9 R = 6–12	M = 91.2 SD = 17.4 R = 55–120	88%	PDD-NOS research criteria. ADOS on 93.6% of the children.	Consecutive referrals (2 years); outpatients of child and adolescent psychiatry department.	DISC-IV; Parent report
Gjevik et al. (2011)	71	–	M = 11.8 SD = 3.3 R = 6.2–17.9	NVIQ: M = 65.2 SD = 29.6 R = 30–129	82%	Research ADI-R	Attending selected special education needs school	K-SADS; parent report
Green et al. (2000)	20	20 CD	AS: M = 13.8 R = 11–19 CD: M = 14.5 R = 11–18	AS: M = 92.2 SD = 17.7 R = 71–141 CD: M = 91.2 SD = 9.1 R = 74–107	100%	ICD-10 clinical criteria for AS	Clinical referral	Modified Isle of Wight Semi-structured Informant and Child Interviews. Parent- and self-report

Study	N	N	Age	IQ	%	Diagnostic criteria	Recruitment	Measure; informant
Joshi et al. (2010)	217	217	ASD: M = 9.7, SD = 3.6, Non-ASD: M = 10.9, SD = 3.5	—	ASD: 87% Non-ASD: 72%	DSM-III checklist. AD: n = 25; PDD-NOS: n = 192	Consecutive referrals to pediatric clinic (N = 2323); 217 meeting ASD criteria and 217 not meeting criteria.	K-SADS; parent report
Mukaddes et al. (2010)	60	—	HFA: M = 10.3, R = 6.2–14.4, AS: M = 11.0, R = 7.0–15.5	HFA: M = 90.5, R = 70–127, AS: M = 106.5, R = 82–138	—	DSM-IV criteria; 30 children and adolescents with diagnosis of HFA and 30 with diagnosis of AS.	Selected from 454 children and adolescents referred to ASD clinic	K-SADS; unclear informant
Mukaddes and Fateh (2010)	37	—	M = 10.9, R = 6–20	M = 116	87%	AS according to DSM-IV criteria	Recruited from private clinic for general psychiatry	K-SADS; unclear informant
Muris et al. (1998)	44	—	M = 9.7, SD = 4.8, R = 2–18	M = 79.5, SD = 14.0, R = 59–116	—	Clinical diagnosis of AD (n = 15) or PDD-NOS (n = 29)	Clinical sample	DISC (version 2.3); parent report
Witwer and Lecavalier (2010)	61	—	M = 11.2, SD = 3.8, R = 6–17	M = 68.4, SD = 23.3, R = 42–150	82%	ADI-R: 16 AS, 17 AD, 26 PDD-NOS.	Advertisements to those receiving services	P-ChIPS; parent report
Subclinical symptoms								
Caamaño et al. (2013)	25	25	ASD: M = 12.8, SD = 2.9, Non-ASD: M = 12.5, SD = 2.9	ASD: M = 97.9, SD = 27.6, Non-ASD: M = 114.4, SD = 16.1	ASD: 96% Non-ASD: 92%	Developmental history and medical reports were scored according to DSM-IV or Gillberg's criteria. The ADOS was used if the two sets of criteria did not match (35%).	Volunteer sample	K-SADS-PL; Parent- and self-report
Adults								
Hofvander et al. (2009)	122	—	Med = 29, R = 16–60	—	67%	DSM-IV AD criteria and the Gillberg & Gillberg Asperger criteria. Used ASDI: 5 AD; 67 AS; 50 PDD-NOS	Referrals to two ASD clinics	SCID-I; unclear informant

(Continued)

Table 2.1 (Continued)

Study	# ASD	Control group	Age	Ability level[a]	Gender; % males	Diagnosis of ASD	Sampling technique (ASD)	Anxiety measure
Joshi et al. (2013)	63	63	**ASD:** M = 29.2, R = 18–63; **Non-ASD:** M = 29.3, R = 18–65	**ASD:** M = 104.4, R = 55–136; **Non-ASD:** M = 106.8, R = 77.5–133	**ASD:** 65% **Non-ASD:** 65%	Clinical structured diagnostic interview: 41 AD; 16 AS; 6 PDD-NOS	Clinical referrals to ASD clinic (ASD group) or general psychopharmacology program (control group; age and sex matched)	SCID-I; self-report
Lever and Geurts (2016)	138	170	**ASD:** M = 46.5, **Non-ASD:** M = 45.9	**ASD:** M = 113.8, **Non-ASD:** M = 113.3	**ASD:** 70% **Non-ASD:** 57%	Clinical diagnoses: 21 Autistic Disorder; 69 AS; 43 PDD-NOS; 5 ASD. ADOS module 4	ASD group: Advertisements to those accessing clinical services. Comparison group advertisements at university and on social media	MINIPlus; self-report
Lugnegård, Hallerbäck, and Gillberg (2011)	54	–	M = 6, SD = 3.9	M = 102, SD = 12	48%	AS diagnosis confirmed using the DISCO and clinical judgment	Current or previous patients of ASD clinics	SCID-I; self-report

Social anxiety disorder (SAD) only

Study	# ASD	Control group	Age	Ability level[a]	Gender; % males	Diagnosis of ASD	Sampling technique (ASD)	Anxiety measure
Maddox and White (2015)	28	26 SAD, 25 TD	**ASD:** M = 23.9, SD = 6.9, R = 16–42; **SAD:** M = 25.9, SD = 7.1, R = 16–42; **TD:** M = 24.8, SD = 7.3, R = 17–44	**ASD:** M = 107, SD = 16.5, R = 80–141; **SAD:** M = 109, SD = 10.5, R = 88–127; **TD:** M = 114, SD = 10.8, R = 91–133	ASD: 54% SAD: 50% TD: 48%	ASD: ADOS-2 and clinical interview; SAD: ADIS-IV-C/P criteria for SAD	Volunteer sample	ADIS-IV-C/P; self-report

[a]Full Scale IQ unless otherwise stated. NVIQ = Non-verbal IQ, M = mean, Med = median, SD = standard deviation, R = range, AD = autistic disorder, PDD-NOS = pervasive developmental disorder not otherwise specified, AS = Asperger syndrome, CD = conduct disorder, HFA = high-functioning autism. CAPA: Child and Adolescent Psychiatric Assessment (Angold and Costello, 2000); K-SADS: Kiddie – Schedule for Affective Disorders and Schizophrenia for School-Age Children (Puig-Antich and Chambers, 1978); ACI: Autism Comorbidity Interview (Leyfer et al., 2006); PAPA: Preschool Age Psychiatric Assessment (Egger and Angold, 2004); DISC: Diagnostic Interview Schedule for Children (Shafer et al., 1996); P-ChIPS: Children's Interview for Psychiatric Version (Weller et al., 1999); SCID: Structured Clinical Interview for DSM-IV Axis I Disorders (First et al., 2002); MINIPlus: the mini International neuropsychiatric interview (Sheehan et al., 1998); ADIS-IV-C/P: anxiety disorder interview schedule for DSM-IV (Silverman and Albano, 1996); ADI-R: Autism Diagnostic Interview – Revised (Rutter et al., 2003); ADOS: Autism Diagnostic Observation Schedule (Lord et al., 2012); ASSQ: Autism Spectrum Screening Questionnaire (Ehlers et al., 1999); 3di: developmental, dimensional and diagnostic interview (Skuse, 2013); DISCO: diagnostic interview for social and communication disorders (Wing et al., 2002); ASDI: the Asperger syndrome diagnostic interview (Gillberg et al., 2001).

Table 2.2 Table showing the prevalence rates (%) for DSM-IV specific anxiety disorders in ASD across the reviewed studies using diagnostic interviews

	Prevalence period	GAD	Social anxiety disorder	Specific phobia	Panic disorder	Agoraphobia	Separation anxiety	OCD	Any anxiety disorder
Children & adolescents									
Population samples									
Simonoff et al. (2008)	3 months	13.4	29.2	8.5	10.1	7.9	0.5	8.2	41.9
Community samples									
Leyfer et al. (2006)	Lifetime	2.4	7.5	44.3	0	–	11.9	37.2	–
Mattila et al. (2010) Combined sample	Current/lifetime	–	4/6	28/34	2/2	2/2	2/8	22/28	42/56
Community sample	*Current/lifetime*	*–*	*6/6*	*33/39*	*6/6*	*0/0*	*6/17*	*11/11*	*39/50*
Clinic sample	*Current/lifetime*	*–*	*2.5/5*	*28/33*	*2.5/2.5*	*2.5/2.5*	*2.5/5*	*25/33*	*45/58*
Salazar et al. (2015)	3 months	66.5	15.1	52.7	3.1	18.0	18.6	–	78.9
Clinic samples									
de Bruin et al. (2007)	1 year	5.3	11.7	38.3	1.1	6.4	8.5	6.4	55.3
Green et al. (2000)	3 months	35	–	10	–	–	–	25	–
Mukaddes et al. (2010) Combined	Lifetime	10	13.3	53.4	1.7	–	13.4	37.2	78.3
AS	*Lifetime*	*16.7*	*13.3*	*46.7*	*0*	*–*	*10*	*36.7*	*73.3*
HFA	*Lifetime*	*3.3*	*13.3*	*60*	*3.3*	*–*	*16.7*	*37.7*	*83.3*
Mukaddes and Fateh (2010) Combined	Lifetime	5.4	5.4	13	5.4	–	2.7	32	59.5
Children	*Lifetime*	*0*	*0*	*21*	*0*	*–*	*4*	*17*	*43*
Adolescents	*Lifetime*	*14*	*14*	*0*	*14*	*–*	*0*	*57*	*85*
Muris et al. (1998)	6 months	22.7	20.5	63.6	9.1	45.5	27.3	11.4	84.1

(Continued)

Table 2.2 (Continued)

	Prevalence period	GAD	Social anxiety disorder	Specific phobia	Panic disorder	Agoraphobia	Separation anxiety	OCD	Any anxiety disorder
Witwer and Lecavalier (2010)	1 month	24.6	16.4	67.2	–	–	14.8	4.9	–
IQ > 70	*1 month*	*50*	*22.7*	*68.2*	*–*	*–*	*13.6*	*13.6*	*–*
IQ < 70	*1 month*	*8.3*	*13.9*	*67.2*	*–*	*–*	*13.9*	*0*	*–*
Gjevik et al. (2011)	Lifetime	0	7	31	–	–	0	10	42
Joshi et al. (2010)	Lifetime	35	28	37	6	35	37	25	61[a]
Subclinical symptoms									
Caamaño et al. (2013)	*Subclinical*	32	40	36~	20	36~	28	48	–
Adults									
Lugnegård et al. (2011)	Lifetime	22	22	–	13	15	–	7	56
Women	*Lifetime*	*25*	*18*	*–*	*18*	*14*	*–*	*4*	*57*
Men	*Lifetime*	*19*	*27*	*–*	*8*	*15*	*–*	*12*	*54*
Hofvander et al. (2009)	Lifetime	15	13	6	11	11	–	24	50
Lever and Geurts (2016)	Lifetime	15.9	15.2	11.6	15.2	21	–	21.7	53.6
Young (19–38)	*Lifetime*	*17.4*	*21.7*	*10.9*	*23.9*	*21.7*	*–*	*28.3*	*65.2*
Middle (39–54)	*Lifetime*	*19.1*	*21.3*	*14.9*	*12.8*	*19.1*	*–*	*21.3*	*53.2*
Older (55–79)	*Lifetime*	*11.1*	*2.2*	*8.9*	*8.9*	*22.2*	*–*	*15.6*	*42.2*
Joshi et al. (2013)	Current	29	40	18	3	24	3	16	38[a]
	Lifetime	35	56	32	15	35	21	24	59[a]
Social anxiety disorder only									
Maddox and White (2015)—		–	50	–	–	–	–	–	–

[a] 2 or more anxiety disorders; ~agoraphobia and specific phobia combined.

higher than the lifetime prevalence in typically developing adults (28.8%; Kessler et al., 2005). Lever and Geurts (2016) collected questionnaire and interview data on different age subsets of adults with ASD. The adults were split into three age groups: young adults (19—38); middle-aged adults (39—54), and older adults (55—79). In the ASD sample as a whole the prevalence of any anxiety disorder was 54% which was significantly higher than 14.7% of the age and IQ matched comparison group. The young and middle-aged adults had the most anxiety (65.2% and 53.2%, respectively), which is in line with the other studies in adults with ASD, whereas the rate among older adults was lower at 42.2%.

Specific anxiety disorders. *Specific phobia* was the most prevalent diagnosis across 8 of the 12 reviewed studies on children and adolescents with ASD (31—67%). Some studies report lower rates, such as 8.5% in Simonoff et al. (2008); however, in this study evidence of functional impairment was additionally required to receive a diagnosis. In the four studies of adults with ASD specific phobia was still common but not consistently as high; prevalence rates ranged from 6% to 32%. Tentative findings indicate the prevalence of specific phobias may decrease as age increases: Mukaddes and Fateh (2010) found that while the majority of children in their sample met criteria none of the adolescents did; Salazar et al. (2015) also found a trend that specific phobia decreases from 62% in those 7.5 years old and under to 44.6% in those older than 7.5 years.

The rates of *OCD* across the reviewed studies are variable (4.9—37.2% in children and adolescents and 7—24% in adults) but consistently reported at moderate rates. The highest prevalence was reported by Leyfer et al. (2006) who applied modified diagnostic criteria such that a diagnosis of OCD could be made on observable signs and symptoms only rather than caregivers being asked to infer children's subjective mental experiences. They argued without this adjustment only a minority of children in their sample would have met criteria. The difference between repetitive behaviors in OCD and ASD is typically considered a qualitative one; in ASD, repetitive behaviors are a source of pleasure whereas in OCD they are associated with distress and anxiety. However, eliciting the associated feelings is often extremely difficult. The anxiety related to repetitive behaviors could be overlooked in ASD and this may explain the variable rates across studies.

The prevalence of *social anxiety disorder* across children and adolescents was also common, although rates varied from 4% to 29.2%. Interpretation of the symptom descriptions, such as social avoidance being coded as either core to ASD or as part of distinct social anxiety, may again help to explain the discrepancies in diagnostic rates. The description adopted by Gjevik et al. (2011) required observable and expressed symptoms such that social avoidance would not be sufficient in and of itself to meet diagnostic criteria. Such descriptions could pose a particular problem in ASD because of reduced emotional literacy and poorer communication. Leyfer et al. (2006) argue that individuals with ASD may try to avoid the non-social aspects of interactions such as noise and that social anxiety disorder per se is less prevalent. The lower prevalence rate reported by Leyfer et al. (2006) may, therefore, reflect the modifications to the criteria applied, which specifically distinguish between fear and avoidance of either the social or the non-social aspects of social situations.

Generalized anxiety disorder (GAD) was found to be prevalent across the four studies of adults (6—32%) and although the rates were more variable in children and adolescents, GAD was also a common anxiety disorder (0—66.5%) in most studies. In contrast to the high rates (e.g., Joshi et al., 2010; Green et al., 2000; Salazer et al., 2015), none of the parents in Gjevik et al. (2011) reported subjective anxiety symptoms required for a diagnosis of GAD. One explanation may be the substantial number of lower cognitive ability participants in the sample. This is supported by the findings of Witwer and Lecavalier (2010) who found GAD was significantly less prevalent in the low-functioning group (8.3%; IQ < 70) than the high-functioning ASD group (50%; IQ > 70). *Panic disorder* was the least common anxiety disorder in children and adolescents with rates ranging from 0% to 10.1%, but appears to be more prevalent in adults (11—15%). Overall, the findings of the current review are in line with a meta-analysis of children and adolescents with ASD conducted by van Steensel et al. (2011), which included both standardized interviews and questionnaires ($N = 2,121$). The meta-analysis found specific phobia to be the most common anxiety disorder in ASD (30%), then OCD (17%), social anxiety disorder and agoraphobia (17%) followed by GAD (15%), separation anxiety (9%), and panic disorder (2%).

FACTORS ASSOCIATED WITH ANXIETY IN ASD

The diagnostic interview studies reviewed above are limited in their inclusion of comparison groups and range of age or ability level within any one sample. The addition of questionnaire studies in the following section is used to be able to draw conclusions about risk factors and correlates of anxiety in ASD.

Anxiety symptomatology in ASD and comparison groups.
Of the reviewed diagnostic interview studies that did include comparison groups, individuals with ASD were found to be significantly more likely to meet diagnostic criteria for anxiety: children with AS had significantly more anxiety symptoms than children with conduct disorder (Green et al., 2000) and adults with ASD had significantly higher rates of multiple anxiety disorders (two or more), agoraphobia, OCD, and social anxiety disorder than non-ASD referrals to a general psychiatric clinic (Joshi et al., 2013).

A substantial proportion of the studies using questionnaires to measure anxiety symptoms, rather than diagnostic rates, compare groups of individuals with ASD to groups of typically developing individuals and those with other clinical conditions. These studies have found individuals with ASD to score significantly higher than individuals with typical development (Bellini, 2004; Kim et al., 2000; Lopata et al., 2010; Thede and Coolidge, 2007; Weisbrot et al., 2005), ID without ASD (e.g., Brereton et al., 2006; Gillott and Standen, 2007), Down's syndrome (Evans et al., 2005), Williams syndrome (Rodgers et al., 2012), and specific language impairment (Gillott et al., 2001). Individuals with ASD have also been found to have comparable levels of anxiety to non-ASD individuals with a clinical anxiety disorder (Farrugia and Hudson, 2006) and parents of children with ASD reported higher total levels of anxiety, OCD symptoms, and fear of injury anxiety than parents of clinically anxious children (Russell and Sofronoff, 2005).

Anxiety in ASD subgroups. The main ASD diagnostic subgroup comparisons have been conducted between individuals with a clinical diagnosis of AS and HFA. Using a clinical diagnostic interview no significant differences in anxiety diagnoses were found between groups of adolescents with AS or HFA, who were diagnosed according to the DSM-IV criteria (Mukaddes et al., 2010). In addition, no significant differences were found on a questionnaire measure of anxiety symptoms in 9- to 14-year-old children with AS or HFA (Kim et al., 2000) who were categorized according to the presence (AS) or absence (HFA) of spontaneous phrase speech by 36 months of age and presence (HFA) or absence (AS) of persistent deviant language development. In contrast, Thede and Coolidge (2007) found children with AS (no parent reported language delays) had significantly higher scores on an anxiety questionnaire than the HFA group and when Tonge et al. (1999) controlled the effects of age and cognitive level across children and adolescents with HFA and AS, diagnosed according to DSM-IV criteria, they found the AS group to be significantly more anxious.

When examining all ASD subgroups Weisbrot et al. (2005) found school age children with autistic disorder (AD) were reported by parents and teachers to have the lowest levels of anxiety, whereas children with a diagnosis of AS or PDD-NOS were rated to have significantly more obsessional symptoms than children with AD and those with AS had more severe generalized anxiety than both other groups. It is important to note, however, that the assignment of diagnostic labels under the DSM-IV was not consistent across professionals or clinical sites (e.g., Lord et al., 2012). It may, therefore, be more beneficial to look for additional explanatory factors such as IQ level rather than diagnostic subsets. For example, Muris et al. (1998) found some anxiety disorders were more frequently seen in children with PDD-NOS than in those with AD (e.g., simple phobia, separation anxiety disorder). However, the children who were labeled as PDD-NOS were both older and had significantly higher IQ scores than the AD group.

Anxiety and ASD severity. It has been suggested that increased ASD symptoms may increase individual's risk of developing anxiety (Wood and Gadow, 2010) but the evidence has been inconsistent. Whereas Mayes et al. (2011) found ASD severity as rated by parents was the best predictor of level of anxiety in children, Eussen et al. (2013) found lower ASD symptom severity was related to higher anxiety symptoms. Furthermore, Rieske et al. (2012) investigated the role of social impairments in predicting co-occurring anxiety and found the addition of this information to a regression model only explained an additional 1.3% of the variance (the full model explained 56%).

One methodological factor may have a large impact on interpreting the results regarding ASD severity. Most studies have looked at an overall rating of ASD severity when it is possible that the social and communication symptoms and the restricted and repetitive behavior symptoms may have differential effects on anxiety. Magiati et al. (2016) found that in contrast to the social and communication score, the repetitive speech and stereotyped behavior score was found to predict overall anxiety scores. Hallett et al. (2013) found children with higher restricted and repetitive behavior scores had more panic and OCD symptoms whereas higher social and communication symptoms were associated with higher separation anxiety symptoms and lower social anxiety symptoms. Such studies are not designed, however, to disentangle different manifestations of the same underlying phenomenology, e.g., repetitive speech from seeking reassurance, lack of social interest from social avoidance, and more sensitive measurement strategies are needed to further explore these findings.

Anxiety across age. The studies that have attempted to explore anxiety in ASD across ages have been inconsistent, with some studies finding no association between chronological age and anxiety (Farrugia and Hudson, 2006; Hallett et al., 2013; Strang et al., 2012; Sukhodolsky et al., 2008) and other studies suggesting that anxiety severity increases with age across children and adolescents (e.g., Green et al., 2012; Kuusikko et al., 2008; Vasa et al., 2013). Davis et al. (2011) used a cross-sectional approach to compare anxiety across ages in 131 toddlers (aged 17—36 months), children (aged 3—16 years), and adults (aged 20—65 years) with ASD. They found anxiety levels increased from toddlerhood to childhood, decreased from childhood to young adulthood, and increased again from young adulthood into older adulthood. However, different anxiety measures were used in the different age groups. Lever and Geurts (2016) also used a cross-sectional design in adults and found a slight decrease in older adults (aged 55—79) but these adults were older again than those in Davis et al. (2011).

Some research has indicated that the trajectory of anxiety across ages may depend on the specific anxiety disorder being measured. The findings from a meta-analysis found that OCD and separation anxiety were more common in younger children with ASD and that GAD and overall levels of anxiety were higher in older children and adolescents with ASD (van Steensel et al., 2011). More recent findings may support the idea of anxiety specific age-effects as Magiati et al. (2016) found age was positively (although weakly) associated only with social anxiety and OCD. Lever and Geurts (2016) found specific phobia to significantly decrease (22% to 2%) in a sample of young, middle-aged, and older adults. Using a diagnostic interview, Salazar et al. (2015) found agoraphobia, GAD, and separation anxiety all had significantly higher prevalence in the older children (over 7.5 years old) than the younger children (below 7.5 years old). Mukaddes and Fateh (2010) also found the prevalence of specific anxiety disorders to differ between children and adolescents; e.g., 57% of adolescents met criteria for OCD but only 17% of children, and 14% of adolescents met criteria for social anxiety which was not present in any children.

In contrast 21% of children met criteria for specific phobia but no adolescents met the criteria. It may be misleading, therefore, to look at prevalence rates in anxiety disorders, especially for each specific disorder across a large age range.

In their review Kerns and Kendall (2012) suggested anxiety patterns may follow two trajectories depending on the type of anxiety: anxiety symptoms strongly related to ASD such as specific phobia, social anxiety disorder, and compulsions may remain constant across the lifespan whereas anxiety symptoms that are similar to those seen in the general population like GAD may follow the same developmental course of being variable across time and more prevalent in older children and adolescents. This requires further exploration.

Anxiety and ability level. A large majority of the work on anxiety in ASD has been conducted with high-functioning individuals (IQ > 70) as assessing anxiety in lower functioning individuals is more complex due to the limited ability of individuals with ASD to express their emotions, and parents and caregivers' difficulty in distinguishing anxiety behaviors from other negative emotions. Studies that have included participants with ASD and ID have found a range of rates of anxiety using parental questionnaires (11–48%; Bakken et al., 2010; Lecavalier, 2006; Sukhodolsky et al., 2008); Bradley et al. (2004) compared samples of individuals with ID and found anxiety to be present more often in individuals with ASD and ID than in individuals with just ID alone.

Studies comparing IQ groups have found inconsistent results. Two reviewed studies utilizing diagnostic interviews found no significant IQ differences in those who did or did not have a co-occurring anxiety disorder across samples with a wide range of IQ scores (de Bruin et al., 2007; Simonoff et al., 2008). However, questionnaire measures of anxiety symptoms have found more variation in findings across IQ. Higher anxiety symptoms have been shown to be more frequent in children with an IQ above 70 and functional language (Gadow et al., 2005; Hallett et al., 2013; Weisbrot et al., 2005) leading Gadow et al. (2005) to hypothesize that high-functioning individuals with ASD have an increased awareness of their differences and this in turn will lead to more anxiety. It may also be that questionnaire measures are better at capturing the presentation of anxiety in higher rather than lower functioning individuals. In contrast, Brereton et al. (2006) found overall psychopathology including anxiety, as measured using questionnaires, was not affected by age, sex or IQ in 381 young people with ASD who ranged from normal IQ to severe intellectual disability.

Witwer and Lecavalier (2010) found diagnostic rates of specific anxiety disorders, based on diagnostic interviews, did vary according to IQ. GAD was significantly more common in the high-functioning (IQ > 70) than low-functioning ASD group (IQ < 70). Although not significant 13.6% of the high-functioning group also met criteria for OCD but none of the low-functioning group did. Whereas prevalence rates for specific phobia and separation anxiety were nearly identical across the two IQ groups. Using questionnaire measures Sukhodolsky et al. (2008) also reported anxiety symptoms related to specific phobia and social anxiety disorder were prevalent across the whole IQ range but symptoms related to, generalized anxiety were significantly more prevalent in higher functioning children and adolescents with ASD (IQ > 70) than the lower functioning group with ASD (IQ < 70).

IMPLICATIONS

Clinical implications. The current review indicates that a large proportion of individuals with ASD also meet diagnostic criteria for at least one anxiety disorder. Existing research suggests that anxiety is the most common reason for clinical referral (Ghaziuddin, 2002). It has also been shown that having anxiety as well as ASD may cause additional burden to the individual and lead to worse functional outcomes (Wood and Gadow, 2010). In combination, these findings indicate that the assessment and diagnosis of anxiety disorders should be a priority for clinicians caring for those with ASD as the diagnosis of an additional co-occurring disorder such as anxiety may lead to a more informed management plan and specific intervention programs.

The importance of assessment and diagnosis is even greater given that interventions used to treat anxiety in the general population have also been shown to improve anxiety in ASD, with some modification to the intervention (Sukhodolsky et al., 2013). Clinicians may also need to be aware of the high level of anxiety symptoms in individuals with ASD that may not meet diagnostic cut-offs. Many children and adolescents with ASD present with subclinical anxiety; Caamaño et al. (2013) found 76% of children and adolescents with ASD were at threshold or subthreshold level for diagnosis. In addition, a considerable percentage of children show impairment in relation to a specific anxiety disorder but do not always meet diagnostic cut-offs (Witwer and Lecavalier, 2010).

Research implications. To gain the most accurate understanding of the prevalence of anxiety disorders in ASD, consensus on a number of conceptual and methodological questions needs to be reached. These questions and avenues for future research are presented below.

Firstly, in contrast to the general population in which prevalence rates are based on population samples, only one study has used a diagnostic interview to measure prevalence rates in a population based study of individuals with ASD (Simonoff et al., 2008). The majority of studies used clinically referred samples, which could inflate prevalence rates due to these individuals being those that require clinical services. Estimates of prevalence rates also need to consider which informants are involved and how to combine responses across different informants, as well as the assessment period.

Anxiety disorders as a whole were prevalent across the age ranges sampled but investigation into specific anxiety disorders highlights that the prevalence of these disorders may vary across the lifespan (e.g., Davis et al., 2011; Lever and Geurts, 2016). Currently, these findings are limited to cross-sectional studies. Longitudinal studies will allow a better understanding of the developmental changes in anxiety disorders in ASD and the bidirectional effects of risk factors. These studies should also measure specific anxiety diagnoses across time as differences in trajectories for different disorders may obscure overall developmental effects.

Diagnostic interviews that apply DSM or ICD criteria are currently the favored method for estimating the prevalence of anxiety disorders; however, the measurement of anxiety symptoms and clinical cut-offs for diagnoses vary across studies with different research groups using different ways to describe anxiety symptoms. One study made modifications to an existing interview to better capture the presentation of anxiety in ASD (Leyfer et al., 2006), and Witwer and Lecavalier (2010) excluded questions that asked about functioning communication, e.g., worry in separation anxiety and GAD as well as thoughts in OCD for participants with lower IQ or language ability. These interviews are limited in providing information about anxiety in ASD. None of the diagnostic interviews have been validated in an ASD sample and this is a necessary first step in obtaining accurate prevalence data. Validation is challenging as there is no single set of biomarkers that accurately index anxiety disorders. Hence, a multimodal approach is required and should include discriminant and convergent validity, as well as longitudinal studies and evaluation of treatment response. It will also be beneficial to distinguish between the symptoms of ASD and anxiety which are similar, e.g., social avoidance and social anxiety; and also to question whether diagnostic criteria or symptom descriptions of anxiety should be modified in ASD.

The triggers or causes and presentation of anxiety in individuals with ASD can be different from the general population; anxieties centered around changes in routines, for example, do not currently fit easily into the diagnostic criteria (Ozsivadjian et al., 2012). Clinicians also face challenges in differentiating anxiety from other syndromes involving the regulation of emotion such as anger, low mood, or oppositionality (Muris et al., 1998). Ozsivadjian et al. (2012) highlight the main differences in presentation of anxiety in ASD. Parents frequently reported that changes to routines, social difficulties such as difficulties with perspective taking and social expectations as well as sensory sensitivities were common triggers in their children and that the presentation of anxiety was usually through challenging behavior or avoidance rather than verbally. These observational reports require confirmation with more experimental studies.

The introduction detailed the main changes in diagnostic criteria between DSM-IV-TR and DSM-5 for anxiety disorders. Little work has been published using the new criteria and therefore it is unknown what impact these changes may have on the prevalence rates in the general population but especially in ASD. For example, the onset of separation anxiety disorder no longer needs to be before 18 years of age, and the awareness of the individual in viewing their anxiety as excessive to receive a diagnosis of phobias may lead to further individuals with ASD meeting criteria as according to DSM-IV they would need to provide some insight into their anxious feelings which they may find difficult.

Future directions for research should include gaining a better understanding of how these two disorders overlap. This will require comparison of genetic markers, neurophysiological and brain-based measures to identify unique and shared mechanisms. We can also ask research questions about whether having both anxiety and ASD impacts on the individual beyond having one disorder of either ASD or anxiety. It has been suggested that anxiety may mediate difficulties already found in ASD such as social avoidance when individuals with ASD have difficulties initiating social contact which encourages social anxiety and prevents any attempts or improvements in social interaction (e.g., Bellini, 2004). The pathways and causal nature of these relationships need further exploration.

Individuals with ASD may find it difficult to recognize and describe their emotions. One avenue for future research should be on methodology which aids individuals with ASD and especially children or lower functioning individuals to report feelings of anxiety. Instead of questionnaire methods, picture-based rating scales could be an alternative. However, May et al. (2015) found that neither parent nor child questionnaire anxiety ratings were correlated to children's "worry thermometer" ratings in which the children rated their anxiety on a picture scale. In addition to modifying methods of self-report, another way to overcome the reporting difficulties would be to use objective measures such as physiological or cognitive markers of anxiety. Indices such as heart rate variability (e.g., Appelhans and Luecken, 2006; Schmitz et al., 2011), galvanic skin response, or cortisol levels (e.g., van West, Claes, Sulon, and Deboutte, 2008) have been used to measure anxiety levels. For example, in a sample of children with ASD, anxiety, or both, the ASD plus anxiety group showed blunted cortisol and heart rate response to psychosocial stress compared to the other groups and these responses were also related to increased anxiety symptoms (Hollocks et al., 2014). Such physiological approaches may improve our understanding of anxiety presentation with and without ID, although measurement biases such as state anxiety due to research participation would need to be controlled for.

In conclusion, the best estimate prevalence rates of DSM-IV anxiety diagnoses in ASD are high. The variability in prevalence rates is likely explained by the different methodologies adopted across studies. Future work on validating measures for individuals with ASD and an understanding of the ascertainment and measurement of samples will further the understanding on the co-occurrence of ASD and anxiety.

REFERENCES

Achenbach, T.M., McConaughy, S.H., Howell, C.T., 1987. Child/adolescent behavioral and emotional problems: implications of cross-informant correlations for situational specificity. Psychol. Bull. 101 (2), 213.

Alonso, J., Angermeyer, M.C., Bernert, S., Bruffaerts, R., Brugha, T., Bryson, H., et al., 2004. Prevalence of mental disorders in Europe: results from the European Study of the Epidemiology of Mental Disorders (ESEMeD) project. Acta Psychiatrica Scandinavica 109 (s420), 21–27.

Angold, A., Costello, E.J., 2000. The child and adolescent psychiatric assessment (CAPA). J. Am. Acad.Child Adoles. Psych. 39 (1), 39–48.

Appelhans, B.M., Luecken, L.J., 2006. Heart rate variability as an index of regulated emotional responding. Rev. General Psychol. 10 (3), 229.

Bailey, N., 2007. Prevalence of psychiatric disorders in adults with moderate to profound learning disabilities. Adv. Mental Health Learn. Disabil. 1 (2), 36–44.

Bakken, T.L., Helverschou, S.B., Eilertsen, D.E., Heggelund, T., Myrbakk, E., Martinsen, H., 2010. Psychiatric disorders in adolescents and adults with autism and intellectual disability: A representative study in one county in Norway. Res. Develop. Disabil. 31 (6), 1669–1677.

Bellini, S., 2004. Social skill deficits and anxiety in high-functioning adolescents with autism spectrum disorders. Focus Autism Other Develop. Disabil. 19 (2), 78–86.

Bradley, E.A., Summers, J.A., Wood, H.L., Bryson, S.E., 2004. Comparing rates of psychiatric and behavior disorders in adolescents and young adults with severe intellectual disability with and without autism. J. Autism Develop. Dis. 34 (2), 151–161.

Brereton, A.V., Tonge, B.J., Einfeld, S.L., 2006. Psychopathology in children and adolescents with autism compared to young people with intellectual disability. J. Autism Develop. Dis. 36 (7), 863–870.

Breton, J.-J., Bergeron, L., Valla, J.-P., Lépine, S., Houde, L., Gaudet, N., 1995. Do children aged 9 through 11 years understand the DISC version 2.25 questions? J. Am. Acad. Child Adoles. Psych. 34 (7), 946–956.

Caamaño, M., Boada, L., Merchán-Naranjo, J., Moreno, C., Llorente, C., Moreno, D., et al., 2013. Psychopathology in children and adolescents with ASD without mental retardation. J. Autism Develop. Dis. 43 (10), 2442–2449.

Charman, T., Pickles, A., Simonoff, E., Chandler, S., Loucas, T., Baird, G., 2011. IQ in children with autism spectrum disorders: data from the Special Needs and Autism Project (SNAP). Psychol. Med. 41 (03), 619–627.

Christensen, D.L., Baio, J., Braun, K.V., Bilder, D., Charles, J., Constantino, J.N., et al., 2016. Prevalence and Characteristics of Autism Spectrum Disorder Among Children Aged 8 Years—Autism and Developmental Disabilities Monitoring Network, 11 Sites, United States, 2012. MMWR Surveill Summ 2016 65 (SS-3), 1–23.

Comer, J.S., Kendall, P.C., 2004. A symptom-level examination of parent–child agreement in the diagnosis of anxious youths. J. Am. Acad. Child Adoles. Psych. 43 (7), 878–886.

Costello, E.J., Egger, H.L., Angold, A., 2005. The Developmental Epidemiology of Anxiety Disorders: Phenomenology, Prevalence, and Comorbidity. Child Adoles. Psych. Clin. North Am. 14 (4), 631–648.

Davis, T.E., Hess, J.A., Moree, B.N., Fodstad, J.C., Dempsey, T., Jenkins, W.S., et al., 2011. Anxiety symptoms across the lifespan in people diagnosed with autistic disorder. Res. Autism Spect. Dis. 5 (1), 112–118.

de Bruin, E.I., Ferdinand, R.F., Meester, S., de Nijs, P.F., Verheij, F., 2007. High rates of psychiatric co-morbidity in PDD-NOS. J. Autism Develop. Dis. 37 (5), 877–886.

Dekker, M.C., Koot, H.M., 2003. DSM-IV disorders in children with borderline to moderate intellectual disability. I: Prevalence and impact. J. Am. Acad. Child Adoles. Psych. 42 (8), 915–922.

Dykens, E., Lense, M., 2011. Intellectual disabilities and autism spectrum disorder: A cautionary note. In In: In: Amaral, D., Dawson, G., Geschwind, D. (Eds.), Autism Spectrum Disorders. Oxford University Press, Oxford, pp. 261–269.

Dziuk, M., Larson, J., Apostu, A., Mahone, E., Denckla, M., Mostofsky, S., 2007. Dyspraxia in autism: association with motor, social, and communicative deficits. Develop. Med. Child Neurol. 49 (10), 734–739.

Edelbrock, C., Costello, A.J., Dulcan, M.K., Conover, N.C., Kala, R., 1986. Parent-child agreement on child psychiatric symptoms assessed via structured interview. J. Child Psychol. Psych. 27 (2), 181–190.

Egger, H.L., Angold, A., 2004. The Preschool Age Psychiatric Assessment (PAPA): A structured parent interview for diagnosing psychiatric disorders in preschool children. In: DelCarmen-Wiggins, R., Carter, A. (Eds.), Handbook of Infant, Toddler, and Preschool Mental Assessment. Oxford University Press, New York, pp. 223–243.

Egger, H.L., Angold, A., 2006. Common emotional and behavioral disorders in preschool children: presentation, nosology, and epidemiology. J. Child Psychol. Psych. 47 (3-4), 313–337.

Ehlers, S., Gillberg, C., Wing, L., 1999. A screening questionnaire for Asperger syndrome and other high-functioning autism spectrum disorders in school age children. J. Autism Develop. Dis. 29 (2), 129–141.

Emerson, E., Hatton, C., 2007. Mental health of children and adolescents with intellectual disabilities in Britain. Brit. J. Psych. 191 (6), 493–499.

Eussen, M.L., Van Gool, A.R., Verheij, F., De Nijs, P.F., Verhulst, F.C., Greaves-Lord, K., 2013. The association of quality of social relations, symptom severity and intelligence with anxiety in children with autism spectrum disorders. Autism 17 (6), 723–735.

Evans, D.W., Canavera, K., Kleinpeter, F.L., Maccubbin, E., Taga, K., 2005. The fears, phobias and anxieties of children with autism spectrum disorders and down syndrome: Comparisons with developmentally and chronologically age matched children. Child Psych. Human Develop. 36 (1), 3–26.

Farrugia, S., Hudson, J., 2006. Anxiety in adolescents with Asperger syndrome: Negative thoughts, behavioral problems, and life interference. Focus Autism Other Develop. Disabil. 21 (1), 25–35.

First, M.B., Spitzer, R.L., Gibbon, M., Williams, J.B.W., 2002. Structured Clinical Interview for DSM-IV-TR Axis I Disorders, Research Version, Patient Edition. (SCID-I/P). Biometrics Research, New York.

Frith, U., 1991. Autism and Asperger Syndrome. Cambridge University Press, Cambridge, UK.

Gadow, K.D., Devincent, C.J., Pomeroy, J., Azizian, A., 2005. Comparison of DSM-IV symptoms in elementary school-age children with PDD versus clinic and community samples. Autism 9 (4), 392–415.

Ghaziuddin, M., 2002. Asperger syndrome associated psychiatric and medical conditions. Focus Autism Other Develop. Disabil. 17 (3), 138–144.

Gillberg, C., Gillberg, C., Råstam, M., Wentz, E., 2001. The Asperger Syndrome (and high-functioning autism) Diagnostic Interview (ASDI): a preliminary study of a new structured clinical interview. Autism 5 (1), 57–66.

Gillott, A., Furniss, F., Walter, A., 2001. Anxiety in high-functioning children with autism. Autism 5 (3), 277–286.

Gillott, A., Standen, P., 2007. Levels of anxiety and sources of stress in adults with autism. J. Intellect. Disabil. 11 (4), 359–370.

Gjevik, E., Eldevik, S., Fjæran-Granum, T., Sponheim, E., 2011. Kiddie-SADS reveals high rates of DSM-IV disorders in children and adolescents with autism spectrum disorders. J. Autism Develop. Dis. 41 (6), 761–769.

Green, S.A., Ben-Sasson, A., Soto, T.W., Carter, A.S., 2012. Anxiety and sensory over-responsivity in toddlers with autism spectrum disorders: Bidirectional effects across time. J. Autism Develop. Dis. 42 (6), 1112–1119.

Green, J., Gilchrist, A., Burton, D., Cox, A., 2000. Social and psychiatric functioning in adolescents with Asperger syndrome compared with conduct disorder. J. Autism Develop. Dis. 30 (4), 279–293.

Grills, A.E., Ollendick, T.H., 2003. Multiple informant agreement and the anxiety disorders interview schedule for parents and children. J. Am. Acad. Child Adoles. Psych. 42 (1), 30–40.

Hallett, V., Ronald, A., Colvert, E., Ames, C., Woodhouse, E., Lietz, S., et al., 2013. Exploring anxiety symptoms in a large-scale twin study of children with autism spectrum disorders, their co-twins and controls. J. Child Psychol. Psych. 54 (11), 1176−1185.

Hofvander, B., Delorme, R., Chaste, P., Nydén, A., Wentz, E., Ståhlberg, O., et al., 2009. Psychiatric and psychosocial problems in adults with normal-intelligence autism spectrum disorders. BMC Psych. 9 (1), 1.

Hollocks, M.J., Howlin, P., Papadopoulos, A.S., Khondoker, M., Simonoff, E., 2014. Differences in HPA-axis and heart rate responsiveness to psychosocial stress in children with autism spectrum disorders with and without co-morbid anxiety. Psychoneuroendocrinology 46, 32−45.

Joshi, G., Petty, C., Wozniak, J., Henin, A., Fried, R., Galdo, M., et al., 2010. The heavy burden of psychiatric comorbidity in youth with autism spectrum disorders: A large comparative study of a psychiatrically referred population. J. Autism Develop. Dis. 40 (11), 1361−1370.

Joshi, G., Wozniak, J., Petty, C., Martelon, M.K., Fried, R., Bolfek, A., et al., 2013. Psychiatric comorbidity and functioning in a clinically referred population of adults with autism spectrum disorders: a comparative study. J. Autism Develop. Dis. 43 (6), 1314−1325.

Kanner, L., 1943. Autistic disturbances of affective contact. Nervous child 2, 217−250.

Kerns, C.M., Kendall, P.C., 2012. The presentation and classification of anxiety in autism spectrum disorder. Clin. Psychol. Sci. Pract. 19 (4), 323−347.

Kessler, R.C., Berglund, P., Demler, O., Jin, R., Merikangas, K.R., Walters, E.E., 2005. Lifetime prevalence and age-of-onset distributions of DSM-IV disorders in the National Comorbidity Survey Replication. Arch. General Psych. 62 (6), 593−602.

Kessler, R.C., Chiu, W.T., Demler, O., Walters, E.E., 2005. Prevalence, severity, and comorbidity of 12-month DSM-IV disorders in the National Comorbidity Survey Replication. Arch. General Psych. 62 (6), 617−627.

Kim, J.A., Szatmari, P., Bryson, S.E., Streiner, D.L., Wilson, F.J., 2000. The prevalence of anxiety and mood problems among children with autism and Asperger syndrome. Autism 4 (2), 117−132.

Kuusikko, S., Pollock-Wurman, R., Jussila, K., Carter, A.S., Mattila, M.-L., Ebeling, H., et al., 2008. Social anxiety in high-functioning children and adolescents with autism and Asperger syndrome. J. Autism Develop. Dis. 38 (9), 1697−1709.

Lecavalier, L., 2006. Behavioral and emotional problems in young people with pervasive developmental disorders: Relative prevalence, effects of subject characteristics, and empirical classification. J. Autism Develop. Dis. 36 (8), 1101−1114.

Lever, A.G., Geurts, H.M., 2016. Psychiatric Co-occurring Symptoms and Disorders in Young, Middle-Aged, and Older Adults with Autism Spectrum Disorder. J. Autism Develop. Dis. 46 (6), 1916−1930.

Leyfer, O.T., Folstein, S.E., Bacalman, S., Davis, N.O., Dinh, E., Morgan, J., et al., 2006. Comorbid psychiatric disorders in children with autism: Interview development and rates of disorders. J. Autism Develop. Dis. 36 (7), 849−861.

Lopata, C., Toomey, J.A., Fox, J.D., Volker, M.A., Chow, S.Y., Thomeer, M.L., et al., 2010. Anxiety and depression in children with HFASDs: Symptom levels and source differences. J. Abnormal Child Psychol. 38 (6), 765−776.

Lord, C., Rutter, M., DiLavore, P.C., Risi, S., Gotham, K., Bishop, S., 2012. Autism Diagnostic Observation Schedule: ADOS-2. Western Psychological Services, Los Angeles, CA.

Loucas, T., Charman, T., Pickles, A., Simonoff, E., Chandler, S., Meldrum, D., et al., 2008. Autistic symptomatology and language ability in autism spectrum disorder and specific language impairment. J. Child Psychol. Psych. 49 (11), 1184−1192.

Lugnegård, T., Hallerbäck, M.U., Gillberg, C., 2011. Psychiatric comorbidity in young adults with a clinical diagnosis of Asperger syndrome. Res. Develop. Disabil. 32 (5), 1910–1917.

Maddox, B.B., White, S.W., 2015. Comorbid Social Anxiety Disorder in Adults with Autism Spectrum Disorder. J. Autism Develop. Dis. 45 (12), 3949–3960.

Magiati, I., Ong, C., Lim, X.Y., Tan, J.W.-L., Ong, A.Y.L., Patrycia, F., et al., 2016. Anxiety symptoms in young people with autism spectrum disorder attending special schools: Associations with gender, adaptive functioning and autism symptomatology. Autism 20 (3), 306–320.

Mattila, M.-L., Hurtig, T., Haapsamo, H., Jussila, K., Kuusikko-Gauffin, S., Kielinen, M., et al., 2010. Comorbid psychiatric disorders associated with Asperger syndrome/high-functioning autism: A community-and clinic-based study. J. Autism Develop. Dis. 40 (9), 1080–1093.

Mayes, S.D., Calhoun, S.L., Murray, M.J., Ahuja, M., Smith, L.A., 2011. Anxiety, depression, and irritability in children with autism relative to other neuropsychiatric disorders and typical development. Res. Autism Spect. Dis. 5 (1), 474–485.

Mukaddes, N.M., Fateh, R., 2010. High rates of psychiatric co-morbidity in individuals with Asperger's disorder. World J. Biol. Psych. 11 (2-2), 486–492.

Mukaddes, N.M., Hergüner, S., Tanidir, C., 2010. Psychiatric disorders in individuals with high-functioning autism and Asperger's disorder: similarities and differences. World J. Biol. Psych. 11 (8), 964–971.

Muris, P., Steerneman, P., Merckelbach, H., Holdrinet, I., Meesters, C., 1998. Comorbid anxiety symptoms in children with pervasive developmental disorders. J. Anxiety Dis. 12 (4), 387–393.

Ozsivadjian, A., Knott, F., Magiati, I., 2012. Parent and child perspectives on the nature of anxiety in children and young people with autism spectrum disorders: a focus group study. Autism 16 (2), 107–121.

Puig-Antich, J., Chambers, W., 1978. The Schedule for Affective Disorders and Schizophrenia for School-age Children (Kiddie-SADS). New York State Psychiatric Institute, New York.

Reid, K., Smiley, E., Cooper, S.A., 2011. Prevalence and associations of anxiety disorders in adults with intellectual disabilities. J. Intellect. Disabil. Res. 55 (2), 172–181.

Rey, J.M., Schrader, E., Morris-Yates, A., 1992. Parent-child agreement on children's behaviours reported by the child behaviour checklist (CBCL). J. Adoles. 15 (3), 219–230.

Rieske, R.D., Matson, J.L., May, A.C., Kozlowski, A.M., 2012. Anxiety in children with high-functioning autism spectrum disorders: significant differences and the moderating effects of social impairments. J. Develop. Phys. Disabil. 24 (2), 167–180.

Rodgers, J., Riby, D.M., Janes, E., Connolly, B., McConachie, H., 2012. Anxiety and repetitive behaviours in autism spectrum disorders and Williams syndrome: A cross-syndrome comparison. J. Autism Develop. Dis. 42 (2), 175–180.

Russell, E., Sofronoff, K., 2005. Anxiety and social worries in children with Asperger syndrome. Aust. NZ J. Psych. 39 (7), 633–638.

Rutter, M., Le Couteur, A., Lord, C., 2003. Autism Diagnostic Interview-Revised. Western Psychological Services, Los Angeles, CA.

Salazar, F., Baird, G., Chandler, S., Tseng, E., O'sullivan, T., Howlin, P., et al., 2015. Co-occurring psychiatric disorders in preschool and elementary school-aged children with Autism Spectrum Disorder. J. Autism Develop. Dis. 45 (8), 2283–2294.

Schmitz, J., Krämer, M., Tuschen-Caffier, B., Heinrichs, N., Blechert, J., 2011. Restricted autonomic flexibility in children with social phobia. J. Child Psychol. Psych. 52 (11), 1203–1211.

Shaffer, D., Fisher, P., Dulcan, M.K., Davies, M., Piacentini, J., Schwab-Stone, M.E., et al., 1996. The NIMH Diagnostic Interview Schedule for Children Version 2.3 (DISC-2.3): Description, acceptability, prevalence rates, and performance in the MECA study. J. Am. Acad. Child Adoles. Psych. 35 (7), 865–877.

Sheehan, D.V., Lecrubier, Y., Sheehan, K.H., Amorim, P., Janavs, J., Weiller, E., et al., 1998. The Mini-International Neuropsychiatric Interview (MINI): the development and validation of a structured diagnostic psychiatric interview for DSM-IV and ICD-10. J. Clin. Psych. 59 (20), 22–33.

Silverman, W.K., Albano, A.M., 1996. Anxiety Disorders Interview Schedule for DSM-IV.: Parent interview schedule. Oxford University Press, New York.

Simonoff, E., Pickles, A., Charman, T., Chandler, S., Loucas, T., Baird, G., 2008. Psychiatric disorders in children with autism spectrum disorders: prevalence, comorbidity, and associated factors in a population-derived sample. J. Am. Acad. Child Adoles. Psych. 47 (8), 921–929.

Skuse, D., 2013. Developmental, Dimensional and Diagnostic Interview. In: Volkmar, F.R. (Ed.), Encyclopedia of Autism Spectrum Disorders. Springer, New York, pp. 2211–2215.

Somers, J.M., Goldner, E.M., Waraich, P., Hsu, L., 2006. Prevalence and incidence studies of anxiety disorders: a systematic review of the literature. Can. J. Psych. 51 (2), 100.

Strang, J.F., Kenworthy, L., Daniolos, P., Case, L., Wills, M.C., Martin, A., et al., 2012. Depression and anxiety symptoms in children and adolescents with autism spectrum disorders without intellectual disability. Res. Autism Spect. Dis. 6 (1), 406–412.

Sukhodolsky, D.G., Bloch, M.H., Panza, K.E., Reichow, B., 2013. Cognitive-behavioral therapy for anxiety in children with high-functioning autism: a meta-analysis. Pediatrics 132 (5), 1341–1350.

Sukhodolsky, D.G., Scahill, L., Gadow, K.D., Arnold, L.E., Aman, M.G., McDougle, C.J., et al., 2008. Parent-rated anxiety symptoms in children with pervasive developmental disorders: Frequency and association with core autism symptoms and cognitive functioning. J. Abnormal Child Psychol. 36 (1), 117–128.

Thede, L.L., Coolidge, F.L., 2007. Psychological and neurobehavioral comparisons of children with Asperger's disorder versus high-functioning autism. J. Autism Develop. Dis. 37 (5), 847–854.

Tonge, B.J., Brereton, A.V., Gray, K.M., Einfeld, S.L., 1999. Behavioural and emotional disturbance in high-functioning autism and Asperger syndrome. Autism 3 (2), 117–130.

van Steensel, F.J., Bögels, S.M., Perrin, S., 2011. Anxiety disorders in children and adolescents with autistic spectrum disorders: A meta-analysis. Clin. Child Family Psychol. Rev. 14 (3), 302–317.

van West, D., Claes, S., Sulon, J., Deboutte, D., 2008. Hypothalamic-pituitary-adrenal reactivity in prepubertal children with social phobia. J Affect. Dis. 111 (2–3), 281–290.

Vasa, R.A., Kalb, L., Mazurek, M., Kanne, S., Freedman, B., Keefer, A., et al., 2013. Age-related differences in the prevalence and correlates of anxiety in youth with autism spectrum disorders. Res. Autism Spect. Dis. 7 (11), 1358–1369.

Weisbrot, D.M., Gadow, K.D., DeVincent, C.J., Pomeroy, J., 2005. The presentation of anxiety in children with pervasive developmental disorders. J. Child Adoles. Psychopharmacol. 15 (3), 477–496.

Weller, E.B., Weller, R.A., Rooney, M.T., Fristad, M.A., 1999. Children's interview for psychiatric syndromes: ChIPS. American Psychiatric Press, Washington, DC.

Wing, L., Leekam, S.R., Libby, S.J., Gould, J., Larcombe, M., 2002. The diagnostic interview for social and communication disorders: Background, inter-rater reliability and clinical use. J. Child Psychol. Psych. 43 (3), 307–325.

Witwer, A.N., Lecavalier, L., 2010. Validity of comorbid psychiatric disorders in youngsters with autism spectrum disorders. J. Develop. Phys. Disabil. 22 (4), 367–380.

Wood, J.J., Gadow, K.D., 2010. Exploring the nature and function of anxiety in youth with autism spectrum disorders. Clin. Psychol. Sci. Pract. 17 (4), 281–292.

CHAPTER 3

Phenomenology and Presentation of Anxiety in Autism Spectrum Disorder

Iliana Magiati[1], Ann Ozsivadjian[2] and Connor M. Kerns[3]
[1]National University of Singapore, Singapore
[2]Guy's and St. Thomas Foundation Trust, London, United Kingdom
[3]Drexel University, Philadelphia, PA, United States

Anxiety has been recognized as a significant presenting feature associated with autism spectrum disorder (ASD) since the first clinical descriptions of ASD, with more recent prevalence studies confirming elevated rates of anxiety in this population across the lifespan compared with the general population. However, elevated anxiety symptoms do not form part of the core ASD diagnostic criteria and clinically significant anxiety is not universally present in all individuals with ASD. Clinically, practitioners working with people with ASD and anxiety have often noted that aspects of their clients' anxiety presentations appear to be distinct to ASD and often different to presenting symptoms typically seen in anxious individuals without ASD. However, systematic research investigating this was until recently lacking, leaving key questions unanswered. For example, which anxiety presentations are more/less common in ASD, and to what extent do these mirror or differ from those typically seen in clinically anxious individuals without ASD? Further, how might these qualitative differences inform assessment, formulation, and treatment? In this chapter, we summarize and draw upon the growing empirical literature to consider the similar and distinct ways in which anxiety presents in ASD and make recommendations for clinical practice and future research.

METHODOLOGIES EMPLOYED IN STUDYING THE PHENOMENOLOGY AND PRESENTATION OF ANXIETY IN ASD

Quantitative studies have attempted to disentangle "traditional" anxiety (i.e., shared and commonly present in clinically anxious individuals without ASD)

Anxiety in Children and Adolescents with Autism Spectrum Disorder.
DOI: http://dx.doi.org/10.1016/B978-0-12-805122-1.00003-X
© 2017 Elsevier Inc.
All rights reserved.

from more ASD-distinct anxiety, using standardized measures (i.e., Renno and Wood, 2013; White et al., 2012). A limitation of this method, however, is that the measures employed were developed for individuals without ASD and as such may be likely more useful in establishing the "shared" rather than the "distinct/ASD-related" anxiety manifestations.

To address this, a small number of quantitative studies have adapted existing measures for use specifically with participants with ASD in order to broaden the scope and range of symptomatology explored (e.g., Kerns et al., 2014; Mayes et al., 2012, 2013; Rodgers et al., 2016). Other studies have used qualitative "bottom-up" studies, in which the participants discuss open-ended questions and thus are not restricted to a potentially unrepresentative range of anxiety experiences. The themes from such analyses can then be thematically organized and established as shared or more distinct to ASD, based on existing theoretical and empirical understanding of anxiety in typically developing young people (i.e., Ollendick and Benoit, 2012).

FINDINGS FROM QUALITATIVE STUDIES

Ozsivadjian et al. (2012) reported on a series of five focus groups involving 17 caregivers of 7- to 18-year old cognitively able children and young people with ASD and significant anxiety concerns in the UK. Caregivers discussed triggers, settings, or situations that precipitated anxiety in their children with ASD, and their observations of their children's somatic/physiological, cognitive, behavioral, or other anxiety presentations. Stressors and triggers identified included "traditional" sources of anxiety commonly identified in individuals without ASD (i.e., worries about social situations and being evaluated/judged; worries about not being able to meet high demands and expectations); as well as more atypical, ASD-related triggers (i.e., disruptions to routine and change; confusion about social situations; over-stimulating sensory stimuli; being prevented from engaging in preferred repetitive behaviors or circumscribed interests). Similarly, a pattern of both "traditional" and more ASD-related features of anxiety presentation emerged: traditional physiological manifestations of anxiety were consistently reported (i.e., increases in arousal and physical sensations typically associated with anxiety in individuals without ASD), while behavioral manifestations of anxiety included both "typical" anxiety-related behaviors (i.e., escape, avoidance, reassurance, safety behaviors), as well as more ASD-related presentations including increases in sensory, repetitive, and ritualistic behaviors or increases in socially inappropriate behaviors (e.g., giggling when anxious).

Ozsivadjian et al.'s (2012) findings have also been largely replicated in a culturally and ethnically diverse sample of children and young people with ASD from special schools in Singapore with a range of intellectual and verbal abilities (Magiati et al., 2016).

Also of relevance, Trembath and colleagues (2012) extended these qualitative findings in Australian young adults (18—35 years old) with ASD and their caregivers. Again, both shared and ASD-related sources of anxiety were identified and these were very similar to those reported by Ozsivadjian et al. (2012) and Magiati et al. (2016) in children and adolescents. More developmentally relevant to young adulthood anxiety precipitants were also identified, including "normative" precipitants (i.e., leaving school, managing finances, public speaking, making important future decisions, news reports, and meeting deadlines) and more ASD-related triggers (i.e., anxiety about explaining their diagnosis or understanding complex social etiquette). Anxiety manifesting itself through increases in challenging and repetitive behaviors was also identified in adults, indicating that these behaviors do not necessarily lessen with age.

Finally, Bearss and colleagues (2016) thematically analyzed focus group discussions to guide the generation of ASD-specific candidate items for the development of an "ASD-friendly" caregiver-reported measure of anxiety symptoms. Forty-five US caregivers of 3—17 year old children with ASD and at least some mild anxiety discussed what anxiety looks like in their children and what situations bring about anxiety. Similar themes and subthemes to those identified in the earlier studies were identified. "Traditional" anxiety triggers identified included separation, crowds, negative (mis)interpretation of events, high academic demands, unwanted social attention, and being teased. More ASD-related triggers were unexpected changes or transitions, others' failure to follow rules and stick to schedules, and sensory stimuli (i.e., toilets, vacuum cleaners).

In summary, four qualitative studies carried out in the UK, USA, Singapore, and Australia involving caregivers, young adults with ASD, and specialist school teachers have yielded consistent and remarkably similar findings strongly pointing towards evidence for shared *and* distinct ASD-related features of anxiety presentation in ASD.

FINDINGS FROM QUANTITATIVE STUDIES

Table 3.1 summarizes key findings from both qualitative and quantitative studies with regards to shared and ASD-related presentations of anxiety.

Table 3.1 Summary of shared and ASD-related precipitants and manifestations of anxiety in ASD identified in qualitative and quantitative studies to date

	Shared/"traditional"/ common in individuals without ASD	More ASD-related/specific/ more common in individuals with ASD
Precipitants/ triggers/setting events or experiences	• Specific fears (i.e., animals, insects, doctors, germs) • Separation from caregiver(s)/significant others • Crowds • Excessive/ overwhelming academic or other demands and expectations • Being teased/bullied/ unwanted social attention • Worried about what others will think • Meeting deadlines	• Idiosyncratic specific fears (i.e., chocolate buttons, men with beards, toilets) • Transitions/change/ disruption to routine • Sensory over-sensitivity and over-stimulation (i.e., sound, light, smell, tactile) • Confusion about social etiquette and situations • Prevention from engaging in circumscribed behaviors/interests

Manifestations/presentation of anxiety

Physiological/ somatic	• Arousal • Heart beating fast • Sweating • "Edgy"/shaking/restless • Tearful/overwhelmed • Anxious facial expressions/body language • Crying/screaming • Sleep/eating disturbances	
Cognitive	• Cognitive distortions (i.e., catastrophizing, all, or nothing thinking) • Dwelling on perceived threat or consequences	• No clearly identifiable threat cognitions
Behavioral	• Avoidance/escape/ withdrawal • Reassurance seeking • Distraction	• Increases/changes in repetitive and/or ritualistic behaviors and interests • Increases in sensory behaviors • Increases in challenging behaviors/acting out

In a study designed to address more systematically the specific question of differential anxiety presentation and diagnosis in ASD to date, Kerns et al. (2014) assessed "traditional" and distinct ASD anxiety presentations in 59 children and young people with ASD using self and parent reports and the clinician-rated Anxiety Disorders Interview Schedule Child and Parent version (ADIS-IV-C/P; Silverman and Albano, 1996). The interview was expanded with additional prompts and sections to capture anxiety symptoms that did not meet "traditional" Diagnostic and Statistical Manual (DSM) criteria, but which were distressing or interfering with the children's development or functioning (as well as more traditional DSM-consistent anxiety disorders). Following findings from earlier studies (i.e., Leyfer et al., 2006), additional items/sections included interfering worries about change or routine disruption, worries relating to ASD preoccupations and interests, social anxiety without a clearly indicated fear of social evaluation, and unusual specific phobias not captured in traditional measures. Sixty-three percent of the participants obtained adapted ADIS-IV-C/P scores in the clinical range, of whom 31% presented with both traditional and ASD-related anxiety symptoms, 17% with traditional DSM-oriented anxiety disorders only, and 15% with impairing ASD-specific anxiety symptoms only. The four most commonly identified atypical clinically significant anxiety difficulties related to anxiety over (1) routine disruption and change; (2) social fears (without clearly articulated social rejection or evaluation concerns); (3) compulsive or ritualistic behaviors not being completed "appropriately" (without a clear indication of wishing to prevent distress or a feared outcome); and (4) unusual specific fears. Results from this study informed the development of the Autism Spectrum Addendum to the ADIS-IV-C/P, the ADIS/ASA (Kerns et al., in press), which provides a systematic approach to differentiating anxiety and ASD symptoms and specifically queries for distinct manifestations of anxiety in ASD, including fears about social etiquette and predictability, fears of change, fears related to unique sensory experiences, and fears related to circumscribed or special interests. A recent study of the ADIS/ASA in a sample of youth with ASD seeking treatment for anxiety supported the validity and reliability of this tool in identifying both traditional and distinct manifestations of anxiety in ASD (see Kerns et al., in press).

White and colleagues' (2015) work examined the factorial equivalence of the Multidimensional Anxiety Scale for Children child and parent report (MASC; March et al., 1997) in 465 children with anxiety problems with and without ASD drawn from anxiety intervention trial studies. Although the MASC anxiety subscales had a similar latent structure in anxious youth with and without ASD at a broad level, the underlying factor structure and the relationships between factors were both similar to and different in ASD as compared to typically developing children without ASD. Four factors were identified, of which three had similar item groupings to the original MASC structure. However, the social anxiety factor items separated into two factors in the ASD group, one concerned with humiliation/rejection and the second with performance anxiety, while the MASC harm avoidance subscale disappeared altogether. Some items on the parent-reported MASC loaded onto different factors compared to the original MASC factor structure. White and colleagues (2015) speculated that this may be because although the same factors emerge, pointing towards shared experiences and presentations of anxiety, the items and factors do not relate to each other in the same way as in non-ASD children, likely because of atypical experiences and presentations of anxiety in ASD. Their findings provide further support for the view that youth with ASD also experience and express anxiety in ways that are different from those without ASD and not captured in "traditional" measures and existing factor structures. Two case vignettes (names changed to protect confidentiality) are presented at the end of this chapter to further illustrate traditional and ASD-related presentations of anxiety in youth on the spectrum.

SHARED AND DISTINCT ANXIETY PRESENTATIONS IN ASD BY ANXIETY TYPE

Specific Phobias/Fears

A meta-analysis of 31 studies involving over 2000 children and young people with ASD by van Steensel et al. (2011) reported that specific phobias were the most commonly reported in 30% of the total sample. All four qualitative studies summarized earlier reported that caregivers spontaneously discussed fears commonly present in individuals without ASD (i.e., relating to germs, spiders, animals), a finding also reflected in studies using quantitative methods (i.e., Evans et al., 2005; Mayes et al., 2013; Magiati et al., 2016; Turner and Romanczyk, 2012). Using a semi-structured diagnostic interview, Kerns et al. (2014) also found that 30% of young people with ASD in their study reported common phobias, such as fears of dogs or spiders.

However, research also suggests variation in the quality and focus of phobias in ASD. Evans and colleagues (2005) found that children with ASD had more fears of specific situations (such as the school bus) and medical situations, but significantly fewer fears of harm/injury compared to developmentally age-matched children, children with Down's syndrome, and chronologically age-matched children. Leyfer et al. (2006)

also reported that many specific fears more commonly reported in normative samples (i.e., fear of flying, tunnels, bridges) were rarely endorsed in their sample of children in ASD, whereas relatively rare phobias of loud noises were more common. Mayes et al. (2013) also reported a high prevalence of unusual/more ASD-idiosyncratic fears in children with ASD (i.e., fears of toilets, vacuum cleaners, and other mechanical things) as well as other fears which appeared unusual in their intensity, obsessiveness, irrationality, or quality (such as fears of walking up stairs, open doors, an irrational fear of dying through bone breaking into chest, and so on). Kerns et al. (2014) also found 12% of their sample reported unusual specific fears, such as the happy birthday song, bubbles, super-markets, or running water.

Social Anxiety

Social anxiety is also a commonly reported anxiety disorder in ASD across studies (16.6% in the van Steensel et al., 2011 meta-analysis). There is clear evidence that a number of individuals with ASD, particularly more cognitively able and socially motivated individuals with ASD, do experience social anxiety as "traditionally" defined to involve heightened arousal and worry in, as well as avoidance of, social situations driven by social humiliation or performance fears (i.e., Bellini, 2004). Their motivation for interpersonal relationships may over time lead to increased social anxiety and avoidance of social situations for fear of repeated social failure, being ridiculed, misunderstood, or rejected (White et al., 2012; see also Kuusikko et al., 2008; Maddox and White, 2015).

At the same time, a key difference in the presentation of social anxiety in ASD may be that social avoidance may present in ASD without an accompanying fear of negative evaluation or worry about social performance, with more ASD-related fears possibly being driven by other social worries relating to ASD impairments, such as not understanding social "rules" and etiquette resulting in social confusion, or fears of causing offence by being too direct or honest (Gillot et al., 2001). In the Kerns et al. (2014) study, 8.5% of the sample reported social fearfulness without any explicit awareness of social judgment or negative perceived social evaluation.

Adopting a dimensional perspective to the study of ASD and anxiety symptomatology, White et al. (2012) examined the structure and construct overlap of 24 items from the Autism Quotient (AQ; Baron-Cohen et al., 2001) and the Social Phobia subscale of the Social Phobia and Anxiety Inventory (SPAI-23; Roberson-Nay et al., 2007) in 623 young adult university students without ASD (of whom 2% scored above ASD cut-off on the AQ). They found two separate, but correlated, factors: one relating to "traditional" social anxiety (i.e., anxiety about speaking in front of others, initiating conversation, entering social situations); and another relating to more ASD-distinct social difficulties (i.e., finding social situations hard, not being good at meeting new people) which included items describing preference for less social activities. Thus, both shared and distinct ASD factors were identified (for more on this, see Tyson and Cruess, 2012) which the authors posited as providing additional support for social anxiety being a "true comorbidity" in ASD, as opposed to being entirely attributable to diagnostic overlap.

Separation Anxiety

Existing literature so far suggests that the presentation of separation anxiety in children and young people with ASD is mostly similar to that of children without ASD. In factor analytic studies of existing anxiety measures developed for typically developing children but used with children with ASD, separation anxiety arises consistently as an internally reliable factor in exploratory or confirmatory derived factor structures (i.e., Evans et al., 2005, using a 69-item survey of fears and phobias developed for their study; Hallett et al., 2013a, using the parent-rated Childhood Anxiety Sensitivity Index scale; Magiati et al., 2016, using the Spence Children's Anxiety Scale-Parent; White et al., 2015, using the MASC-Parent report), and caregivers, young people, and adults with ASD often endorse the "traditional" separation anxiety symptoms in existing scales (i.e., Gillott and Standen, 2007, using the SCAS; Hallett et al., 2013a,b, using the Revised-Child Anxiety and Depression Scale child and parent report). No qualitative or quantitative studies to date have identified any atypical separation anxiety presentations. However, caregivers and clinicians often anecdotally describe intense anxiety in children with ASD associated with unusual attachments to objects (such as bottle caps, elastic bands, rocks, or pieces of string). It is also plausible that separation anxiety may be driven by similar, ASD-related worries as those observed in social anxiety, such as "I won't know what to say, so I need my mum/dad'" as well as more typical fears of something bad happening to themselves or a caregiver (see Vignette 1).

Generalized Anxiety

Generalized anxiety rates in ASD vary from 13.4% (Simonoff et al., 2008) to 25% in clinically anxious young people with ASD (Ung et al., 2013), and 15% in the van Steensel et al. (2011) meta-analysis. Items relating to general or excessive every day worries about school, family, the weather, health, finances, or other general worries are often endorsed by caregivers or self-report (i.e., Blakeley-Smith et al., 2012; Hallett et al., 2013a,b; Mazefsky et al., 2011; Storch et al., 2012; see Vignette 1).

A generalized anxiety factor has also been identified in one factor analytic study (Evans et al., 2005; Hallett et al., 2013a,b; White et al., 2015 used measures which did not include "traditional" generalized anxiety items), although in preliminary findings from a large international pooled dataset of more than 700 6–18-year old children with ASD from the US, UK, and Singapore, Magiati et al. (under review) found that there was no "clear" generalized anxiety factor in this population, but rather a mixed social/generalized anxiety factor. These findings point towards considerable overlap in the presentation of generalized anxiety in children with and without ASD, with perhaps a more blended presentation of mixed symptomatology in ASD, which will need to be further examined in larger factor analytic studies.

Panic/Agoraphobia

In contrast to most other anxiety subtypes, where higher rates of presenting symptoms have consistently been reported in ASD, panic/agoraphobia symptoms were found to be the lowest in van Steensel et al.'s (2011) meta-analysis at 1.8%, on par with prevalence rates of panic disorder of 1–4% in neurotypical adults (Kessler et al., 2006). There is currently no evidence to suggest distinct ASD presentations of panic disorder and associated agoraphobia. It is possible that the lower rates may be due to communication difficulties verbalizing internal physiological experiences often associated with panic attacks. Sukhodolsky and colleagues (2008) found higher rates of panic disorder symptomatology in children and young people with ASD and higher IQ as compared to those with IQ < 70, which suggests that to some extent these internal experiences or the cognitions typically associated with panic disorder (i.e., the misinterpretation of a physiological experience as a sign that something dreadful will happen) either are not experienced by individuals with ASD and intellectual disabilities or cannot be verbally expressed to the same extent as other types of anxiety. Hofvander et al. (2009) also found higher rates of panic disorder in cognitively able adults with ASD (11%), suggesting that perhaps intact intellectual abilities/developmental maturity may be a prerequisite for the development of traditionally-defined panic disorder. Individuals with ASD have been reported to often present with physiological over-arousal seen in panic disorder, but without associated threatening misinterpretations (i.e., Hallett et al., 2013a,b; Storch et al., 2012).

OCD

Although Obsessive Compulsive Disorder (OCD) is no longer included in the DSM-5 anxiety disorders, it has been examined in most studies of anxiety in ASD prior to the publication of the DSM-5 in 2013 and is included as a subscale of symptoms in many existing DSM-IV informed anxiety measures. A number of studies using existing anxiety checklists or clinical interviews designed for typically developing individuals have shown that rates of endorsement of OCD symptoms or meeting criteria for a diagnosis of OCD are much higher in individuals with ASD compared to those without (e.g., 37.2%, Leyfer et al., 2006; see reviews by White et al., 2009; van Steensel et al., 2011). However, in many of these studies there were no systematic efforts to tease out ASD-related repetitive or compulsive behaviors from OCD-related obsessions and compulsions, nor efforts to examine whether the individuals felt compelled to perform certain rituals to reduce anxiety or to prevent a dreaded outcome. In other studies, where specific guidelines for distinguishing OCD and ASD were applied, lower rates have been reported (i.e., 8.2% in Simonoff et al., 2008). Some studies have reported differences in the presentation of obsessive compulsive behaviors in ASD and/or different rates or types of obsession endorsement in children with ASD as compared to those with OCD without ASD (i.e., Cath et al., 2008; McDougle et al., 1995; Ruta et al., 2010). In adults with ASD, McDougle and colleagues (1995) found that repeating, touching, and hoarding were endorsed more frequently, while cleaning, checking, counting obsessive thoughts, and compulsions were much less frequently endorsed compared to adults with OCD only, although there were differences in the two groups in terms of their intellectual functioning. Others have reported no differences (Russell et al., 2005). When considering both traditional and more ASD-related presentations, Kerns et al. (2014) reported ASD-specific compulsive and ritualistic behaviors in 8.5% of children with ASD in their sample, characterized by similar behaviors to those seen in OCD but in the absence of a clear desire to prevent a feared outcome (e.g., having mealtime or bedtime rituals or insisting that doors are closed or sleeves rolled up without articulating a feared outcome to be avoided through these rituals).

In a recent study with adults with ASD + OCD, ASD alone, OCD alone, and without OCD or ASD, individuals with diagnoses of both ASD and OCD self-reported more OCD symptoms than those with ASD alone, suggesting that despite some potential overlap in ASD and OCD symptom presentation and endorsement which may be due to challenges in disentangling the two, OCD behaviors also manifest distinctly from ASD repetitive behaviors (Cadman et al., 2015). Individuals with ASD + OCD were not significantly different to their comparison group of individuals with OCD only in checking, washing, neutralizing, or obsessing, while the 6-factor structure of the Obsessive Compulsive Inventory-Revised (Foa et al., 2002) was confirmed, pointing towards similar presentation of OCD symptoms in individuals with and without ASD. Again, the evidence from the Kerns et al. (2014) and Cadman et al. (2015) in particular point towards both shared and distinct OCD presentations in ASD, with differences in the types of obsessions and ritualistic behaviors and the presence of a clear desire to prevent a dreaded outcome.

PTSD

Similarly to OCD, Post-Traumatic Stress Disorder (PTSD) is part of Trauma and Stressor-related disorders in DSM-5. There has been relatively less focus on examining traumatic experiences and associated PTSD symptomatology in ASD (see Kerns et al., 2015b). To our knowledge, only one study has to date examined the rates and presentation of PTSD symptoms in children and young people with ASD (Mehtar and Mukaddes, 2011). They reported that 12 out of the 69 children with ASD and varying levels of average to severely impaired intellectual abilities in their sample met criteria for PTSD following a semi-structured clinical interview. They also reported a presentation of PTSD symptomatology similar to that traditionally observed in typically developing children (i.e., sleep disturbances, agitation) and children with developmental disabilities (i.e., manifesting PTSD-related distress through deterioration in social behaviors, increases in stereotyped, or challenging behaviors).

ANXIETY/FEARS/WORRIES ASSOCIATED WITH CORE ASD SYMPTOMATOLOGY

Anxiety Around Change or Disruption of Routine/Predictability

One "hallmark" feature of ASD is insistence on sameness and related to this insistence, worries about changes in routines, rules, and novelty. Examples of related worries reported in qualitative studies include difficulty with transitions, such as getting changed for Physical Education (PE) classes or having a substitute teacher, and non-routine school events, such as sports days (i.e., Ozsivadjian et al., 2012). In Kerns et al. study (2014), 22% of the sample reported fears of change and novelty, including changing or taking new traveling routes, or changes in daily schedules (see Vignette 2).

Gotham and colleagues (2013) reported a modest significant positive association of $r = .27$ between anxiety and insistence on sameness, but also found that despite the relationship the two constructs were largely distinct. An interesting body of research has further examined the relationship between anxiety and Intolerance of Uncertainty (IU) in ASD. IU is considered to be a key feature of Generalized Anxiety Disorder (GAD; Dugas et al., 1998) and has been implicated in a number of other anxiety disorders in clinically anxious individuals without ASD (e.g., Carleton et al., 2012). Boulter et al. (2014) noted the resonance of this trans-diagnostic feature with some of the core characteristics of ASD and found that IU was not only significantly related to anxiety severity in a group of young people with ASD, but also accounted for increased levels of anxiety in this group. Thus, IU may be an important driving feature of anxiety functioning similarly in children with and without ASD.

Anxiety Relating to Sensory Oversensitivity

Sensory over- and under-responsivity are known to be common in young people with ASD, yet the relationship between sensory sensitivity and anxiety has received little attention. A number of the atypical fears reported in Kerns et al. (2014), Mayes et al. (2013) and the qualitative studies reviewed earlier may be sensory in origin, although in Kerns et al. (2014) such fears were identified in the absence of a generalized sensitivity to noise. Sasson et al. (2008) and Uljarevic et al. (2016) identified children and adolescents with ASD with adaptive, moderate, and severe sensory related symptomatology based on parent report and found that participants with moderate and severe sensory symptoms had significantly higher anxiety scores than those with less severe sensory symptoms.

Anxiety Presenting as Increases in Challenging or Stereotyped/Repetitive Behaviors

In all four qualitative studies, participants reported anxiety being expressed in the form of observable increases in repetitive/stereotyped or challenging behaviors. In a large clinically referred sample of 445 children and young people with ASD, Hallett et al. (2013a,b) found that items such as restlessness, tension, and sleep difficulties were most frequently endorsed at the clinical level on the caregiver-rated Child and Adolescent Symptom Inventory (CASI) Anxiety scale as manifestations of anxiety compared to other anxiety symptoms. Storch et al. (2012) also found that children with ASD and anxiety presented with more co-occurring disruptive behavior problems that further exacerbated functional impairment. Similarly, Niditch et al. (2012) reported that a positive relationship between IQ and anxiety symptoms was mediated by the presence of aggression. In an earlier study, Evans et al. (2005) found that the association between increased behavioral problems and anxieties and fears was significantly higher in children with ASD compared to the same relationship in children with Down syndrome or typically developing children (see also Farrugia and Hudson, 2006). Rodgers et al. (2012) found that children with ASD and higher anxiety displayed more repetitive behaviors that those with fewer anxiety symptoms. Spiker et al. (2012) also found that symbolic enactment of restricted interests in play was associated with greater anxiety symptoms in youth with ASD. Collectively, these findings suggest that increased externalizing/challenging or repetitive and restricted behaviors may be a way of expressing or coping with anxiety in youth with ASD resulting in a distinct anxiety presentation consistently identified in both qualitative and quantitative studies.

Reduced Verbal Reporting of Anxiety and Anxiety-related Cognitions

In Ozsivadjian et al.'s study (2012), parents reported that their children had great difficulty in telling them about their worries. In line with this, Hallett and colleagues (2013a,b), using the caregiver-rated CASI-Anxiety scale, found that items requiring verbal expression of worries (i.e., "worries about physical health"; "complains about feeling sick or heart pounding") were rarely endorsed at the clinical level by caregivers, suggesting that questionnaires, especially carer- or teacher-reports, may fail to capture such important features of anxiety. However, when physical and social threat-related cognitions were specifically examined using self-report measures, Farrugia and Hudson (2006) found that adolescents with ASD reported more anxious cognitions and dysfunctional attitudes than clinically anxious adolescents without ASD despite equivalent overall anxiety using the CATS (Children's Automatic Thoughts Scale). Similarly, using the same measure, Ozsivadjian et al. (2014) also found that child-rated scores on the CATS were positively correlated with anxiety symptoms, whereas the typically developing comparison group did not show this association. Elevated dysfunctional attitudes in ASD compared to those reported by typically developing children were also found by Greenaway and Howlin (2010). Kerns et al. (2014) also found that anxious cognitions (reported by youth via a questionnaire) predicted both traditional and ASD-related anxiety in their sample. These studies suggest that cognitively and verbally more able children with ASD may in fact be able to accurately report their cognitions, but possibly only with certain supports (e.g., via a structured questionnaire, which offsets difficulties with generation, verbal processing, and conversational to and fro skills typically required in clinical interviews or informal questioning by caregivers).

In the study by Ozsivadjian et al. (2012), when parents were able to make comments about their children's cognitive processing style, some interesting patterns emerged. A few typical cognitive distortions or "thinking errors" were described, such as "I'm totally useless" or "The world's against me". More commonly reported were more ASD-related cognitive processes, such as a delay between a stressful experience occurring and the verbalization of the worries related to the event, and also disorganized, piecemeal, or negatively biased verbal reporting of events and worries.

FACTORS ASSOCIATED WITH TRADITIONAL AND DISTINCT ANXIETY SYMPTOMATOLOGY

Although numerous studies have examined factors associated with the presentation of anxiety in ASD (i.e., gender, chronological age, IQ, adaptive functioning, ASD symptom severity, and others; see, e.g., Dubin et al., 2015; Hallett et al., 2013a,b; Magiati et al., 2016; van Steensel et al., 2011; Vasa and Mazurek, 2015 for reviews; see also Chapter 1: Introduction), to date only Kerns et al. (2014) have explored whether child characteristics may be *differentially* associated with traditional *versus* ASD-related anxiety presentations. They found that a more anxious cognitive style, higher language ability, and hypersensitivity were positively associated with traditional anxiety, while ASD symptom severity was not. In contrast, only ASD symptom severity and an anxious cognitive style predicted ASD-related anxiety. These findings suggest two qualitatively and phenomenologically distinct mechanisms of anxiety in ASD—one which is similar in processes and presentation to the anxiety of youth without ASD, and another wherein anxiety and ASD-related vulnerabilities and symptoms may interact. Previous research examining the relationship between ASD symptom severity and anxiety has been inconsistent, with some studies finding no association (e.g., Hallett et al., 2013a,b; Renno and Wood, 2013; Simonoff et al., 2008) and others reporting a significant correlational or predictive positive relationship (i.e., Magiati et al., 2016; Mayes et al., 2011; Sukhodolsky et al., 2008). Findings by Kerns et al. (2014) suggest that there may be a stronger relationship between ASD symptom severity and ASD-related anxiety as compared to traditional anxiety symptoms, lending some insight to these inconsistent findings.

FUTURE DIRECTIONS AND IMPLICATIONS FOR RESEARCH AND PRACTICE

Implications for Conceptualizing Anxiety in ASD

A number of models have been proposed, conceptualizing anxiety in ASD, summarizing current knowledge, and offering future directions for research. One of the earliest ones was that of Wood and Gadow (2010), who proposed hypothetical pathways between ASD-related stressors and anxiety (which could in turn, it was proposed, lead to an increase in ASD-related behaviors, such as social avoidance). Ollendick and White (2012) proposed a theoretically informed model of shared and unique processes of anxiety in ASD: shared processes likely include negative bias, unhelpful automatic thoughts, and physiological arousal, while more ASD-specific processes likely include social confusion, difficulties "reading" emotions in others, sensory sensitivity, negative social interactions with others, rigidity, and insistence on sameness. Kerns and Kendall (2014) also presented the first review of the differences and similarities between anxiety in youth with and without ASD and suggested the presence of both traditional and more ambiguous or ASD-related anxiety presentations with distinct phenomenologies.

Our critical review of the literature to date in this Chapter largely supports the hypotheses put forth in these models, particularly the distinction of shared and distinct presentations of anxiety in ASD and their potentially different etiological pathways. Nonetheless, future research is needed. Whereas more traditional anxiety presentations may be true co-occurring mental health conditions in individuals with ASD, reflecting "true" psychiatric comorbidity, more distinct symptoms may reflect a distinct anxiety sub-type relating to the severity and impact of the individual's core ASD challenges or, alternatively, core symptoms of ASD (see Kerns and Kendall, 2014; Wood and Gadow, 2010).

In keeping with Kerns and Kendall (2014), the discourse relating to how anxiety problems should be conceptualized in ASD should thus potentially not be a comorbidity *or* ASD variance dichotomy, but rather a comorbidity *and* ASD variance explanation, depending on the nature of the presenting anxiety difficulties. Further studies are needed to examine factors associated with and predicting traditional as compared to ASD-related anxiety symptoms. True comorbidity of anxiety disorders with ASD will require evidence of not only phenotypical similarities, but also common pathways to traditional anxiety in individuals with and without

ASD, such as cognitive factors (e.g., attentional bias), environmental factors (e.g., conditioning, adverse experiences, parenting), and genetic factors. Anxiety-like presentations specifically associated with core ASD features may, in contrast, be better predicted by ASD-specific factors, such as weaker central coherence, social impairments, and sensory oversensitivity. Direct tests of these hypotheses are needed.

Implications for the Measurement and Assessment of Anxiety in ASD

A primary challenge in the identification of anxiety in ASD is the overlap between anxiety and ASD features. Disentangling overlapping presentations requires very careful, comprehensive assessment by experienced professionals with expertise in ASD and the presentation of mental health problems in this population. Furthermore, the diagnostic identification of comorbid anxiety in ASD was not previously aided by earlier classification systems, such as DSM-IV-TR (APA, 2000), which prohibited the diagnosis of some anxiety disorders if ASD was also present. These prohibitions are no longer included in DSM-5, which instead encourages clinicians to disentangle anxiety symptoms as much as possible from ASD symptomatology when considering a comorbid diagnosis. Nonetheless, the actual process of assessing and differentiating anxiety symptoms in youth with ASD is still very much reliant on clinical opinion, in the absence of specific, widely-available measures for this target population (although see Chapter 5: Assessment of Anxiety in Youth with Autism Spectrum Disorder and Chapter 6: Cognitive-Behavioral Principles and Their Applications Within ASD for advances in the assessment of anxiety; and recommendations by Kerns et al., 2016 and Vasa et al., 2016). Existing anxiety measures developed for use with typically developing children appear useful to some extent, but are likely not sufficient to capture the full range of anxiety presentations in ASD. Data on the varied presentation of anxiety in ASD underscore the importance of evaluating the reliability, validity, and clinical utility of existing measures (i.e., see Magiati et al., 2014; van Steensel et al., 2014; Zainal et al., 2014), while also systematically piloting expanded versions of such measures that include items for the more distinct manifestations of anxiety in ASD (see Bearss et al., 2016; Kerns et al., 2014; Rodgers et al., 2016). The ADIS/ASA has demonstrated valid and reliable measurement of traditional and more distinct manifestations of anxiety in ASD, but is time intensive with regard to training and administration and thus may be most useful when careful and comprehensive description of anxiety symptoms is needed for research or clinical practice (Kerns et al., in press). Future studies may enrich our understanding of anxiety in ASD by reporting not only total or subscale anxiety scores, but also item-level analyses. As demonstrated by Hallett et al. (2013a,b), this level of detail can be extremely informative, particularly in the development or adaptation of existing measures for use in ASD.

Implications for Anxiety Interventions in ASD

Existing evaluations of anxiety interventions for young people with ASD (see Ung et al., 2015; Vasa et al., 2014 for reviews) have focused on adapting existing CBT-oriented anxiety interventions developed for children without ASD (see Moree and Davis, 2010), however less attention has been paid to examining whether different adaptations or approaches may be more effective in treating "traditional" as compared to ASD-related anxiety. It may be that traditional anxiety will respond better in interventions informed by existing traditional anxiety programs, while targeting core ASD symptomatology (especially reducing insistence on sameness or managing sensory sensitivity) may be more effective treatment targets in interventions for ASD-related anxiety problems. Future intervention studies would benefit from describing their participants' anxiety presentations within frameworks conceptualizing the full range of traditional and ASD-distinct presentations and evaluating their differential treatment response.

In conclusion, both traditional and distinct aspects of the phenomenology of anxiety in ASD should be considered in our future clinical and research efforts to define, measure, understand, and treat anxiety more comprehensively and effectively in ASD.

ACKNOWLEDGMENTS

We would like to give thanks to Hannah Long for her invaluable help in compiling the reference list. This work was also supported by grant funding awarded to C. Kerns (K23 HD087472).

VIGNETTE 1—"TRADITIONAL" PRESENTATION: SEPARATION AND GENERALIZED ANXIETY

Sophie was an 11-year old cognitively able young woman with ASD. She had a longstanding history of peer rejection at school and did not have friends. She was very reluctant to go places without her parents or allow them to go anywhere without her. If they did, she would call them repeatedly, up to 20 times per day. She carried with her when out bags containing "security items", as she believed she might need them in case she was kidnapped or her parents were killed, which she often worried about. She often went to sleep in her parents' bed at night due to anxiety. She worried about her performance at school, her health and her family's health, and the war in Iraq.

VIGNETTE 2—"DISTINCT" PRESENTATION: ANXIETY AROUND CHANGE

James was a 4-year old minimally verbal boy with ASD and moderate intellectual disability, with strengths in visual processing. He was attending preschool daily and had been very happy and settled there. He was using visual schedules with real photos of objects or activities to communicate with others at home and pre-school. Part way through the year, however, he demonstrated a behavioral change, becoming increasingly more irritable, and with increased echolalia and stereotyped speech. He started to show extreme anxiety when separating from his mother for pre-school. The teachers have in the last month switched to a communication system with symbols rather than photos of real objects and a new substitute teacher has been teaching his class, because his regular teacher has been unwell.

REFERENCES

American Pyschiatric Association, 2000. Diagnostic and Statistical Manual of Mental Disorders IV. Author, Washington DC.

Baron-Cohen, S., Wheelwright, S., Skinner, R., Martin, J., Clubley, E., 2001. The autism-spectrum quotient (AQ): evidence from Asperger Syndrome/high-functioning autism, males and females, scientists and mathematicians. J. Autism Dev. Disord. 31 (1), 5−17.

Bearss, K., Taylor, C.A., Aman, M.G., Whittemore, R., Lecavalier, L., Miller, J., et al., 2016. Using qualitative methods to guide scale development for anxiety in youth with autism spectrum disorder. Autism 20 (6), 663−672.

Bellini, S., 2004. Social skill deficits and anxiety in high-functioning adolescents with autism spectrum disorders. Focus Autism Other Dev Disabil. 19 (2), 78−86.

Blakeley-Smith, A., Reaven, J., Ridge, K., Hepburn, S., 2012. Parent−child agreement of anxiety symptoms in youth with autism spectrum disorders. Res Autism Spectr. Disord. 6 (2), 707−716.

Boulter, C., Freeston, M., South, M., Rodgers, J., 2014. Intolerance of uncertainty as a framework for understanding anxiety in children and adolescents with Autism Spectrum Disorders. J Autism Dev Disord. 44 (6), 1391−1402.

Cadman, T., Spain, D., Johnston, P., Russell, A., Mataix-Cols, D., Craig, M., et al., 2015. Obsessive−compulsive disorder in adults with high-functioning Autism Spectrum Disorder: what does self-report with the OCI-R tell us?. Autism Res. 8 (5), 477−485.

Carleton, R.N., Mulvogue, M.K., Thibodeau, M.A., McCabe, R.E., Antony, M.M., Asmundson, G.J.G., 2012. Increasingly certain about uncertainty: intolerance of uncertainty across anxiety and depression. J Anxiety Disord. 26 (3), 468−479.

Cath, D.C., Ran, N., Smit, J.H., van Balkom, A.J.L.M., Comijs, H.C., 2008. Symptom overlap between autism spectrum disorder, generalized social anxiety disorder and obsessive−compulsive disorder in adults: a preliminary case-controlled study. Psychopathology 41 (2), 101−110.

Dubin, A.H., Lieberman-Betz, R., Michele Lease, A., 2015. Investigation of individual factors associated with anxiety in youth with Autism Spectrum Disorders. J. Autism Dev. Disord. 45 (9), 2947—2960.

Dugas, M.J., Gagnon, F., Ladouceur, R., Freeston, M.H., 1998. Generalized anxiety disorder: a preliminary test of a conceptual model. Behav. Res. Ther. 36 (2), 215—226.

Evans, D.W., Canavera, K., Kleinpeter, F.L., Maccubbin, E., Taga, K., 2005. The fears, phobias and anxieties of children with autism spectrum disorders and down syndrome: comparisons with developmentally and chronologically age matched children. Child Psychiat. Human Dev. 36 (1), 3—26.

Farrugia, S., Hudson, J., 2006. Anxiety in adolescents with Asperger Syndrome: negative thoughts, behavioral problems, and life interference. Focus Autism Other Dev. Disabil. 21 (1), 25—35.

Foa, E.B., Huppert, J.D., Leiberg, S., Langner, R., Kichic, R., Hajcak, G., et al., 2002. The obsessive—compulsive inventory: development and validation of a short version. Psychol. Assessment 14 (4), 485—496.

Gillott, A., Standen, P.J., 2007. Levels of anxiety and sources of stress in adults with autism. J. Intellectual Disabil. 11 (4), 359—370.

Gillott, A., Furniss, F., Walter, A., 2001. Anxiety in high-functioning children with autism. Autism 5 (3), 277—286.

Gotham, K., Bishop, S.L., Hus, V., Huerta, M., Lund, S., Buja, A., et al., 2013. Exploring the relationship between anxiety and insistence on sameness in autism spectrum disorders. Autism Res. 6 (1), 33—41.

Greenaway, R., Howlin, P., 2010. Dysfunctional attitudes and perfectionism and their relationship to anxious and depressive symptoms in boys with autism spectrum disorders. J. Autism Dev. Disord. 40 (10), 1179—1187.

Hallett, V., Lecavalier, L., Sukhodolsky, D.G., Cipriano, N., Aman, M.G., McCracken, J. T., et al., 2013a. Exploring the manifestations of anxiety in children with autism spectrum disorders. J. Autism Dev. Disord. 43 (10), 2341—2352.

Hallett, V., Ronald, A., Colvert, E., Ames, C., Woodhouse, E., Lietz, S., et al., 2013b. Exploring anxiety symptoms in a large-scale twin study of children with autism spectrum disorders, their co-twins and controls. J. Child Psychol. Psychiatry 54 (11), 1176—1185.

Hofvander, B., Delorme, R., Chaste, P., Nyden, A., Wentz, E., Stahlberg, O., et al., 2009. Psychiatric and psychosocial problems in adults with normal-intelligence autism spectrum disorders. BMC Psychiatry 9, doi:Artn 3510.1186/1471-244x-9-35.

Kerns, C.M., Kendall, P.C., Berry, L., Souders, M.C., Franklin, M.E., Schultz, R.T., et al., 2014. Traditional and atypical presentations of anxiety in youth with Autism Spectrum Disorder. J.Autism Dev. Disord. 44 (11), 2851—2861.

Kerns, C.M., Maddox, B.B., Kendall, P.C., Rump, K., Berry, L., Schultz, R.T., et al., 2015a. Brief measures of anxiety in non-treatment-seeking youth with autism spectrum disorder. Autism 19 (8), 969—979.

Kerns, C.M., Newschaffer, C.J., Berkowitz, S.J., 2015b. Traumatic childhood events and Autism Spectrum Disorder. J. Autism Dev. Disord. 45 (11), 3475—3486.

Kerns, C.M., Kendall, P.C.,, 2014. Autism and anxiety: overlap, similarities, and differences. In: White, S.W., Ollendick, T.H., Davis III, T.E. (Eds.), Handbook of Autism and Anxiety. Springer, New York, NY, pp. 75—89.

Kerns, C.M., Renno, P., Kendall, P.C., Wood, J.J., Storch, E.A. (in press). Anxiety Disorders Interview Schedule-Autism Addendum: Reliability and validity in children with autism spectrum disorder. *Journal of Clinical Child and Adolescent Psychology.*

Kessler, R.C., Adler, L., Barkley, R., Biederman, J., Conners, C.K., Demler, O., et al., 2006. The prevalence and correlates of adult ADHD in the United States: results from the National Comorbidity Survey Replication. Am. J. Psychiatry 163 (4), 716—723.

Kerns, C.M., Rump, K., Worley, J., Kratz, H., McVey, A., Herrington, J., et al., 2016. The Differential Diagnosis of Anxiety Disorders in Cognitively-Able Youth With Autism. Cogn. Behav. Pract. 23 (4), 530−547.

Kuusikko, S., Pollock-Wurman, R., Jussila, K., Carter, A.S., Mattila, M.L., Ebeling, H., et al., 2008. Social anxiety in high-functioning children and adolescents with autism and Asperger syndrome. J. Autism Dev Disord. 38 (9), 1697−1709.

Leyfer, O.T., Folstein, S.E., Bacalman, S., Davis, N.O., Dinh, E., Morgan, J., et al., 2006. Comorbid psychiatric disorders in children with autism: interview development and rates of disorders. J. of Autism Dev.Disord. 36 (7), 849−861.

Maddox, B.B., White, S.W., 2015. Comorbid Social Anxiety Disorder in adults with Autism Spectrum Disorder. J. Autism Dev. Disord. 45 (12), 3949−3960.

Magiati, I., Chan, J.Y., Tan, W.L.J., Poon, K.K., 2014. Do non-referred young people with Autism Spectrum Disorders and their caregivers agree when reporting anxiety symptoms? A preliminary investigation using the Spence Children's Anxiety Scale. Res. Autism Spectrum Disord. 8 (5), 546−558.

Magiati, I., Ong, C., Lim, X.Y., Tan, J.W., Ong, A.Y., Patrycia, F., et al., 2016. Anxiety symptoms in young people with autism spectrum disorder attending special schools: associations with gender, adaptive functioning and autism symptomatology. Autism 20 (3), 306−320. Available from: http://dx.doi.org/10.1177/1362361315577519.

Magiati, I., Tan, W.-L.J., Chen, A., Knott, F., Ozsivadjian, A. 2016. A qualitative study of the factors associated with anxiety in children and young people with Autism Spectrum Disorder: further evidence for shared and autism-specific triggers and signs. Unpublished manuscript.

March, J.S., Parker, J.D.A., Sullivan, K., Stallings, P., Conners, C.K., 1997. The multidimensional anxiety scale for children (MASC): factor structure, reliability, and validity. J. Am. Acad. Child Adolesc. Psychiatry 36 (4), 554−565.

Mayes, S.D., Calhoun, S.L., Mayes, R.D., Molitoris, S., 2012. Autism and ADHD: overlapping and discriminating symptoms. Res. Autism Spectrum Disord. 6 (1), 277−285.

Mayes, D.S., Calhoun, S.L., Murray, M.J., Ahuja, M., Smith, L.A., 2011. Anxiety, depression and irritability in children with autism relative to other neuropsychiatric disorders and typical development. Res. Autism. Spectr. Discord. 5 (1), 474−485.

Mayes, S.D., Calhoun, S.L., Aggarwal, R., Baker, C., Mathapati, S., Molitoris, S., et al., 2013. Unusual fears in children with autism. Res. Autism Spectrum Disord. 7 (1), 151−158.

Mazefsky, C.A., Kao, J., Oswald, D.P., 2011. Preliminary evidence suggesting caution in the use of psychiatric self-report measures with adolescents with high-functioning autism spectrum disorders. Res Autism Spectrum Disord. 5 (1), 164−174.

McDougle, C.J., Kresch, L.E., Goodman, W.K., Naylor, S.T., Volkmar, F.R., Cohen, D. J., et al., 1995. A case-controlled study of repetitive thoughts and behavior in adults with autistic disorder and obsessive−compulsive disorder. Am. J. Psychiatry 152 (5), 772−777.

Mehtar, M., Mukaddes, N.M., 2011. Posttraumatic Stress Disorder in individuals with diagnosis of Autistic Spectrum Disorders. Res. Autism Spectrum Disord. 5 (1), 539−546.

Moree, B.N., Davis III, T.E., 2010. Cognitive-behavioral therapy for anxiety in children diagnosed with autism spectrum disorders: modification trends. Res. Autism Spectrum Disord. 4, 346−354.

Niditch, L.A., Varela, R.E., Kamps, J.L., Hill, T., 2012. Exploring the association between cognitive functioning and anxiety in children with Autism Spectrum Disorders: the role of social understanding and aggression. J. Clin. Child Adolesc. Psychol. 41 (2), 127−137.

Ollendick, T.H., Benoit, K.E., 2012. A parent−child interactional model of Social Anxiety Disorder in youth. Clin. Child Family Psychol. Rev. 15 (1), 81−91.

Ollendick, T.H., White, S.W., 2012. The presentation and classification of anxiety in Autism Spectrum Disorder: where to from here? Clin. Psychol. Sci. Practice 19 (4), 352–355.

Ozsivadjian, A., Knott, F., Magiati, I., 2012. Parent and child perspectives on the nature of anxiety in children and young people with autism spectrum disorders: a focus group study. Autism 16 (2), 107–121.

Ozsivadjian, A., Hibberd, C., Hollocks, M.J., 2014. Brief report: the use of self-report measures in young people with Autism Spectrum Disorder to access symptoms of anxiety, depression and negative thoughts. J. Autism Dev. Disord. 44 (4), 969–974.

Renno, P., Wood, J.J., 2013. Discriminant and convergent validity of the anxiety construct in children with Autism Spectrum Disorders. J. Autism Dev. Disord. 43 (9), 2135–2146.

Roberson-Nay, R., Strong, D.R., Nay, W.T., Beidel, D.C., Turner, S.M., 2007. Development of an abbreviated Social Phobia and Anxiety Inventory (SPAI) using item response theory: the SPAI-23. Psychol. Assessment 19 (1), 133–145.

Rodgers, J., Riby, D.M., Janes, E., Connolly, B., McConachie, H., 2012. Anxiety and repetitive behaviours in autism spectrum disorders and williams syndrome: a cross-syndrome comparison. J. Autism Dev. Disord. 42 (2), 175–180.

Rodgers, J., Wigham, S., McConachie, H., Freeston, M., Honey, E., Parr, J.R., 2016. Development of the anxiety scale for children with autism spectrum disorder (ASC-ASD). Autism Res. Available from: http://dx.doi.org/10.1002/aur.1603.

Russell, A.J., Mataix-Cols, D., Anson, M., Murphy, D.G., 2005. Obsessions and compulsions in Asperger syndrome and high-functioning autism. Br. J. Psychiatry 186, 525–528.

Ruta, L., Mugno, D., D'Arrigo, V.G., Vitiello, B., Mazzone, L., 2010. Obsessive–compulsive traits in children and adolescents with Asperger syndrome. Eur. Child Adolesc. Psychiatry 19 (1), 17–24.

Sasson, N.J., Turner-Brown, L.M., Holtzclaw, T.N., Lam, K.S.L., Bodfish, J.W., 2008. Children with autism demonstrate circumscribed attention during passive viewing of complex social and nonsocial picture arrays. Autism Res. 1 (1), 31–42.

Silverman, W.K., Albano, A.M., 1996. The Anxiety Interview Schedule for DSM-IV – Child and Parent Versions. Graywing, San Antonio, TX.

Simonoff, E., Pickles, A., Charman, T., Chandler, S., Loucas, T., Baird, G., 2008. Psychiatric disorders in children with autism spectrum disorders: prevalence, comorbidity, and associated factors in a population-derived sample. J. Am. Acad. Child Adolesc. Psychiatry 47 (8), 921–929.

Spiker, M.A., Lin, C.E., Van Dyke, M., Wood, J.J., 2012. Restricted interests and anxiety in children with autism. Autism 16, 306–320.

Storch, E.A., May, J.E., Wood, J.J., Jones, A.M., De Nadai, A.S., Lewin, A.B., et al., 2012. Multiple informant agreement on the Anxiety Disorders Interview Schedule in youth with Autism Spectrum Disorders. J. Child Adolesc. Psychopharmacol. 22 (4), 292–299.

Sukhodolsky, D.G., Scahill, L., Gadow, K.D., Arnold, L.E., Aman, M.G., McDougle, C.J., et al., 2008. Parent-rated anxiety symptoms in children with pervasive developmental disorders: frequency and association with core autism symptoms and cognitive functioning. J. Abnormal Child Psychol. 36 (1), 117–128.

Trembath, D., Germano, C., Johanson, G., Dissanayake, C., 2012. The experience of anxiety in young adults with Autism Spectrum Disorders. Focus Autism Other Dev. Disabil. 27 (4), 213–224.

Turner, L.B., Romanczyk, R.G., 2012. Assessment of fear in children with an autism spectrum disorder. Res. Autism Spectrum Disord. 6 (3), 1203–1210.

Tyson, K.E., Cruess, D.G., 2012. Differentiating high-functioning autism and social phobia. J. Autism Dev. Disord. 42 (7), 1477–1490.

Uljarevic, M., Carrington, S., Leekam, S., 2016. Brief report: effects of sensory sensitivity and intolerance of uncertainty on anxiety in mothers of children with Autism Spectrum Disorder. J. Autism Dev. Disord. 46 (1), 315—319.

Ung, D., Wood, J.J., Ehrenreich-May, J., Arnold, E.B., Fujii, C., Renno, P., et al., 2013. Clinical characteristics of high-functioning youth with autism spectrum disorder and anxiety. Neuropsychiatry 3 (2), 147—157.

Ung, D., Selles, R., Small, B.J., Storch, E.A., 2015. A systematic review and meta-analysis of Cognitive-Behavioral Therapy for anxiety in youth with High-Functioning Autism Spectrum Disorders. Child Psychiatry Human Dev. 46 (4), 533—547.

van Steensel, F.J., Bogels, S.M., Perrin, S., 2011. Anxiety disorders in children and adolescents with autistic spectrum disorders: a meta-analysis. Clin. Child Family Psychol. Rev. 14 (3), 302—317.

van Steensel, F.J.A., Dirksen, C.D., Bogels, S.M., 2014. Cost-effectiveness of cognitive-behavioral therapy versus treatment as usual for anxiety disorders in children with autism spectrum disorder. Res. Autism Spectrum Disord. 8 (2), 127—137.

Vasa, R.A., Mazurek, M.O., 2015. An update on anxiety in youth with autism spectrum disorders. Curr. Opin. Psychiatry 28 (2), 83—90.

Vasa, R.A., Carroll, L.M., Nozzolillo, A.A., Mahajan, R., Mazurek, M.O., Bennett, A.E., et al., 2014. A systematic review of treatments for anxiety in youth with autism spectrum disorders. J Autism Dev. Disord. 44 (12), 3215—3229.

Vasa, R.A., Mazurek, M.O., Mahajan, R., Bennett, A.E., Bernal, M.P., Nozzolillo, A.A., et al., 2016. Assessment and treatment of anxiety in youth with Autism Spectrum Disorders. Pediatrics 137 (2).

White, S.W., Oswald, D., Ollendick, T., Scahill, L., 2009. Anxiety in children and adolescents with autism spectrum disorders. Clin. Psychol. Rev. 29 (3), 216—229.

White, S.W., Bray, B.C., Ollendick, T.H., 2012. Examining shared and unique aspects of Social Anxiety Disorder and Autism Spectrum Disorder using factor analysis. J. Autism Dev. Disord. 42 (5), 874—884.

White, S.W., Lerner, M.D., McLeod, B.D., Wood, J.J., Ginsburg, G.S., Kerns, C., et al., 2015. Anxiety in youth with and without Autism Spectrum Disorder: examination of factorial equivalence. Behav. Therapy 46 (1), 40—53.

Wood, J.J., Gadow, K.D., 2010. Exploring the nature and function of anxiety in youth with Autism Spectrum Disorders. Clin. Psychol. Sci. Practice 17 (4), 281—292.

Zainal, H., Magiati, I., Tan, J.W.L., Sung, M., Fung, D.S.S., Howlin, P., 2014. A preliminary investigation of the Spence Children's Anxiety Parent Scale as a screening tool for anxiety in young people with Autism Spectrum Disorders. J. Autism Dev. Disord. 44 (8), 1982—1994.

CHAPTER 4

Neurobiological Mechanisms of Anxiety in ASD

John D. Herrington[1,2], Valentina Parma[3] and Judith S. Miller[1,2]
[1]The Children's Hospital of Philadelphia, Philadelphia, PA, United States
[2]University of Pennsylvania, Philadelphia, PA, United States
[3]Scuola Internazionale Superiore di Studi Avanzati, Trieste, Italy

INTRODUCTION

The majority of the existing literature on the cognitive neuroscience of ASD has focused on key diagnostic features—namely, social function, communication, and the systems that support these (e.g., visual perception and language). As a result, one might presume that we know very little about emotion systems in ASD, as affective processes do not figure prominently in the ASD diagnostic criteria. Then again, a strong case could be made that much of the existing literature on social information processing in ASD directly informs our understanding of affective processes in ASD, should we choose to view it that way. Indeed, the line between what is "social" and what is "emotional" is thin at best. This is clearly evident when one examines the kind of methodologies in widespread use to examine putative social information processes in ASD. For example, numerous experiments have been conducted in which an individual with ASD is asked to identify the emotion portrayed by an image of a face. What does it mean that most of these studies have interpreted the results in terms of social information processing and Theory of Mind, rather than affective processes? This choice of interpretation will often come as a surprise to an affective neuroscientist studying anxiety, who may conduct the identical experiment in a sample without ASD, without making any reference to Theory of Mind or social information processes. The bottom line is that most meaningful social interaction is also emotional.

It is therefore probable that findings of different patterns of "social brain" activity in ASD represent important clues as to why difficulties with emotion processes are so common. This chapter will review evidence from central and peripheral nervous system research on why

Anxiety in Children and Adolescents with Autism Spectrum Disorder.
DOI: http://dx.doi.org/10.1016/B978-0-12-805122-1.00004-1

© 2017 Elsevier Inc.
All rights reserved.

anxiety may occur so frequently in the context of ASD. First, we will start with a review of amygdala involvement in anxiety and social information processes in ASD, covering prominent theories of function, structure, and integration between the two. In addition to being perhaps the most widely studied brain region in the cognitive neuroscience of both ASD and anxiety disorders, emerging evidence indicates that it may be the most important place to look when trying to understand their comorbidity. Second, we will review amygdala within the context of other brain structures — namely prefrontal cortex — as evidence implicates differences in amygdala/prefrontal cortex connectivity in both ASD and anxiety. Lastly, we will review the relationship between amygdala function and autonomic nervous system findings (electrodermal and cardiac autonomic activity). For a variety of reasons, the autonomic nervous system may prove more amenable to the large-scale research required to address the co-occurrence of anxiety in ASD.

THE RELATIONSHIP BETWEEN AMYGDALA, ANXIETY, AND ASD

Amygdala function. The most salient neurobiological account of the high rates of anxiety in ASD has to do with amygdala. This brain structure is among the most studied in all of human cognitive neuroscience; most of the content that follows is elaborated upon in much more detail in one of many review books and chapters (for example, see Whalen and Phelps, 2009). Amygdala has been implicated in a variety of processes related to emotional and social function. It is of great interest to our understanding of the human brain because it appears to function across a wide swath of human life—from the engagement of pervasive instincts and reactions ("fight or flight") to the interpretation of the most subtle of social cues.

Ongoing, advanced theoretical work continues to shape our understanding of the role of amygdala in humans and non-humans (for reviews see Amaral et al., 2003a; Davidson, 2002; Phelps and LeDoux, 2005; Whalen, 1998). We find, however, that the literature on human amygdala function can be coarsely divided into two overlapping but somewhat distinct perspectives. The first perspective focuses on the role of amygdala in the "surveillance" of the environment for emotional and socially relevant information (henceforth, called the surveillance perspective). The second focuses on the role of amygdala in the experience and encoding of emotion (henceforth, called the emotion learning perspective).

The surveillance perspective. Amygdala is viewed as critical in coordinating biological systems to orient toward, process, and respond to significant external events. Much of the evidence in favor of this perspective comes from studies indicating that amygdala can be especially sensitive to degraded or peripheral socio-emotional information (e.g., detecting a "snake in the grass"; Whalen, 2007). Although controversial (see Pessoa and Adolphs, 2010), multiple lines of research indicate that amygdala receives some input from the external environment ahead of low-level perceptual structures (particularly those in visual cortex), suggesting that it has a privileged role in processing social and affective information (Morris et al., 1999; Pasley et al., 2004; Troiani et al., 2012). The surveillance perspective on amygdala function readily encompasses emotional as well as social information processes.

Most of the existing research on amygdala function in ASD is rooted in the surveillance perspective. These studies typically share a unidirectional perspective on amygdala activity in ASD—that it is underactive in situations where individuals rely on it to process social and emotional information (for reviews see Baron-Cohen et al., 2000; Herrington and Schultz, 2010; Pelphrey et al., 2011). The underactive amygdala narrative is probably the most ubiquitous of all narratives in the cognitive neuroscience literature on ASD.

The emotion learning perspective. A robust and longstanding literature suggests that amygdala plays a critical role in fear learning across species (Davis, 1992; Kalin et al., 2004; Wilensky et al., 2006). Amygdala has been shown to coordinate with prefrontal cortex during the encoding and experience of emotion-based learning, and to coordinate with memory structures (i.e. hippocampus) in the consolidation and retention of that learning (for example Shaw et al., 2005). Although most of this literature focuses on negatively valenced emotions (i.e., fear), the human amygdala also appears to play a role in positive emotions as well (Hamann et al., 2002; Herrington et al., 2010). Not surprisingly, increased amygdala activity is one of the most widely agreed upon theories of the neurobiology of anxiety disorders—whereby the increased amygdala activity leads to elevated levels of worry and fear, and diminished habituation to feared stimuli and events (in the absence of sufficient coordination with other regulatory structures; Davis, 1992; Pine et al., 2008; Rauch et al., 2006).

Of course, individuals with ASD have higher rates of anxiety than the general population (Gadow, Devincent et al., 2005; Lecavalier, 2006; Sukhodolsky et al., 2008). Thus, we are faced with reconciling the fact that ASD is associated with *underactivity* of the amygdala, but that anxiety is associated with *overactivity*. We contend that the single most pressing issue in the cognitive neuroscience of anxiety in ASD concerns how we integrate these two empirical findings on amygdala function, and the two broader perspectives from which they are drawn.

To illustrate from our own data: in a large child sample (N = 81 ASD and 67 typically developing controls, or TDC; mean age = 12.5 years for both groups), symptoms of anxiety and ASD are correlated with amygdala function in opposite directions (Herrington, Miller, Pandey, and Schultz, 2016). Participants in this study completed a face identity task that elicits robust amygdala activity in both ASD and non-ASD samples. The parents of all participants completed the Social Communication Questionnaire (SCQ, a measure of core ASD symptoms; Chandler et al., 2007) and the parent-report version of the Screen for Child Anxiety Related Emotional Disorders (SCARED; Birmaher et al., 1997). The right panel of Fig 4.1 shows the correlations between each of these two questionnaire measures

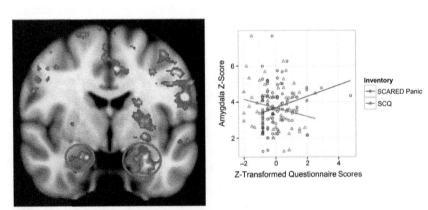

Figure 4.1 Anxiety and core ASD symptoms correlate with amygdala activity in opposite directions. Left panel: increased bilateral amygdala activity (circled) in control children (N = 67) compared to children with ASD matched for anxiety symptoms (i.e., low anxiety levels; N = 24). Right panel: correlations between right amygdala activity, the Panic/Somatic subscale of the Screen for Child Anxiety Related Emotional Disorders (SCARED; Birmaher et al., 1997), and the Social Communication Questionnaire (SCQ; Chandler et al., 2007). Questionnaire scores were z-transformed for illustration because the two inventories have very different ranges.

and peak activity within left amygdala in the ASD group (the questionnaires have different ranges and are therefore plotted as z-scores, using the ASD group mean and standard deviation for each). Although data from the Panic/Somatic subdomain of the SCARED are depicted in Fig. 4.1, the findings are nearly identical for the Separation Anxiety subscale and overall scale as well (relationships between amygdala activation and both social and generalized anxiety were less strong). Fig. 4.1 left panel illustrates significantly increased amygdala activity in the TDC group relative to individuals in the bottom quartile of SCARED scores (i.e., matched with the TDC group in anxiety). When comparing the TDC group to the other ASD quartiles, no significant difference was found within bilateral amygdala. These data point to two conclusions. First, social deficits and anxiety symptoms are associated with amygdala activity in opposite directions. Second, the longstanding findings of decreased amygdala activity only hold for those individuals with ASD and low levels of anxiety.

These data raise the question: how do we reconcile the association between *decreased* amygdala activation and social deficits in ASD with findings of *increased* amygdala activation and anxiety in ASD? And, by extension, what do the seminal findings of decreased amygdala activity as a putative biomarker of ASD have to say to the alarmingly high rates of anxiety symptoms in this population? Sadly, there is a striking lack of data available to address these questions. At the time this chapter was written, we knew of two functional imaging studies other than our own that formally integrated data on anxiety symptoms, with mixed findings. Whereas Weng et al. (2011) reported no relationship between amygdala activity and anxiety scores on the Spence Child Anxiety Scale (Spence, 1998), Kleinhans et al. (2010) reported a significant correlation between social anxiety and amygdala activity (measured via the Social Avoidance and Distress Scale). Clearly these results are in need of replication, ideally using a variety of dimensional and categorical measures of anxiety in ASD in large samples of children with ASD.

Amygdala structure. In addition to studies of amygdala function, research on amygdala structure in ASD is also likely to play a role in our understanding of the co-occurrence of anxiety in ASD. This brief review focuses primarily on lesion studies in non-human primates and neuroimaging studies of morphometry (for a review of cytoarchitectural and postmortem studies, see Schumann and Nordahl, 2011).

Lesion studies relate to brain structure and function; we have chosen somewhat arbitrarily to review it in this section on structure.

The non-human primate lesion work of David Amaral, Margaret Baumann, and Cindy Schumann provides a vivid representation of the relationship between amygdala structure and anxiety in ASD. Although nearly a century of amygdala lesion studies in non-human primates have been cited as evidence of amygdala-mediated social deficits in ASD, a series of experiments conducted by Amaral et al. cast these studies in a new light (Amaral, 2002; Amaral et al., 2003b; Bauman et al., 2004a,b). Their experiments involved rhesus monkeys that were monitored in a seminaturalistic environment (a field cage permitting communication between conspecifics). They found that highly selective amygdala lesions did not appear to diminish the nature or quality of social interaction in adult monkeys. In fact, they reported that social behavior actually increased (due to the absence of typical social inhibition processes implemented by amygdala). In subsequent studies, they examined the effect of amygdala lesions earlier in development; they found that monkeys with amygdala lesions who were reared by their mothers demonstrated typical primate social behavior across a variety of metrics (i.e., postures, vocalizations, facial expression, etc.). Furthermore, their interest in conspecifics did not appear diminished (i.e., intact social motivation; see Chevallier et al., 2012).

Conversely, monkeys with amygdala lesions demonstrated behaviors consistent with abnormal fear processes. These behaviors include the inconsistent and inaccurate evaluation of threats in the environment, and hyperresponsivity to these threats. These and other results led the authors to the striking conclusion that the relationship between amygdala and social deficits in ASD may in fact be mediated by anxiety (Amaral et al., 2003b).

The relationship between these findings and human imaging studies of amygdala structure are presently unclear. Findings on amygdala structure in ASD have been notoriously ambiguous, with multiple studies showing decreased volume (Aylward et al., 1999; Nacewicz et al., 2006; Pierce et al., 2001), increased volume (Howard et al., 2000; Mosconi et al., 2009; Munson et al., 2006), and null results (Haznedar et al., 2000). As pointed out by Schumann et al. (2010, 2011), discrepancies between findings are driven by multiple factors, among which two appear critical. First, it is likely that differences in amygdala structure are not specific to ASD, and may therefore relate to only part of the ASD phenotype (for instance, they have been associated with mood and anxiety disorders; Milham et al., 2005; J. C. Pfeifer et al., 2008). Second, amygdala growth follows a developmental progression that may prove more informative than cross-sectional differences in volume. In one of the only longitudinal studies of amygdala volume in ASD, Schumann et al. reported that individuals with ASD showed amygdala overgrowth earlier in development, but a later deceleration in this growth, yielding a null volume difference between ASD and control participants at adolescence (Schumann et al., 2004). The implication is that the observation of amygdala volume differences in ASD may turn critically on the age of the cohort under consideration.

Given the compelling findings from the non-human primate research connecting anxiety to amygdala function, it is surprising that there are no published studies formally testing the relationship between amygdala volume and anxiety disorders in ASD (though Juranek et al., 2006, identified a positive correlation between amygdala volume and the anxious/depressed subscale of the Child Behavior Checklist). We recently completed data collection among 63 children with ASD and 37 non-anxious TDC children (mean age = 12 years) who underwent extensive psychodiagnostic assessment for anxiety disorders (including the Anxiety Disorder Interview Schedule developed by Silverman et al., 2001, and the ASD-specific addendum developed by Kerns et al., 2014). As predicted by Schumann et al., we did not see a significant difference between ASD and TDC groups in amygdala volume as a whole at this age. However, volume differences emerged when the co-occurrence of anxiety disorders were factored into the analysis. When breaking down the ASD group into children with and without a co-occurring anxiety disorder, we found a significant decrease in right amygdala volume for ASD children with anxiety relative to the TDC group. This result raises the intriguing possibility that previous studies examining the relationship between amygdala volume and the core symptoms of ASD missed out on an extremely important piece of information—the presence or absence of co-occurring anxiety.

Amygdala: Integration and future research. It is often difficult to integrate findings on brain function and structure, as they do not always show a reciprocal relationship. Structural differences may manifest clearly in signals from functional imaging, and differences in functional activation magnitude may be closely related or entirely unrelated to structural differences (at least at the scale where we can observe them with modern neuroimaging). Furthermore, functional and structural imaging do not always have analogous relationships with psychological variables. Nevertheless, the available data relating differences in amygdala function and structure to the co-occurrence of anxiety in ASD seem compelling, though nascent.

In reviewing these data, we are drawn to two lines of inquiry as future directions. The first concerns a deeper understanding of possible differential roles of amygdala subregions. Although frequently overlooked in human imaging research, a compelling case can be made that amygdala is not actually a single structure, but rather, a constellation of nuclei with putatively diverse functions (Swanson and Petrovich, 1998). Functional heterogeneity within amygdala has long been a focus of preclinical work; but, due to multiple limitations of MRI technology and methodology, it is extremely difficult to examine non-invasively in humans. There are nevertheless emerging theories regarding functional heterogeneity that could have a major impact on how we understand the neurobiology of anxiety in ASD. For example, recent data and methodological work by Bickart et al. (Bickart et al., 2014; Bickart et al., Hollenbeck et al., 2012) indicate that amygdala may be functionally subdivided into regions implementing socio-emotional perception, social approach/affiliation, and aversion/fear. Data such as these point to the hypothesis that the etiology of ASD involves differences in amygdala structure and function, and whether those differences relate to symptoms of anxiety as well as social deficits turns critically on the portions of amygdala affected in any given individual (and/or the connections between distinct portions of amygdala and other cortical structures).

A second important line of inquiry is more theoretical in nature. There is a pressing need to arrive at a clear understanding of precisely how amygdala simultaneously supports what might be categorized as approach (prosocial, affiliative) and avoidance (fear, aversion) tendencies in humans. There is a reason that the review above refers to two "perspectives" on amygdala function and not, say, two "theories." It is improbable that these surveillance and emotion learning perspectives are genuinely distinct (to take one straightforward example, humans clearly leverage fear learning in the context of social information processing). But, when examining why anxiety occurs so often in ASD, how we resolve this distinction matters. To frame the debate in constructs that will be familiar to both ASD and anxiety disorder researchers: we need a better understanding of how this structure plays a simultaneous role in social motivation, social understanding, and in the experience of emotion (particularly negative emotion).

AMYGDALA, PREFRONTAL CORTEX, AND BRAIN CONNECTIVITY IN ASD

Although amygdala has assumed particular importance in our understanding of social and emotional functions, it works in concert with other brain systems that may prove very important in our understanding of anxiety in ASD. These areas include portions of prefrontal cortex (PFC) that have long been implicated in affect and the regulation of affect. The identification of different roles for these structures is an active area of research (Blackford and Pine, 2012; Engels et al., 2007; Mohanty et al., 2007). Here we highlight some of these structures and how they relate to the etiology of ASD, and of anxiety within ASD.

Ventral PFC (i.e., the bottom portion of the frontal lobes) shares (primarily inhibitory) connections with amygdala and adjacent medial temporal cortex. This area can be further subdivided into ventrolateral and ventromedial PFC (vlPFC and vmPFC), with the latter corresponding to subgenual anterior cingulate cortex. vmPFC has been shown to coordinate with amygdala during fear learning, and appears to play a particular role in fear extinction (Delgado et al., 2008; Milad et al., 2007). Aberrant vmPFC activation has been observed in studies of multiple mood and anxiety disorders (for review see Davidson, 2002; Myers-Schulz and Koenigs, 2012).

Existing evidence indicates that vlPFC has a somewhat distinct role in emotion processes vis-à-vis vmPFC. vlPFC has been implicated in attentional biases toward emotional information (Britton et al., 2012; Waters et al., 2010). Anxiety disorders have long been associated with increased attentional capture by affective stimuli; this process is in fact interpreted as part of the etiology of anxiety (Bar-Haim et al., 2007; Heeren et al., 2011).

Support is accumulating for differences in attentional bias patterns toward and away from social and emotional information in ASD (Chawarska et al., 2010; Chevallier et al., in press; Isomura, Ogawa, Yamada et al., 2014). We nevertheless have very little data to speak to whether these effects are moderated by anxiety, as would be predicted by the anxiety disorder attentional bias literature. This is unfortunate, because attentional bias paradigms hold promise as potential non-verbal assessments of anxiety in ASD. However, there are now two studies suggesting that measures of attentional bias may *not* in fact be sensitive to anxiety symptoms in ASD (Hollocks et al., 2013; May et al., 2015). The question of whether anxiety-related attentional bias mechanisms are indeed different in ASD and non-ASD populations (and not a result of experimental confounds) is a pressing one, as it may help us determine the extent to which anxiety in ASD is a distinct phenomenon (Isomura et al., 2014).

The anxiety disorder literature on ventral PFC and anxiety raises the questions: are differences in ventral PFC function generally observed in ASD, and are these related to anxiety? At present, the available data speaking to either question are sparse. More dorsal portions of PFC have been much more carefully studied in ASD, as these are implicated in Theory of Mind processes (see Herrington and Schultz, 2010). Watanabe et al. (2012) reported decreased vmPFC activity in ASD during the perception of social stimuli in ASD. Conversely, Dalton et al. (2005) reported increased ventral PFC activation in ASD during a face processing task.

Examinations of ventral PFC/amygdala connectivity may prove more valuable in understanding anxiety in ASD than studies of ventral PFC alone. A recurring theme in the developmental neuroimaging literature is the role of these areas in regulating amygdala function in the context of social and emotional processes. For example, it appears likely that the development of enhanced cognitive control and emotion regulation in adolescence is accompanied by enhanced regulation of amygdala by these structures (Giedd and Rapoport, 2010; though see J.H. Pfeifer and Allen, 2012, for counterarguments to this perspective). In this context, emotion regulation emerges from a balance between amygdala activity (which may in fact be "bottom up") and PFC regulatory processes (which would be more "top down"). We and others often refer to this informally as the "balance model" of amygdala/PFC connectivity. Abnormalities in the development of this reciprocal relationship may in fact represent trans-diagnostic biomarkers of psychopathology, encompassing ASD, mood and anxiety disorders, attention deficit-hyperactivity disorder, and others (Arnsten and Rubia, 2012; Heatherton and Wagner, 2011; Passarotti et al., 2010; Pine et al., 2008).

A case can be made that the balance model has particular explanatory power in ASD, and in the context of co-occurring anxiety in ASD. This case is based on emerging findings of differences in both short and long-range brain connectivity in ASD (for review see Minshew and Williams, 2007). Although these findings have been reported among neuronal cell bodies and their connecting fibers (i.e., gray and white matter), some evidence exists to indicate that white matter may be particularly vulnerable (Barnea-Goraly et al., 2004; Cheon et al., 2011; Ke et al., 2009). These findings point to the largely untested hypothesis that individuals with ASD and co-occurring anxiety in ASD have differences in fibers that connect amygdala and adjacent temporal lobe areas to prefrontal cortex (white matter tracks of particular interest include the arcuate and uncinate fasciculus and the cingulum). Again, we may be presented with a situation where a relatively broad neurodevelopmental progression leads to symptoms of ASD, but only leads to symptoms of anxiety in those individuals where this progression affects specific areas (i.e., tissue spanning amygdala and PFC). Although the structural evidence for diminished PFC/amygdala connectivity has yet to fully emerge, a growing number of studies show abnormal functional connectivity between these regions (Bachevalier and Loveland, 2006; Murphy et al., 2012; Swartz et al., 2013).

THE BRAIN IN CONTEXT: THE AUTONOMIC NERVOUS SYSTEM IN ANXIETY AND ASD

Brain imaging research promises to play an important role in our emerging understanding of the etiology of anxiety in ASD. However, there are limitations to what we can learn from brain imaging. The separation of the inherently overlapping symptom profiles of anxiety and ASD may require rather large numbers of well-characterized research participants to accomplish—a problem, given the difficulty and expense of both characterization and imaging. Furthermore, brain imaging studies are generally skewed toward more mildly affected individuals due to the inherent difficulty of the recording procedures (staying very still for an extended period of time inside an MRI machine). As a result, brain imaging research often runs the risk of yielding results that do not generalize well across the entire autism spectrum.

There are of course many ways to examine the neurobiology of anxiety in ASD that do not rely on imaging. Here we discuss the growing field of research on the autonomic nervous system (ANS) in ASD, for several reasons. ANS is considered a primary behavioral regulation system (Porges, 2001), controlling multiple organs and glands throughout the body via complex afferent—efferent pathways. There are multiple ANS manifestations of anxiety, some of which relate to amygdala function (Porges, 2001; Thayer et al., 2012). Given the complexity of the afferent/efferent interactions, dysfunction of the ANS is hypothesized as a possible etiological factor in social information processing differences in ASD. Fortunately, ANS measurement is tractable across the whole spectrum, irrespective of developmental and functional levels, given the relative ease of recording procedures (for this and other reasons, it also has significant appeal as a marker of treatment outcome). Last, but not least, recent technological advancements permit the recording of ANS functions in naturalistic settings outside of the laboratory.

Although there are now a fair number of studies on ANS function in ASD (reviewed briefly here), only a handful of them formally consider the co-occurrence of anxiety.

The ANS can be divided in two main branches: the sympathetic nervous system (SNS, mediating "fight or flight" behavior, resulting in increased heart rate and hyperarousal), and the parasympathetic nervous system (PNS, responsible for "rest-and-digest" responses, characterized by bradycardia and lower arousal). Recent studies support ANS dysregulation in the majority of individuals with ASD, as evidenced by patterns of sympathetic hyperarousal and blunted parasympathetic vagal tone (Klusek et al., 2015; Patriquin et al., 2011). However, findings are still mixed, as revealed by the analysis of SNS and PNS indices such as electrodermal activity (EDA) and cardiac activity, respectively.

Electrodermal activity, anxiety, and ASD

Research on EDA (sometimes referred to as skin conductance, or the older term galvanic skin response) in ASD has increased in recent years. Greater EDA has long been associated with attentional orienting as well as increased anxiety (Dawson et al., 2007). Indeed, hyperarousal—an elevated state of physiological activation—is a defining feature of anxiety.

There is considerable variability in reports of tonic baseline measures of EDA among children with ASD (Hirstein et al., 2001; Joseph et al., 2008; McCormick et al., 2014; Schoen, Miller et al., 2009; van Engeland, 1984). Similarly mixed results are also found when analyzing phasic EDA to different sensory stimuli (Schoen et al., 2009; van Engeland, 1984). There is general agreement that this variability is driven in no small part by variability across samples (e.g., age, symptom severity), experimental parameters, and recording procedures (Hirstein et al., 2001; McCormick et al., 2014). However, this variability is also very likely related to clinically relevant variables with known relationships to EDA—namely, anxiety and arousal.

We recently tested this hypothesis among a group of 75 children with and without ASD and a comorbid anxiety diagnosis (i.e., a 2 X 2 design with presence/absence of ASD and anxiety diagnoses as factors; Parma et al., in preparation). We found that ASD and anxiety contributed uniquely to tonic EDA; whereas anxiety is associated with hyperarousal (increased EDA) in the typically developing group, the opposite pattern was evident when studying participants with ASD and anxiety (however, it should be noted that the difference in tonic EDA did not differ between ASD individuals with and without anxiety).

While baseline, tonic EDA activity provides significant information about ANS function in ASD and anxiety, phasic, time-locked changes in EDA provide additional information regarding how individuals respond to social and emotional stimuli in the environment. The small literature on phasic EDA in response to emotion and social processes do not yet provide a clear pattern. In a study of direct vs. averted gaze identification, ASD showed larger EDA responses while looking at faces (Joseph et al., 2008), suggesting that emotional hyperarousal in ASD is present and may interfere with face processing (also see Dalton et al., 2005). However, opposite results (reduced EDA responses) have been reported when adults with ASD were asked to judge facial emotions (Hubert et al., 2009). Again, the relative role of confounding and clinical relevant variables has yet to be fully explored.

Classical conditioning paradigms measuring EDA provide valuable insight into amygdala-dependent socio-emotional arousal. In the conditioning context, EDA reflects the dynamics of learning to discriminate between threatening and safe stimuli (the greater the EDA, the greater the learning). South et al. (2011) demonstrated the increment in learning by those participants in the ASD group who showed the greater the SCR during conditioning. Interestingly, greater EDA corresponded also to greater social deficits and the most reduced social functioning.

Cardiac activity, anxiety, and ASD

A reliable assessment of PNS function can be obtained from the analysis of cardiac activity. The application of spectral analysis to heart rate yields a metric called heart rate variability (HRV), which refers to the variation in the duration of time intervals between heartbeats. Heart rate and HRV are governed by many components of physiology. One of these is the vagus nerve, a key component of the PNS that interfaces with the brain and the sinoatrial node of the heart (alongside multiple other organs; Berntson et al., 2007). Vagal control over the heart has the effect of increasing HRV (particularly in higher frequency bands, or respiratory sinus arrhythmia [RSA], when the high-frequency component occurs in conjunction with respiratory patterns). Increase HRV indicates a state of physiological calm (Berntson et al., 2007). Conversely, vagal control decreases under conditions of stress, yielding a decrease in HRV (Allen et al., 2014).

Decreased HRV has long been associated with disorders of social and emotional function, and has been shown to track changes in these symptoms in non-ASD samples (Bär et al., 2004; Porges et al., 1975; Tucker et al., 1997; Yeragani et al., 1992). Dozens of studies have examined the relationship between HRV and individual differences in social communication and emotion regulation (for review see Porges, 2001). There is now a large body of evidence indicating that increased HRV is associated with increased social engagement, and that decreased HRV is associated with decreased quality and magnitude of social contact (Bal et al., 2010; Guy et al., 2014; Hallett et al., 2013; Neuhaus et al., 2010; Neuhaus et al., 2013). HRV may in fact provide a much-needed index of social functioning in ASD that is not verbally mediated.

Conversely, increased HRV is viewed as directly and indirectly associated with prosocial behavior. The dominant theories within biopsychosocial research on HRV rely on the premise that it is positively associated with an increased propensity for social engagement, an increase in the quality of that engagement, and better emotion regulation skills (see Porges's Polyvagal Theory [Porges, 2001; Porges et al., 2012], Thayer and Lane's Neurovisceral Integration Model [Thayer and Lane, 2000], and Bertson's Model of Autonomic Space [Berntson et al., 2008]). Most recently, it has been proposed that the Autonomic Space Model and Neurovisceral Integration Model together hold explanatory potential in the proposed socio-emotional deficits in ASD and its cortical, subcortical, autonomic and behavioral correlates (Benevides and Lane, 2015).

While HRV is associated with prosocial engagement behaviors among typically developing individuals, until recently there have been few studies of HRV in ASD. A growing number of recent studies consistently report decreased HRV in ASD (Bal et al., 2010; Guy et al., 2014; Hollocks et al., 2014; Neuhaus et al., 2013; Porges et al., 2012). We recently showed a significant decrease in HRV for a modest sample of youth with ASD compared to age- and IQ-matched controls (Guy et al., 2014), and have now replicated and extended this finding in a larger sample (43 ASD, 26 controls; in preparation). These data indicate a large and replicable effect between ASD and controls, regardless of medication status in ASD participants.

In principle, vagal control of HRV represents a compelling account for the co-occurrence of anxiety in ASD. Specifically, differences in PNS function may simultaneously account for the core social symptoms of ASD and symptoms of anxiety that often accompany them. Data related to HRV, anxiety, and ASD are only beginning to emerge. Neuhaus et al. (Neuhaus et al., 2013) reported a relationship between resting state HRV and internalizing symptoms (measured via the Child Behavior Checklist) in an ASD sample. Hollocks et al. (Hollocks et al., 2014) reported a relationship between higher levels of anxiety in an ASD sample and decreased HRV subsequent to a psychosocial stressor (the Trier Social Stress Test). With the dramatic increase in availability of heart rate measures, we can expect to see much more research in this area in the future, ideally with large samples that permit the parsing of heterogeneity across multiple symptom domains (i.e., anxiety and social functioning).

CONCLUSIONS AND FUTURE DIRECTIONS

When looking back on the remarkable quantity of ASD cognitive neuroscience research from recent decades, it is hard not to get the sense that there has been a missed opportunity to deepen our understanding of why anxiety is so common in ASD. The missed opportunity stems largely from one cause—anxiety has seldom been considered a relevant dimension in ASD neurobiology research, and has therefore not been measured. In a sense this is quite understandable—the valid and reliable measurement of core ASD symptoms is challenging enough by itself. But we have entered an era where ASD is viewed as multidimensional, and transdiagnostic research is increasingly prioritized. We seem poised to develop a much more mature understanding of the neurobiology of anxiety in ASD—one that requires the use of multi-method approaches.

Studies examining amygdala, ventral PFC, and their connectivity will likely be at the forefront of research on the neurobiology in ASD. Large-sample studies of well-characterized participants will be critical. But perhaps more important will be the willingness of cognitive neuroscientists to expand their research perspective beyond traditional ASD constructs (such as Theory of Mind), to encompass the rich literature on the neurobiology of affect.

Another critical area for future research relates to developmental progression. Researchers of anxiety in ASD face an ongoing conundrum: to what extent is anxiety part of the etiology of ASD versus a consequence of the symptoms of ASD? Neurobiology could provide critical insights on this question, especially if more research were to be conducted using younger populations followed longitudinally. Brain imaging is challenging in young children, whereas ANS measures are less so. More data are needed on the progression of peripheral biomarkers of anxiety and arousal in toddlers and preschoolers with ASD.

The proliferation of psychophysiological measures will open up new doors to our understanding of the biological mechanisms of ASD, by allowing for a more nuanced clinical characterization, describing treatment targets, and predicting and measuring responses to intervention. Furthermore, the accessibility and affordability of new technologies allows for the collection of data outside of laboratory settings on an unprecedented scale, thereby increasing our ability to isolate unique and overlapping relationships between psychological dimensions and the neurobiology of ASD. Indeed, biosensors are now often wireless and can stream to devices that are commonplace in many households (like smartphones). However, it is worth noting that many commercially available biosensors do not provide the type, quality, and reliability of data needed to devise anything but the coarsest indices (e.g., beats per minute). Whereas mobile tools for electrocardiography (ECG) may suffer less from movement artifacts, analogous tools for measuring EDA are especially problematic, because the noise introduced by movement is extremely hard to disentangle from the electrodermal signal itself. It is unclear how this particular problem will best be solved. Relatedly, the near absence of empirical, peer-reviewed studies validating mobile heart rate and electrodermal measures against gold-standard equipment is something that needs to be rectified.

And finally, more data are needed involving state manipulations of anxiety in ASD. The development of affective challenge paradigms such as the Laboratory Temperament Assessment Battery (Lab-TAB; Gagne et al., 2011) may provide critical information about the flexibility of affective systems—information that may not be available at rest or during traditional experimental tasks. It will require creativity on the part of cognitive neuroscience to implement these types of paradigms. But the payoff they provide might be very large, allowing us to obtain potentially critical information on the temporal dynamics of anxiety (and emotion regulation more generally) in ASD.

REFERENCES

Allen, A.P., Kennedy, P.J., Cryan, J.F., Dinan, T.G., Clarke, G., 2014. Biological and psychological markers of stress in humans: focus on the Trier Social Stress Test. Neurosci. Biobehav. Rev. 38, 94—124, http://doi.org/10.1016/j.neubiorev.2013.11.005.
Amaral, D.G., 2002. The primate amygdala and the neurobiology of social behavior: implications for understanding social anxiety. Biol. Psychiatry 51 (1), 11—17.
Amaral, D.G., Bauman, M., Capitanio, J., Lavenex, P., Mason, W., Mauldin-Jourdain, M., et al., 2003a. The amygdala: Is it an essential component of the neural network for social cognition? Neuropsychologia Vol 41 (4), 517—522.

Amaral, D.G., Bauman, M.D., Schumann, C.M., 2003b. The amygdala and autism: implications from non-human primate studies. Genes Brain Behav. 2 (5), 295–302.

Arnsten, A.F.T., Rubia, K., 2012. Neurobiological circuits regulating attention, cognitive control, motivation, and emotion: disruptions in neurodevelopmental psychiatric disorders. J. Am. Acad. Child Adolesc. Psychiatry 51 (4), 356–367, http://doi.org/10.1016/j.jaac.2012.01.008.

Aylward, E.H., Minshew, N.J., Goldstein, G., Honeycutt, N.A., Augustine, A.M., Yates, K.O., et al., 1999. MRI volumes of amygdala and hippocampus in non-mentally retarded autistic adolescents and adults. Neurology 53 (9), 2145–2150.

Bachevalier, J., Loveland, K.A., 2006. The orbitofrontal-amygdala circuit and self-regulation of social-emotional behavior in autism. Neurosci. Biobehav. Rev. 30 (1), 97–117, http://doi.org/10.1016/j.neubiorev.2005.07.002.

Bal, E., Harden, E., Lamb, D., Van Hecke, A.V., Denver, J.W., Porges, S.W., 2010. Emotion recognition in children with autism spectrum disorders: relations to eye gaze and autonomic state. J. Autism Dev. Disord. 40 (3), 358–370, http://doi.org/10.1007/s10803-009-0884-3.

Bär, K.-J., Greiner, W., Jochum, T., Friedrich, M., Wagner, G., Sauer, H., 2004. The influence of major depression and its treatment on heart rate variability and pupillary light reflex parameters. J. Affect. Disord. 82 (2), 245–252, http://doi.org/10.1016/j.jad.2003.12.016.

Bar-Haim, Y., Lamy, D., Pergamin, L., Bakermans-Kranenburg, M.J., van IJzendoorn, M.H., 2007. Threat-related attentional bias in anxious and nonanxious individuals: a meta-analytic study. Psychol. Bull. 133 (1), 1–24, http://doi.org/10.1037/0033-2909.133.1.1.

Barnea-Goraly, N., Kwon, H., Menon, V., Eliez, S., Lotspeich, L., Reiss, A.L., 2004. White matter structure in autism: preliminary evidence from diffusion tensor imaging. Biol. Psychiatry 55 (3), 323–326.

Baron-Cohen, S., Ring, H., Bullmore, E., Wheelwright, S., Ashwin, C., Williams, S., 2000. The amygdala theory of autism. Neurosci. Biobehav. Rev. 24 (3), 355–364.

Bauman, M.D., Lavenex, P., Mason, W.A., Capitanio, J.P., Amaral, D.G., 2004a. The development of mother-infant interactions after neonatal amygdala lesions in rhesus monkeys. J. Neurosci. 24 (3), 711–721, http://doi.org/10.1523/JNEUROSCI.3263-03.2004.

Bauman, M.D., Lavenex, P., Mason, W.A., Capitanio, J.P., Amaral, D.G., 2004b. The development of social behavior following neonatal amygdala lesions in rhesus monkeys. J. Cogn. Neurosci. 16 (8), 1388–1411, http://doi.org/10.1162/0898929042304741.

Benevides, T.W., Lane, S.J., 2015. A review of cardiac autonomic measures: considerations for examination of physiological response in children with autism spectrum disorder. J. Autism Dev. Disord. 45 (2), 560–575, http://doi.org/10.1007/s10803-013-1971-z.

Berntson, G.G., Quigley, K.S., Lozano, Da, 2007. Cardiovascular Psychophysiology. In: Cacioppo, J.T., Tassinary, L.G., Berntson, G.G. (Eds.), Handbook of Psychophysiology, 3rd ed Cambridge University Press, New York, NY, USA, p. 182. , -120.

Berntson, G.G., Norman, G.J., Hawkley, L.C., Cacioppo, J.T., 2008. Cardiac autonomic balance versus cardiac regulatory capacity. Psychophysiology 45 (4), 643–652, http://doi.org/10.1111/j.1469-8986.2008.00652.x.

Bickart, K.C., Hollenbeck, M.C., Barrett, L.F., Dickerson, B.C., 2012. Intrinsic amygdala-cortical functional connectivity predicts social network size in humans. J. Neurosci. 32 (42), 14729–14741, http://doi.org/10.1523/JNEUROSCI.1599-12.2012.

Bickart, K.C., Dickerson, B.C., Barrett, L.F., 2014. The amygdala as a hub in brain networks that support social life. Neuropsychologia 63, 235–248, http://doi.org/10.1016/j.neuropsychologia.2014.08.013.

Birmaher, B., Khetarpal, S., Brent, D., Cully, M., Balach, L., Kaufman, J., et al., 1997. The Screen for Child Anxiety Related Emotional Disorders (SCARED): scale construction and psychometric characteristics. J. Am. Acad. Child Adolesc. Psychiatry 36 (4), 545−553, http://doi.org/10.1097/00004583-199704000-00018.

Blackford, J.U., Pine, D.S., 2012. Neural substrates of childhood anxiety disorders: a review of neuroimaging findings. Child Adolesc. Psychiatric Clin. N. Am. 21 (3), 501−525, http://doi.org/10.1016/j.chc.2012.05.002.

Britton, J.C., Bar-Haim, Y., Carver, F.W., Holroyd, T., Norcross, M.A., Detloff, A., et al., 2012. Isolating neural components of threat bias in pediatric anxiety. J. Child Psychol. Psychiatry Allied Dis. 53 (6), 678−686, http://doi.org/10.1111/j.1469-7610.2011.02503.x.

Chandler, S., Charman, T., Baird, G., Simonoff, E., Loucas, T., Meldrum, D., et al., 2007. Validation of the Social Communication Questionnaire in a Population Cohort of Children With Autism Spectrum Disorders. J. Am. Acad. Child Adolesc. Psychiatry 46 (10), 1324−1332, http://doi.org/10.1097/chi.0b013e31812f7d8d.

Chawarska, K., Volkmar, F., Klin, A., 2010. Limited attentional bias for faces in toddlers with autism spectrum disorders. Arch. Gen. Psychiatry 67 (2), 178−185, http://doi.org/10.1001/archgenpsychiatry.2009.194.

Cheon, K.-A., Kim, Y.-S., Oh, S.-H., Park, S.-Y., Yoon, H.-W., Herrington, J., et al., 2011. Involvement of the anterior thalamic radiation in boys with high functioning autism spectrum disorders: a Diffusion Tensor Imaging study. Brain Res. 1417, 77−86, http://doi.org/10.1016/j.brainres.2011.08.020.

Chevallier, C., Kohls, G., Troiani, V., Brodkin, E.S., Schultz, R.T., 2012. The social motivation theory of autism. Trends Cogn. Sci. 16 (4), 231−239, http://doi.org/10.1016/j.tics.2012.02.007.

Chevallier, C., Parish-Morris, J., McVey, A., Rump, K., Sasson, N.J., Herrington, J.D., et al. (In press). Measuring social attention and Motivation in Autism Spectrum Disorder using eye-tracking: Stimulus type matters. Autism Research.

Dalton, K.M., Nacewicz, B.M., Johnstone, T., Schaefer, H.S., Gernsbacher, M.A., Goldsmith, H.H., et al., 2005. Gaze fixation and the neural circuitry of face processing in autism. Nat. Neurosci. 8 (4), 519−526.

Davidson, R., 2002. Anxiety and affective style: Role of prefrontal cortex and amygdala. Biol. Psychiatry 51 (1diss), 68−80.

Davis, M., 1992. The role of the amygdala in fear and anxiety. Annu. Rev. Neurosci. 15, 353−375, http://doi.org/10.1146/annurev.ne.15.030192.002033.

Dawson, M.E., Schell, A.M., Filion, D.L., 2007. The electrodermal system. In: Cacioppo, John T., Tassinary, Louis G., Berntson, Gary G. (Eds.), Handbook of Psychophysiology, 3rd ed. Cambridge University Press, New York, NY, pp. 159−181, x.

Delgado, M.R., Nearing, K.I., Ledoux, J.E., Phelps, E.A., 2008. Neural circuitry underlying the regulation of conditioned fear and its relation to extinction. Neuron 59 (5), 829−838, http://doi.org/10.1016/j.neuron.2008.06.029.

Engels, A.S., Heller, W., Mohanty, A., Herrington, J.D., Banich, M.T., Webb, A.G., et al., 2007. Specificity of regional brain activity in anxiety types during emotion processing. Psychophysiology 44 (3), 352−363, http://doi.org/10.1111/j.1469-8986.2007.00518.x.

Gadow, K.D., Devincent, C.J., Pomeroy, J., Azizian, A., 2005. Comparison of DSM-IV symptoms in elementary school-age children with PDD versus clinic and community samples. Autism 9 (4), 392−415, http://doi.org/10.1177/1362361305056079.

Gagne, J.R., Van Hulle, C.A., Aksan, N., Essex, M.J., Goldsmith, H.H., 2011. Deriving childhood temperament measures from emotion-eliciting behavioral episodes: Scale construction and initial validation. Psychol. Assess. 23 (2), 337−353, http://doi.org/10.1037/a0021746.

Giedd, J.N., Rapoport, J.L., 2010. Structural MRI of pediatric brain development: what have we learned and where are we going? Neuron 67 (5), 728−734, http://doi.org/10.1016/j.neuron.2010.08.040.

Guy, L., Souders, M.C., Bradstreet, L.E., DeLussey, C., Herrington, J.D., 2014. Emotion Regulation and Respiratory Sinus Arrhythmia in Autism Spectrum Disorder. J. Autism Dev. Disord. 44 (10), 2614−2620, http://doi.org/10.1007/s10803-014-2124-8.

Hallett, V., Lecavalier, L., Sukhodolsky, D.G., Cipriano, N., Aman, M.G., McCracken, J.T., et al., 2013. Exploring the Manifestations of Anxiety in Children with Autism Spectrum Disorders. J Autism Dev. Disord. 43 (10), 2341−2352, http://doi.org/10.1007/s10803-013-1775-1.

Hamann, S., Ely, T., Hoffman, J., Kilts, C., 2002. Ecstasy and agony: Activation of human amygdala in positive and negative emotion. Psychol. Sci. 3 (2), 135−141.

Haznedar, M.M., Buchsbaum, M.S., Wei, T.C., Hof, P.R., Cartwright, C., Bienstock, C.A., et al., 2000. Limbic circuitry in patients with autism spectrum disorders studied with positron emission tomography and magnetic resonance imaging. Am. J. Psychiatry 157 (12), 1994−2001, http://doi.org/10.1176/appi.ajp.157.12.1994.

Heatherton, T.F., Wagner, D.D., 2011. Cognitive neuroscience of self-regulation failure. Trends Cogn. Sci. 15 (3), 132−139, http://doi.org/10.1016/j.tics.2010.12.005.

Heeren, A., Peschard, V., Philippot, P., 2011. The causal role of attentional bias for threat cues in social anxiety: a test on a cyber-ostracism task. Cogn. Therapy Res. http://doi.org/10.1007/s10608-011-9394-7.

Herrington, J.D., Schultz, R.T., 2010. Neuroimaging of developmental disorders. In: Shenton, M., Turetsky, B.I. (Eds.), Understanding Neuropsychiatric Disorders: Insights From Neuroimaging. Cambridge University Press, Cambridge.

Herrington, J.D., Heller, W., Mohanty, A., Engels, A.S., Banich, M.T., Webb, A.G., et al., 2010. Localization of asymmetric brain function in emotion and depression. Psychophysiology 47 (3), 442−454, http://doi.org/10.1111/j.1469-8986.2009.00958.x.

Herrington, J.D., Miller, J., Pandey, J., Schultz, R.T., 2016. Anxiety and social deficits have distinct relationships with amygdala function in autism spectrum disorder. Soc. Cogn. Affect. Neurosci. 11 (6), 907−914, http://doi.org/10.1093/scan/nsw015.

Hirstein, W., Iversen, P., Ramachandran, V.S., 2001. Autonomic responses of autistic children to people and objects. Proc. Biol. Sci. 268 (1479), 1883−1888, http://doi.org/10.1098/rspb.2001.1724.

Hollocks, M.J., Ozsivadjian, A., Matthews, C.E., Howlin, P., Simonoff, E., 2013. The relationship between attentional bias and anxiety in children and adolescents with autism spectrum disorders: attentional bias and anxiety in ASD. Autism Res. 6 (4), 237−247, http://doi.org/10.1002/aur.1285.

Hollocks, M.J., Howlin, P., Papadopoulos, A.S., Khondoker, M., Simonoff, E., 2014. Differences in HPA-axis and heart rate responsiveness to psychosocial stress in children with autism spectrum disorders with and without co-morbid anxiety. Psychoneuroendocrinology 46, 32−45, http://doi.org/10.1016/j.psyneuen.2014.04.004.

Howard, M.A., Cowell, P.E., Boucher, J., Broks, P., Mayes, A., Farrant, A., et al., 2000. Convergent neuroanatomical and behavioural evidence of an amygdala hypothesis of autism. Neuroreport 11 (13), 2931−2935.

Hubert, B.E., Wicker, B., Monfardini, E., Deruelle, C., 2009. Electrodermal reactivity to emotion processing in adults with autistic spectrum disorders. Autism 13 (1), 9−19, http://doi.org/10.1177/1362361308091649.

Isomura, T., Ogawa, S., Yamada, S., Shibasaki, M., Masataka, N., 2014. Preliminary evidence that different mechanisms underlie the anger superiority effect in children with and without Autism Spectrum Disorders. Front. Psychol. 5, http://doi.org/10.3389/fpsyg.2014.00461.

Joseph, R.M., Ehrman, K., McNally, R., Keehn, B., 2008. Affective response to eye contact and face recognition ability in children with ASD. J. Int. Neuropsychol. Soc. 14 (6), 947−955, http://doi.org/10.1017/S1355617708081344.

Juranek, J., Filipek, P.A., Berenji, G.R., Modahl, C., Osann, K., Spence, M.A., 2006. Association between amygdala volume and anxiety level: magnetic resonance imaging (MRI) study in autistic children. J. Child Neurol. 21 (12), 1051−1058.

Kalin, N.H., Shelton, S.E., Davidson, R.J., 2004. The role of the central nucleus of the amygdala in mediating fear and anxiety in the primate. J. Neurosci. 24 (24), 5506−5515, http://doi.org/10.1523/JNEUROSCI.0292-04.2004.

Kerns, C.M., Kendall, P.C., Berry, L., Souders, M.C., Franklin, M.E., Schultz, R.T., et al., 2014. Traditional and atypical presentations of anxiety in youth with autism spectrum disorder. J. Autism Dev. Disorders 44 (11), 2851−2861, http://doi.org/10.1007/s10803-014-2141-7.

Ke, X., Tang, T., Hong, S., Hang, Y., Zou, B., Li, H., et al., 2009. White matter impairments in autism, evidence from voxel-based morphometry and diffusion tensor imaging. Brain Res. 1265, 171−177, http://doi.org/10.1016/j.brainres.2009.02.013.

Kleinhans, N.M., Richards, T., Weaver, K., Johnson, L.C., Greenson, J., Dawson, G., et al., 2010. Association between amygdala response to emotional faces and social anxiety in autism spectrum disorders. Neuropsychologia 48 (12), 3665−3670, http://doi.org/10.1016/j.neuropsychologia.2010.07.022.

Klusek, J., Roberts, J.E., Losh, M., 2015. Cardiac autonomic regulation in autism and Fragile X syndrome: a review. Psychol. Bull. 141 (1), 141−175, http://doi.org/10.1037/a0038237.

Lecavalier, L., 2006. Behavioral and emotional problems in young people with pervasive developmental disorders: relative prevalence, effects of subject characteristics, and empirical classification. J Autism Dev. Disord. 36 (8), 1101−1114.

May, T., Cornish, K., Rinehart, N.J., 2015. Mechanisms of anxiety related attentional biases in children with autism spectrum disorder. J. Autism Dev. Disord. 45 (10), 3339−3350, http://doi.org/10.1007/s10803-015-2500-z.

McCormick, C., Hessl, D., Macari, S.L., Ozonoff, S., Green, C., Rogers, S.J., 2014. Electrodermal and behavioral responses of children with autism spectrum disorders to sensory and repetitive stimuli. Autism Res. 7 (4), 468−480, http://doi.org/10.1002/aur.1382.

Milad, M.R., Wright, C.I., Orr, S.P., Pitman, R.K., Quirk, G.J., Rauch, S.L., 2007. Recall of fear extinction in humans activates the ventromedial prefrontal cortex and hippocampus in concert. Biol. Psychiatry 62 (5), 446−454, http://doi.org/10.1016/j.biopsych.2006.10.011.

Milham, M.P., Nugent, A.C., Drevets, W.C., Dickstein, D.P., Leibenluft, E., Ernst, M., et al., 2005. Selective reduction in amygdala volume in pediatric anxiety disorders: a voxel-based morphometry investigation. Biol. Psychiatry 57 (9), 961−966, http://doi.org/10.1016/j.biopsych.2005.01.038.

Minshew, N.J., Williams, D.L., 2007. The new neurobiology of autism: cortex, connectivity, and neuronal organization. Arch. Neurol. 64 (7), 945−950, http://doi.org/64/7/945.

Mohanty, A., Engels, A.S., Herrington, J.D., Heller, W., Ho, M.-H.R., Banich, M.T., et al., 2007. Differential engagement of anterior cingulate cortex subdivisions for cognitive and emotional function. Psychophysiology 44 (3), 343−351.

Morris, J.S., Ohman, A., Dolan, R.J., 1999. A subcortical pathway to the right amygdala mediating "unseen" fear. Proc. Natl. Acad. Sci. USA 96 (4), 1680−1685.

Mosconi, M.W., Cody-Hazlett, H., Poe, M.D., Gerig, G., Gimpel-Smith, R., Piven, J., 2009. Longitudinal Study of Amygdala Volume and Joint Attention in 2- to 4-Year-Old Children With Autism. Arch Gen Psychiatry 66 (5), 509−516, http://doi.org/10.1001/archgenpsychiatry.2009.19.

Munson, J., Dawson, G., Abbott, R., Faja, S., Webb, S.J., Friedman, S.D., et al., 2006. Amygdalar volume and behavioral development in autism. Arch Gen Psychiatry 63 (6), 686–693, http://doi.org/10.1001/archpsyc.63.6.686.

Murphy, E.R., Foss-Feig, J., Kenworthy, L., Gaillard, W.D., Vaidya, C.J., 2012. Atypical Functional Connectivity of the Amygdala in Childhood Autism Spectrum Disorders during Spontaneous Attention to Eye-Gaze. Autism Res. Treat. 2012, 652408, http://doi.org/10.1155/2012/652408.

Myers-Schulz, B., Koenigs, M., 2012. Functional anatomy of ventromedial prefrontal cortex: implications for mood and anxiety disorders. Mol. Psychiatry 17 (2), 132–141, http://doi.org/10.1038/mp.2011.88.

Nacewicz, B.M., Dalton, K.M., Johnstone, T., Long, M.T., McAuliff, E.M., Oakes, T.R., et al., 2006. Amygdala volume and nonverbal social impairment in adolescent and adult males with autism. Arch. Gen. Psychiatry 63 (12), 1417–1428, http://doi.org/63/12/1417.

Neuhaus, E., Beauchaine, T.P., Bernier, R., 2010. Neurobiological correlates of social functioning in autism. Clinical Psychol. Rev. 30 (6), 733–748, http://doi.org/10.1016/j.cpr.2010.05.007.

Neuhaus, E., Bernier, R., Beauchaine, T.P., 2013. Brief report: social skills, internalizing and externalizing symptoms, and respiratory sinus arrhythmia in autism. J. Autism Dev. Disord. http://doi.org/10.1007/s10803-013-1923-7.

Pasley, B., Mayes, L., Schultz, R., 2004. Subcortical discrimination of unperceived objects during binocular rivalry. Neuron 42 (1), 163–172.

Passarotti, A.M., Sweeney, J.A., Pavuluri, M.N., 2010. Neural correlates of response inhibition in pediatric bipolar disorder and attention deficit hyperactivity disorder. Psychiatry Res. 181 (1), 36–43, http://doi.org/10.1016/j.pscychresns.2009.07.002.

Patriquin, M.A., Scarpa, A., Friedman, B.H., Porges, S.W., 2011. Respiratory sinus arrhythmia: A marker for positive social functioning and receptive language skills in children with autism spectrum disorders. Dev. Psychobiol. 55 (2), 101–112, http://doi.org/10.1002/dev.21002.

Pelphrey, K.A., Shultz, S., Hudac, C.M., Vander Wyk, B.C., 2011. Research Review: Constraining heterogeneity: the social brain and its development in autism spectrum disorder. J Child Psychol. Psychiatry 52 (6), 631–644, http://doi.org/10.1111/j.1469-7610.2010.02349.x.

Pessoa, L., Adolphs, R., 2010. Emotion processing and the amygdala: from a "low road" to "many roads" of evaluating biological significance. Nat. Rev. Neurosci. 11 (11), 773–783, http://doi.org/10.1038/nrn2920.

Pfeifer, J.C., Welge, J., Strakowski, S.M., Adler, C.M., DelBello, M.P., 2008. Meta-analysis of amygdala volumes in children and adolescents with bipolar disorder. J. Am. Acad. Child Adolesc. Psychiatry 47 (11), 1289–1298, http://doi.org/10.1097/CHI.0b013e318185d299.

Pfeifer, J.H., Allen, N.B., 2012. Arrested development? Reconsidering dual-systems models of brain function in adolescence and disorders. Trends Cogn. Sci. 16 (6), 322–329, http://doi.org/10.1016/j.tics.2012.04.011.

Phelps, E.A., LeDoux, J.E., 2005. Contributions of the amygdala to emotion processing: from animal models to human behavior. Neuron 48 (2), 175–187, http://doi.org/10.1016/j.neuron.2005.09.025.

Pierce, K., Müller, R.A., Ambrose, J., Allen, G., Courchesne, E., 2001. Face processing occurs outside the fusiform "face area" in autism: evidence from functional MRI. Brain 124 (10), 2059–2073.

Pine, D.S., Guyer, A.E., Leibenluft, E., 2008. Functional magnetic resonance imaging and pediatric anxiety. J. Am. Acad. Child Adolesc. Psychiatry 47 (11), 1217–1221, http://doi.org/10.1097/CHI.0b013e318185dad0.

Porges, S.W., 2001. The polyvagal theory: phylogenetic substrates of a social nervous system. Int. J. Psychophysiol. 42 (2), 123–146.

Porges, S.W., Walter, G.F., Korb, R.J., Sprague, R.L., 1975. The influences of methylphenidate on heart rate and behavioral measures of attention in hyperactive children. Child Dev. 46 (3), 725–733.

Porges, S.W., Macellaio, M., Stanfill, S.D., McCue, K., Lewis, G.F., Harden, E.R., et al., 2012. Respiratory sinus arrhythmia and auditory processing in autism: Modifiable deficits of an integrated social engagement system? Int. J. Psychophysiol. http://doi.org/10.1016/j.ijpsycho.2012.11.009.

Rauch, S.L., Shin, L.M., Phelps, E.A., 2006. Neurocircuitry models of posttraumatic stress disorder and extinction: human neuroimaging research—past, present, and future. Biol. Psychiatry 60 (4), 376–382, http://doi.org/10.1016/j.biopsych.2006.06.004.

Schoen, S.A., Miller, L.J., Brett-Green, B.A., Nielsen, D.M., 2009. Physiological and behavioral differences in sensory processing: a comparison of children with autism spectrum disorder and sensory modulation disorder. Front. Integrative Neurosci. 3, 29, http://doi.org/10.3389/neuro.07.029.2009.

Schumann, C.M., Nordahl, C.W., 2011. Bridging the gap between MRI and postmortem research in autism. Brain Res. 1380, 175–186, http://doi.org/10.1016/j.brainres.2010.09.061.

Schumann, C.M., Hamstra, J., Goodlin-Jones, B.L., Lotspeich, L.J., Kwon, H., Buonocore, M.H., et al., 2004. The amygdala is enlarged in children but not adolescents with autism; the hippocampus is enlarged at all ages. J. Neurosci. 24 (28), 6392–6401, http://doi.org/10.1523/JNEUROSCI.1297-04.2004.

Schumann, C.M., Bloss, C.S., Barnes, C.C., Wideman, G.M., Carper, R.A., Akshoomoff, N., et al., 2010. Longitudinal magnetic resonance imaging study of cortical development through early childhood in autism. J. Neurosci. 30 (12), 4419–4427, http://doi.org/10.1523/JNEUROSCI.5714-09.2010.

Schumann, C.M., Bauman, M.D., Amaral, D.G., 2011. Abnormal structure or function of the amygdala is a common component of neurodevelopmental disorders. Neuropsychologia 49 (4), 745–759, http://doi.org/10.1016/j.neuropsychologia.2010.09.028.

Shaw, P., Brierley, B., David, A.S., 2005. A critical period for the impact of amygdala damage on the emotional enhancement of memory? Neurology 65 (2), 326–328, http://doi.org/10.1212/01.wnl.0000168867.40688.9b.

Silverman, W.K., Saavedra, L.M., Pina, A.A., 2001. Test-retest reliability of anxiety symptoms and diagnoses with the Anxiety Disorders Interview Schedule for DSM-IV: child and parent versions. J Am. Acad. Child Adolesc. Psychiatry 40 (8), 937–944.

South, M., Larson, M.J., White, S.E., Dana, J., Crowley, M.J., 2011. Better fear conditioning is associated with reduced symptom severity in autism spectrum disorders. Autism Res. 4 (6), 412–421, http://doi.org/10.1002/aur.221.

Spence, S., 1998. A measure of anxiety symptoms among children. Behav. Res. Therapy 36 (5), 545–566, http://doi.org/10.1016/S0005-7967(98)00034-5.

Sukhodolsky, D.G., Scahill, L., Gadow, K.D., Arnold, L.E., Aman, M.G., McDougle, C.J., et al., 2008. Parent-rated anxiety symptoms in children with pervasive developmental disorders: frequency and association with core autism symptoms and cognitive functioning. J. Abnormal Child Psychol. 36 (1), 117–128.

Swanson, L.W., Petrovich, G.D., 1998. What is the amygdala? Trends Neurosci. 21 (8), 323–331.

Swartz, J.R., Wiggins, J.L., Carrasco, M., Lord, C., Monk, C.S., 2013. Amygdala habituation and prefrontal functional connectivity in youth with autism spectrum disorders. J. Am. Acad. Child Adolesc. Psychiatry 52 (1), 84–93, http://doi.org/10.1016/j.jaac.2012.10.012.

Thayer, J.F., Lane, R.D., 2000. A model of neurovisceral integration in emotion regulation and dysregulation. J Affect. Disorders 61 (3), 201–216.

Thayer, J.F., Ahs, F., Fredrikson, M., Sollers 3rd, J.J., Wager, T.D., 2012. A meta-analysis of heart rate variability and neuroimaging studies: Implications for heart rate variability as a marker of stress and health. Neurosci. Biobehav. Rev. 36 (2), 747–756, http://doi.org/10.1016/j.neubiorev.2011.11.009.

Troiani, V., Price, E.T., Schultz, R.T., 2012. Unseen fearful faces promote amygdala guidance of attention. Soc. Cogn. Affect. Neurosci. http://doi.org/10.1093/scan/nss116.

Tucker, P., Adamson, P., Miranda, R., Scarborough, A., Williams, D., Groff, J., et al., 1997. Paroxetine increases heart rate variability in panic disorder. J. Clin. Psychopharmacol. 17 (5), 370–376.

van Engeland, H., 1984. The electrodermal orienting response to auditive stimuli in autistic children, normal children, mentally retarded children, and child psychiatric patients. J. Autism Dev. Disorders 14 (3), 261–279.

Watanabe, T., Yahata, N., Abe, O., Kuwabara, H., Inoue, H., Takano, Y., et al., 2012. Diminished medial prefrontal activity behind autistic social judgments of incongruent information. PloS One 7 (6), e39561, http://doi.org/10.1371/journal.pone.0039561.

Waters, A.M., Henry, J., Mogg, K., Bradley, B.P., Pine, D.S., 2010. Attentional bias towards angry faces in childhood anxiety disorders. J. Behav. Therapy Exp. Psychiatry 41 (2), 158–164, http://doi.org/10.1016/j.jbtep.2009.12.001.

Weng, S.-J., Carrasco, M., Swartz, J.R., Wiggins, J.L., Kurapati, N., Liberzon, I., et al., 2011. Neural activation to emotional faces in adolescents with autism spectrum disorders. J. Child Psychol. Psychiatry Allied Discip. 52 (3), 296–305, http://doi.org/10.1111/j.1469-7610.2010.02317.x.

Whalen, P.J., 1998. Fear, vigilance, and ambiguity: Initial neuroimaging studies of the human amygdala. Curr. Directions Psychol. Sci. 7 (6), 177–188.

Whalen, P.J., 2007. The uncertainty of it all. Trends Cogn. Sci. 11 (12), 499–500, http://doi.org/10.1016/j.tics.2007.08.016.

Whalen, P.J., Phelps, E.A. (Eds.), 2009. The Human Amygdala. Guilford Press, New York.

Wilensky, A.E., Schafe, G.E., Kristensen, M.P., LeDoux, J.E., 2006. Rethinking the fear circuit: the central nucleus of the amygdala is required for the acquisition, consolidation, and expression of Pavlovian fear conditioning. J. Neurosci. 26 (48), 12387–12396, http://doi.org/10.1523/JNEUROSCI.4316-06.2006.

Yeragani, V.K.Y., Pohl, R., Balon, R., Ramesh, C., Glitz, D., Weinberg, P., et al., 1992. Effect of imipramine treatment on heart rate variability measures. Neuropsychobiology 26 (1-2), 27–32, http://doi.org/10.1159/000118892.

CHAPTER 5

Assessment of Anxiety in Youth With Autism Spectrum Disorder

Lauren J. Moskowitz[1], Tamara Rosen[2], Matthew D. Lerner[2] and Karen Levine[3]
[1]St. John's University, Queens, NY, United States
[2]Stony Brook University, Stony Brook, NY, United States
[3]Harvard Medical School, Lexington, MA, United States

ASSESSMENT OF ANXIETY IN AUTISM SPECTRUM DISORDER

Background

Anxiety-related concerns are among the most common presenting problems for children and adolescents with autism spectrum disorders (ASDs) (White et al. 2009), with approximately 40% of youth with ASD meeting criteria for at least one anxiety disorder (van Steensel et al. 2011). This is likely an underestimate, given that anxiety is often overlooked in individuals with ASD. This may be due to a general clinical consensus that symptoms of anxiety are "better explained by the ASD itself" (White et al. 2009), a tendency known as diagnostic overshadowing. Another reason anxiety may be overlooked is because, historically, behaviorists have been reluctant to use the construct of "anxiety" to describe or explain behavior when discussing those with ASD (Groden et al. 1994). This may be because, unlike behaviors, the cognitions, affective/subjective state, and physiological arousal that are part of the construct of anxiety often cannot be directly observed in those individuals who cannot self-report (Groden et al., 1994). This perspective highlights the importance of attempting to address the multiple components of anxiety using a multimethod approach as well as the inherent difficulties of assessing anxiety in this population.

Difficulty of Assessing Anxiety in ASD

One reason anxiety is so difficult to assess is due to the inherent communication impairments in ASD. Given that up to one-half of individuals

Anxiety in Children and Adolescents with Autism Spectrum Disorder.
DOI: http://dx.doi.org/10.1016/B978-0-12-805122-1.00005-3
© 2017 Elsevier Inc.
All rights reserved.
79

with ASD are functionally nonverbal and even those *with* verbal language often have difficulty describing their thoughts and feelings (Leyfer et al., 2006), traditional assessment of anxiety using self-report can be difficult or even impossible (Hagopian and Jennett, 2008). These communication deficits might also cause parents to be unaware of their child's thoughts and feelings, limiting the usefulness of other-informant-reports, and underscoring the importance of a multimethod assessment approach. Second, the presence of co-occurring ID in over 50% of children with ASD (CDC, 2014) can further compound these difficulties with assessment, given that youth with ASD and ID often lack the ability to communicate their anxiety to an even greater extent than those with ASD who do not have ID (Davis et al., 2011). Third, symptoms of anxiety may present differently in ASD, making it more difficult for caretakers to identify the symptoms of anxiety. For example, those with ASD are more likely to express fear or anxiety through behaviors such as aggression, self-injury, and tantrums (White et al. 2009). Additionally, the content of the anxiety may differ for youth with ASD, such as fears of an unusual focus (e.g., fear of graffiti) in some youth with ASD (Kerns et al., 2014). Finally, given the symptom overlap in the current diagnostic classification system, clinicians often find it challenging to decide if symptoms such as social avoidance or compulsive checking should be conceptualized as part of the ASD or as a separate comorbid anxiety disorder (White et al. 2009). Ultimately, as Wood and Gadow (2010) suggested, the only way to distinguish between the overlapping symptoms of ASD and anxiety disorders may be to assess the function of the symptom—e.g., to assess the function of the social avoidance (i.e., disliking social interaction *versus* fear of being scrutinized or rejected). Still, it may be difficult or even impossible to assess these functions if a child cannot talk or report his own mental state. Faced with such difficulties, one might take a multistep approach, such as that advocated by Kerns and colleagues (2016) (i.e., consideration of development; assessment of discrete impairment; examination of overlap with candidate ASD symptoms) to identify whether a child may formally meet anxiety comorbidity criteria. Alternatively, one could prioritize a pragmatic approach, and conceptualize and treat patterns of behavior that are "phobia-like" as phobias, even if their derivation may not be fully understood or when it may be suspected that these are from a source such as hyperacusis or sensory over-reactivity (e.g., Koegel et al., 2004). In either case, a methodical and empirically-grounded assessment process, relying on a variety of different measures and informants to converge upon the presence of anxiety, is a vital first step.

CLINICAL ASSESSMENT OF ANXIETY IN ASD

Given the prevalence and difficulties associated with anxiety in ASD, it is important to regularly screen and/or assess for anxiety during clinical evaluations. Toward this end, an array of measures are available that can be useful. We now review available questionnaires/rating scales, clinical interviews, clinician-rated symptom measures, direct observation measures, and physiological measures, and how they might be useful for the assessment of anxiety in ASD.

TOOLS FOR ASSESSING ANXIETY IN ASD

Questionnaires/Rating Scales

Self-report questionnaires

Self-report questionnaires are the most widely-used formal evaluative method for assessing anxiety in youth with and without ASD. However, virtually none of these instruments are specifically designed to assess anxiety in ASD (see Table 5.1 for a summary of questionnaire instruments). Among the most well-researched measures are the Multidimensional Anxiety Scale for Children (MASC-C; March et al., 1997), the Screen for Child Anxiety Related Emotional Disorders (SCARED-C; Birmaher et al., 1997), and the Spence Children's Anxiety Scale (SCAS; Spence, 1998). However, these measures may be more appropriate for higher-functioning youth, given their emphasis on verbally-mediated symptoms. On the other hand, the Revised Child Anxiety and Depression Scale (RCADS; Chorpita et al., 2000) may be useful for lower-functioning youth (i.e., those with ID and/or minimal verbal ability).

Potentially appropriate treatment outcome measures include the MASC, SCARED, and the RCADS, while the Revised Children's Manifest Anxiety Scale (RCMAS; Reynolds and Richmond, 1978) may be more useful as a screening measure. The State–Trait Anxiety Inventory for Children (STAIC; Spielberger, 1973) may be useful for the specific purpose of distinguishing trait and state anxiety in ASD (Lanni et al., 2012), while the Social Anxiety Scale for Children revised (SASC-R; La Greca and Stone, 1993), the Social Anxiety Scale for Adolescents (SAS-A; La Greca and Lopez, 1998), or the Social Worries Questionnaire

Table 5.1 Questionnaires

Form	# of items; time	Age range	Possible raters	Subscales/domains	Reliability in ASD	Validity in ASD	Use in ASD
MASC (March et al., 1997)	39 items; 15 min	8–19 years	Child, Parent	Social anxiety, physical symptoms, harm avoidance, separation anxiety/panic	• Acceptable internal consistency (Wood et al., 2009)	• Modest convergent validity (Storch et al., 2012); • Treatment sensitivity (Wood et al., 2009)	Appropriate with conditions as outcome measure, but emphasis on language may make it limited to high-functioning youth (Lecavalier et al., 2014); self-report scale may be measuring the same anxiety constructs in ASD and TD youth, more so than parent-report (White et al., 2015)
SCARED (Birmaher et al., 1997, 1999)	41 items; 10 min	9–18 years	Child, Parent	Panic/somatic, generalized anxiety, separation anxiety, social phobia, and school phobia	• Moderate internal consistency (Reaven et al., 2009)	• Moderate convergent validity; • Mixed evidence for sensitivity and specificity (Kerns et al., 2015; Stern, Gadgil et al., 2014); • Some evidence for treatment sensitivity (Reaven et al., 2009)	Potentially appropriate for as outcome measure, but emphasis on language may make it limited to higher-functioning youth (Lecavalier et al., 2014); evidence that the SCARED measures anxiety similarly in ASD and TD youth (Stern et al., 2014)
SCAS (Spence, 1998)	44 items; 15 min	7–14 years	Child, Parent	Separation anxiety, social phobia, obsessive-compulsive, panic-agoraphobia, generalized anxiety and physical injury fears	• Acceptable internal consistency, though not strong for all subscales (Kerns et al., 2016)	• Acceptable sensitivity and specificity (Kerns et al., 2016)	• Acceptable to moderate parent-child agreement (Kerns et al., 2016) • May be more appropriate for higher-functioning youth (Grondhuis and Aman, 2012)
RCMAS (Reynolds and Richmond, 1978)	37 items; 10–15 min	6–19 years	Child	Physiological anxiety, worry/oversensitivity, and social concerns	• Good internal consistency (Mazefsky et al., 2011)	• Some evidence for specificity and sensitivity (Mazefsky et al., 2011)	May be useful as screening measure, not appropriate as outcome measure (Lecavalier et al., 2014)
RCADS (Chorpita et al., 2000)	47 items; 20 min	9–18 years	Child, parent	Separation anxiety, social phobia, generalized anxiety, panic, obsessive-compulsive	• Acceptable test-retest reliability (Kaat and Lecavalier, 2015); Poor inter-rater reliability (Kaat and Lecavalier, 2015); • Acceptable internal consistency (Hallett et al., 2013; Sterling et al., 2015)	• Mixed findings regarding divergent validity (Kaat and Lecavalier, 2015; Sterling et al., 2015) • Modest convergent validity (Sterling et al., 2015)	Potentially appropriate as outcome measure (Lecavalier et al., 2014); May be useful for ID, as 33% of individuals in Kaat and Lecavalier (2015) had IQ below 85

Measure	Items; time	Age range	Informant	Constructs	Reliability	Validity	Notes
ASC-ASD (Rodgers et al., 2016)	24 items; 10 min	8–15 years	Child, parent	Performance Anxiety, Uncertainty, AnxiousArousal, Separation Anxiety	Good-to-excellent internal consistency and 1 month test-retest reliability and high parent–child agreement (Rodgers et al., 2016)	• Good convergent, discriminant, and content validity (Rodgers et al., 2016)	May be limited to verbally fluent youth with ASD (Rodgers et al., 2016)
STAIC (Spielberger, 1973)	20 items; 20 min	6–14 years	Child	State anxiety, trait anxiety	Yet to be evaluated	• Yet to be evaluated	May be useful for distinguishing state and trait anxiety (Lanni et al., 2012)
SASC-R (La Greca and Stone, 1993); SAS-A (La Greca and Lopez, 1998)	22 (SASC-R); 26 (SAS-A); 10–15 min	8–18 years	Child	Fear of negative evaluation, generalized and specific social avoidance/distress	Good internal consistency (Kaboski et al., 2015)	• Treatment sensitivity (Kaboski et al., 2015) • Some evidence for convergent validity (Henderson et al., 2006)	When items overlapping with ASD were removed, total scale had good internal consistency (Kuusikko et al., 2008)
CASI-4R (Gadow and Sprafkin, 2002)	26 (anx items); 15–20 min	5–18 years	Parent, teacher	Generalized anxiety disorder, social phobia, separation anxiety disorder, obsessive-compulsive disorder, specific phobia, panic attack	20-item version created to measure anxiety in ASD showed good internal consistency in children with and without cognitive impairment (Sukhodolsky et al., 2008; White et al., 2012)	• Good convergent validity for 20-item version (White et al., 2012)	20-item version is appropriate with conditions for use in ASD as outcome measure (Lecavalier et al., 2014)
SWQ (Spence, 1995)	10; 10 min	8–17 years	Parent, child	Social anxiety	Acceptable internal consistency (Kerns et al., 2016)	• Treatment sensitivity (Kerns et al., 2016)	Weak relation of parent- and child-report; limited psychometric data (Kerns et al., 2016)
ASD-CC (Matson and Gonzalez, 2007)	49 items	2–16 years	Parent	Worry/Depressed and Avoidant subscales	Worry/Depressed and Avoidant subscales of the ASD-CC have demonstrated moderately good internal consistency (Davis et al., 2011)	• Worry/Depressed and Avoidant subscales of the ASD-CC have demonstrated good convergent & discriminant validity (Rieske et al., 2013)	May be useful in assessing anxiety (Rieske et al., 2013)

(Continued)

Table 5.1 (Continued)

Form	# of items; time	Age range	Possible raters	Subscales/domains	Reliability in ASD	Validity in ASD	Use in ASD
ADAMS (Esbensen et al. 2003)[a]	28 items; 10 min	10–79 years	Informant-rating scale	Social avoidance, general anxiety, compulsive behavior	• Excellent internal consistency and test-retest reliability; interrater reliability good for Compulsive Behavior but poor for GAD in ID (Esbensen et al. 2003)	• Valid for screening for OCD in individuals with ID (Esbensen et al. 2003)[a]	• Potentially appropriate as an outcome measure for anxiety in ASD and ID, but only examined in ID, not ASD (Lecavalier et al., 2014)
BISCUIT, Part II (Matson et al., 2009)[a]	11 (anx items); 10 min	17–37 months	Parent or caregiver	Anxiety/Repetitive Behavior Avoidance behavior	• Excellent internal consistency in youth with DD including ASD (Matson et al 2009)[a]	• Yet to be evaluated in ASD	• Cutoffs and norms for each factor established for children with DD including ASD (Matson et al. 2009)
DBC (Brereton et al., 2006)[a]	9 (anx items); 15–20 min	3–24 years	Parent or teacher	Anxiety subscale	• Excellent test-retest reliability, but moderate interrater reliability and internal consistency in youth with ID (Reardon et al., 2015)[a]	• Satisfactory construct, criterion, convergent, divergent, and criterion validity in youth with ID without ASD (Reardon et al., 2015)[a]	• Used to compare psychopathology including anxiety in youth with ASD (73% of whom had ID) to ID alone (Brereton et al., 2006)
NCBRF (Aman et al., 1996)[a]	15 (anx items); 7–8 min	4–18 years	Parent or teacher	Insecure/Anxious subscale and Overly Sensitive subscale	• Good internal consistency and test retest reliability in ID (but not ASD; moderate to poor parent-teacher interrater reliability (Reardon et al., 2015)[a]	• Some support for criterion validity; low convergent validity with DBC–Anxiety in ID, 37% with PDD (Reardon et al., 2015)[a]	• Used to characterize children with ASD, but has not been evaluated as a screen for anxiety disorders in ID or ASD (Reardon et al., 2015); not appropriate as anxiety outcome measure in ASD (Lecavalier et al., 2014)

Note: ASD = autism spectrum disorder. ASC-ASD = Anxiety Scale for Children with ASD. ADAMS = Anxiety, Depression, and Mood Scale. BISCUIT = Baby and Infant Screen for Children with aUtism Traits. DBC = Developmental Behaviour Checklist. MASC = Multidimensional Anxiety Scale for Children. NCBRF = Nisonger Child Behavior Rating Form. SCARED = Screen for Child Anxiety Disorders. RCMAS = Revised Children's Manifest Anxiety Scale. RCADS = Revised Child Anxiety and Depression Scale. STAIC = State–Trait Anxiety Inventory for Children. SASC-R = Social Anxiety Scale for Children revised. SAS-A = Social Anxiety Scale for Adolescents.
[a]Sample includes Intellectual Disability (ID).

(SWQ; Spence, 1995) may be the measures of choice for assessing social anxiety. However, the SWQ is relatively under-researched. Although all of these self-reports were designed for typically developing (TD) children rather than those with ASD, the freely available *Anxiety Scale for Children with ASD, Parent and Child versions (ASC-ASD)*, an adapted version of the RCADS which includes additional items related to sensory anxiety, intolerance of uncertainty and phobias, shows promising psychometric properties for youth with fluent speech (Rodgers et al., 2016).

Self-reports in ASD and ID

Although the RCMAS, SASC, and STAIC have each been used in one study with youth with ID (see Reardon et al., 2015 for a review), the majority of aforementioned self-report questionnaires have only been examined in youth with high-functioning ASD (HFA; i.e., those who have average or above average IQ and/or greater verbal abilities). Traditional self-report questionnaires, which typically require a second- or third-grade reading level, may be inappropriate for some children with ASD and ID due to limitations in cognition, communication, and comprehension. However, there is some evidence that self-reports that are modified can be reliable and valid for some individuals with ID (Hagopian and Jennett, 2008). For example, the Fear Survey Schedule for Children-Revised (FSSC-R) and the Fear Survey for Children With and Without Mental Retardation (FSCMR) have both been psychometrically evaluated with youth with ID (Reardon et al., 2015). Modifications to self-reports for those with ID include both verbal and visual presentation, simpler language, limiting the number of words, pictorial representations of response options (e.g., a visual scale of facial expressions of fear), illustrations/photos to provide visual representations of items, and neutral items to assess acquiescence or choosing the more positive response (Hagopian and Jennett, 2008).

Other Informant Rating Scales

Questionnaires completed by other informants (see Table 5.1), such as parents or teachers, can offer additional information beyond self-reports. First, other-informant-report versions are available for the MASC, SCARED, RCADS, SCAS, and SWQ. However, relations of parent and child report may be weaker for the MASC and SWQ. The Child and Adolescent Symptom Inventory-4th Edition Revised (CASI-4R; Gadow and Sprafkin, 2002) is an additional other-informant-report measure. A 20-item version of the anxiety scale has been created to assess anxiety specifically in ASD samples (Sukhodolsky et al., 2008), which may be appropriate as a treatment outcome measure in ASD (Lecavalier et al., 2014).

Of note, in contrast to the previously mentioned self-reports, most of the youth with ASD in the study by Sukhodolsky et al. (2008) had ID, ranging from mild to severe/profound ID. Finally, the Autism Spectrum Disorders-Comorbidity for Children (ASD-CC; Matson and Gonzalez, 2007) was designed to assess co-occurring disorders in ASD, specifically. The Worry/Depressed and Avoidant subscales of the ASD-CC may be useful for assessing the presence of anxiety in ASD (Rieske et al., 2013). As youth with ASD may evince patterns of elevated self-perceptions when completing self-report measures compared to parent-ratings (Lerner et al., 2012), these other-informant measures may be useful in obtaining a more comprehensive picture of anxiety in ASD.

Other-Informant Rating Scales in ASD and ID

Although almost all of the aforementioned questionnaires (with the exception of the CASI) have only been examined in youth with HFA and there are none designed specifically to assess anxiety in children with ASD and comorbid ID, there are several global measures of emotional and behavioral problems (including anxiety) that have been developed for individuals with ID or DD. Among these broad-based informant questionnaires, the Developmental Behaviour Checklist (DBC; Brereton et al., 2006) and the Nisonger Child Behaviour Rating Form (NCBRF; Aman et al., 1996) have demonstrated the strongest psychometric properties of their subscales measuring anxiety symptoms, although their capacity to screen for anxiety disorders in youth with ID and/or ASD has not been evaluated and they may not be useful as an outcome measure for anxiety in ASD and/or ID. The Anxiety, Depression, and Mood Scale (ADAMS; Esbensen et al. 2003) appears to be a reliable and valid instrument for screening for OCD in individuals with ID, although its use with other anxiety disorders may be limited (Hagopian and Jennett, 2008) and it has not been examined in ASD specifically. The Baby and Infant Screen for Children with aUtism Traits (BISCUIT), Part II (Matson et al., 2009) was developed to screen for comorbid psychopathology—including Anxiety/Repetitive Behavior—in infants and toddlers who have a developmental delay including ASD. One potential limitation is that anxiety is combined with repetitive behaviors. Although there may be overlap, it would be important to differentiate symptoms of comorbid anxiety from repetitive behavior, which is a core ASD symptom, given that repetitive and/or restricted behaviors and interests (RRBIs) are associated with anxiety in ASD but remain distinct constructs (Kerns et al., 2016).

CLINICAL INTERVIEWS

While questionnaires are valuable for screening and assessing a wide variety of symptoms from multiple sources and are less time- and resource-intensive than interviews, diagnoses of anxiety disorders tend to be more accurately made using interviews, which allow the clinician to obtain more detailed information from the child and/or parent's verbal reports as well as from observations of the child's behavior during the interview. Semi-structured interviews can be tailored to the child and/or parent and allow the clinician to provide examples and clarify items. Although most interviews used to assess anxiety in youth with ASD have been designed for TD youth, two interviews have been modified for youth with ASD (Table 5.2).

Of the interviews designed for TD youth, the *Anxiety Disorders Interview Schedule for DSM-IV, Child and Parent Versions (ADIS-IV-C/P*; Silverman and Albano, 1996) is the only interview specifically developed for assessing anxiety disorders, covering multiple dimensions of anxiety, and is generally considered the "gold standard." The *ADIS-IV-CP* is the interview with the most research support in ASD; it has been validated in youth with HFA, used for both diagnosis and treatment outcome, and uses visual prompts to supplement a child's language. Another semi-structured interview, the *Schedule for Affective Disorders and Schizophrenia in School-Aged Children (K-SADS-PL*; Kaufman et al., 1997), has been used less frequently in ASD and is lighter in its coverage of anxiety disorders than the *ADIS*, but has demonstrated reliability in youth with HFA, is free-of-charge, and requires less training than the ADIS. One limitation of both the *ADIS* and *K-SADS* is that they do not have a systematic approach for distinguishing symptoms of anxiety from the core features of ASD and may not capture the unique manifestations of anxiety in ASD; as such, they have been modified for ASD.

The *Autism Comorbidity Interview—Present and Lifetime Version (ACI-PL*; Leyfer et al., 2006) was modified from the *K-SADS* to differentiate between the core symptoms of autism and symptoms of other mental disorders including anxiety, which may make it more stringent than other interviews that do not differentiate (see Mazefsky et al., 2012); however, OCD was the only anxiety disorder to be examined psychometrically. More recently, Kerns and colleagues (2014) developed the *Autism Spectrum Addendum* to the *ADIS-P* (the *ADIS/ASA*), a set of guidelines and supplementary items designed to differentiate traditional

Table 5.2 Interviews and clinician rating scales

Measure	Time to complete	Age range	Possible interviewees	Format	Reliability in ASD	Validity in ASD	Use in ASD
ADIS-IV-C/P (Silverman and Albano, 1996)	1–3 h	7–18	Parent and child	Semi-structured interview (interviewer-based)	Poor agreement between child and parent, but excellent parent and consensus agreement (Storch et al., 2012) and clinician-to-clinician agreement (Ung et al., 2014)	Discriminant validity between anxiety and ASD severity; convergent validity among differing reports of two of the anxiety subdomains (Renno and Wood, 2013)	Used for diagnosis and outcome in several RCTs (e.g., Wood et al., 2009); appropriate with conditions as an outcome measure (Lecavalier et al., 2014), although only examined in youth with HFA (IQ ≥ 70)
ADIS/ASA (Kerns et al., 2014)[a]	15–30 min for ASA (+1–3 h for ADIS)	7–18	Parent and child	Semi-structured interview (addendum to ADIS)	Good-to-excellent interrater agreement and test-retest reliability (Kerns et al., 2014; Kerns et al., in press)	Adequate convergent and discriminant validity with other measures (Kerns et al., in press)	Can aid in differential diagnosis of ASD and anxiety; has not been used for diagnosis or outcome in treatment research (Kerns et al., 2014)
PARS (RUPP, 2002)	20–30 min	6–17	Parent and child	Clinician rating scale	Excellent test-retest reliability and interrater reliability, but low internal consistency (Storch et al., 2012b); IQ > 70	Convergent and divergent validity partially supported (moderately low correlations with other anxiety measures) (Storch et al., 2012b)	Sensitive to treatment (Johnco et al., 2015); Appropriate with conditions as outcome measure; child interview requires fluent language (may limit use to HFA) (Lecavalier et al., 2014)
CY-BOCS-PDD (Scahill et al., 2006)	30 min	6–17	Parent and child	Clinician rating scale	Excellent interrater reliability and internal consistency (Scahill et al., 2006)[b]	Appears distinct from other measures of repetitive behavior (Scahill et al., 2006)[b]	Demonstrated sensitivity to change (McDougle et al., 2005)
K-SADS-PL (Kaufman et al., 1997)	90 min to 2.5 h	6–18	Parent and child	Semi-structured interview (interviewer-based)	Excellent interrater reliability between interviewers in youth with HFA (Mattila et al., 2010; Zainal et al., 2014)	Preliminary evidence of convergent validity between SCAS-P and K-SADS-PL anxiety total score in youth with HFA (Zainal et al., 2014)	Used to assess prevalence of comorbid DSM-IV disorders including anxiety in youth with ASD (e.g., Gjevik et al., 2011) and used for diagnosis in treatment research (Reaven et al., 2009); has not been used as an outcome measure

Measure	Duration	Age range	Informant	Format	Reliability	Validity	Comments
ACI-PL (Leyfer et al., 2006)[a]	1–3 h	5–17	Parent	Semi-structured interview (modified from K-SADS)	Good inter-rater reliability and test-retest reliability for OCD (Leyfer et al., 2006);[b] Mean IQ = 82	Good concurrent validity for OCD, though validity for other anxiety disorders not examined (Leyfer et al., 2006)[b]	Used to assess prevalence of psychiatric disorders including anxiety in ASD (Mazefsky et al., 2011); has not been used as an outcome measure
P-ChIPS (Fristad et al., 1998)	60 min	6–17	Parent	Structured interview (respondent-based)	Good-to-excellent interrater reliability (except for GAD in youth with IQ < 70) Internal consistency good for SoP, fair for SP & SAD, poor for GAD & OCD (Witwer et al., 2012)[b]	Fair concordance between P-ChIPS and CASI (Witwer et al., 2012) in ASD; some challenges related to face and content validity (Witwer and Lecavalier, 2010)[b] ; Mean IQ = 68 (range 42–150)	Used to assess prevalence of comorbid disorders including anxiety in ASD, both with and without ID (Witwer and Lecavalier, 2010; Witwer et al., 2012); has not been used as an outcome measure
DISC-IV (Shaffer et al., 2000)	70–120 min per informant	2–18	Parent and child	Structured interview (respondent-based)	Reliability not examined in youth with ASD	Validity not examined in youth with ASD	Used to assess prevalence of psychiatric disorders including anxiety in youth with ASD (deBruin et al., 2007); has not been used as an outcome measure
CAPA (Angold et al., 1995)	60 minutes per informant	9–17	Parent and Child	Combines interviewer-based & respondent-based format	Reliability not examined in youth with ASD	Validity not examined in youth with ASD	Used to assess prevalence of psychiatric disorders including anxiety in ASD (Simonoff et al., 2008); has not been used as an outcome measure
PAPA (Egger et al., 1999)	1.5–2 h	2–5- year old	Parent	Combines interviewer and respondent-based format	Reliability not examined in youth with ASD	Validity not examined in youth with ASD	Used to assess prevalence of psychiatric disorders including anxiety in ASD (Salazar et al., 2015)[b]

Note: ADIS-IV-C/P = Anxiety Disorders Interview Schedule for DSM-IV, Child and Parent Versions. ACI-PL = Autism Comorbidity Interview – Present and Lifetime Version. ADIS/ASA = Autism Spectrum Addendum to the ADIS-P. CAPA = Child and Adolescent Psychiatric Assessment. CY-BOCS-PDD = Children's Yale-Brown Obsessive Compulsive Scale for Pervasive Developmental Disorders. DISC = Diagnostic Interview Schedule for Children. K-SADS = Schedule for Affective Disorders and Schizophrenia in School-Aged Children. PAPA = Preschool Age Psychiatric Assessment. PARS = Pediatric Anxiety Rating Scale. P-ChIPS = Children's Interview for Psychiatric Syndromes – Parent Version.
[a]Designed for ASD.
[b]Includes ID.

DSM anxiety disorders in ASD from the more ambiguous symptoms (e.g., worries regarding schedule or environmental changes) often present in ASD. Recent findings show strong psychometric properties of the ADIS/ASA (Kerns, in press), which is the only measure designed to probe for more varied symptoms of anxiety in ASD.

Structured, or respondent-based, interviews—such as the *Children's Interview for Psychiatric Syndromes − Parent Version* (*P-ChIPS*; Fristad et al., 1998) and *Diagnostic Interview Schedule for Children, Version IV* (*DISC-IV*; Shaffer et al., 2000)—and interviews that combine respondent-based and interviewer-based approaches—such as the *Child and Adolescent Psychiatric Assessment* (*CAPA*; Angold et al., 1995) and *Preschool Age Psychiatric Assessment* (*PAPA*; Egger et al. 1999)—have also been used to assess comorbid psychiatric disorders including anxiety in youth with ASD. The only one of these that has reported reliability and validity in ASD is the *P-ChIPS* (Witwer et al., 2012). Although these four interviews allow for direct comparison with TD populations and are briefer and require less training than the *ADIS* and *ACI*, these interviews may inflate the prevalence of anxiety in ASD by not discriminating symptoms of anxiety from symptoms of ASD (Mazefsky et al., 2012), or underestimate anxiety in ASD by capturing only those symptoms that present in a similar manner as in typically developing youth (Kerns and Kendal, 2012). In sum, although the *ADIS/ASA*, *ACI-PL*, and *P-ChIPS* are promising interviews, we need further examination of psychometric properties of these measures in youth with ASD (Kerns et al., 2016).

Interviews in ASD and ID

Most of the interviews designed to assess anxiety in TD youth have only been examined in research studies with youth with ASD whose IQ > 70. However, Witwer et al. (2012) examined the reliability and validity of the *P-ChIPS* in parents of youth with ASD whose IQs ranged from 42 to 150. Although overall interrater agreement for GAD was excellent, IQ < 70 impacted interrater agreement for GAD, suggesting that some modifications to the *P-ChIPS* may be necessary in youth with ASD and ID (Witwer et al., 2012). For individuals with ASD and ID, informant reports that were designed for TD children may need to be modified to take into account that caregivers may not know what their children are thinking or feeling. For example, Cordeiro, Ballinger, Hagerman, and Hessl (2011) modified the *ADIS*-P for the parents of individuals with fragile X syndrome by eliminating the screening question criteria, which allowed for a diagnosis of social phobia in individuals who exhibited clinically significant impairment as a result of social phobia symptoms but were unable to verbalize "a worry that they might do something embarrassing."

CLINICIAN-RATED SYMPTOM MEASURES

The *Pediatric Anxiety Rating Scale (PARS*; RUPP, 2002) is a clinician-rated measure of anxiety symptoms severity that was designed to rate the current frequency, severity, and associated impairment of anxiety symptoms across a range of anxiety disorders. The *ADIS* and *PARS*, which both have strong psychometric properties in youth with HFA, were the only clinician interviews that were classified as "appropriate with conditions" for use as an outcome measure in ASD, although their use may be limited to those who are more verbal and/or have a higher IQ (Lecavalier et al., 2014). Another semi-structured clinician-rated instrument is the *Children's Yale-Brown Obsessive Compulsive Scale for Pervasive Developmental Disorders* (CY-BOCS-PDD; Scahill et al., 2006) which was designed to assess the symptoms and severity of OCD in youth with ASD, 61% of whom had ID. The CY-BOCS-PDD only includes the Compulsions checklist from the original CY-BOCS (obsessions were dropped because of cognitive and communication limitations in ASD) and added repetitive behaviors common to youth with ASD. Although the CY-BOCS-PDD demonstrates strong psychometric properties, it can be difficult to truly ascertain the presence of OCD by only relying on compulsions, without assessing obsessions, given the functional relationship between obsessions and compulsions. Of note, although the CY-BOCS-PDD performed somewhat differently for children in the normal IQ range (IQ $\geq$ 70) *versus* those with ID (IQ $<$ 70), most differences were not significant.

DIRECT OBSERVATION

As a result of difficulties with self-report and other-informant-report, anxiety in individuals with ASD, particularly those with comorbid ID and/or minimal verbal abilities, must often be inferred from the individual's overt behavior or "fear responses" *via* direct observation (Rosen et al., 2016). Although information collected from interviews and questionnaires can narrow the focus and help clinicians to formulate hypotheses regarding the controlling variables of anxiety, direct behavioral observation is often needed to clarify and validate these findings in children with ASD, particularly those with both ASD and ID (Hagopian and Jennett, 2008). Direct observations may generate more detailed and likely more accurate information than questionnaires/interviews about the situations that evoke anxiety in youth with ASD, the behaviors they display when they are anxious, and the antecedents and consequences related to their anxiety. Important variables that are overlooked in questionnaires and interviews are sometimes uncovered during direct observation. However, observation requires more time and financial commitment, and may restrict the opportunity to observe a range of anxious behaviors and anxiety-provoking situations.

One approach to direct observation is the Behavioral Avoidance Test (BAT), which involves progressively exposing the child to the feared stimulus while assessing the child's avoidance response, subjective level of anxiety, physiological reactions, and/or behavioral responses (Hagopian and Jennett, 2008). BATs can be used to observe levels of anxiety during assessment as well as during and after intervention to evaluate treatment outcomes. While certain anxiety disorders lend themselves to this design (e.g., phobias, OCD), it may be more challenging to identify or control stimuli that evoke anxiety in children with more generalized anxiety (Hagopian and Jennett, 2008). Although the BAT has been widely used for assessing anxiety disorders, it may be particularly important to include a BAT in the assessment of anxiety in youth with ASD and ID, given the limits of self-report and interview in this population (Hagopian and Jennett, 2008). When a BAT is not feasible, naturalistic observations can still be used to assess anxiety during the interview and/or in the child's home, school, or community. Practically, having caretakers record children's anxious behavior may be a better option (Hagopian and Jennett, 2008). However, due to the limited verbal abilities of many individuals with ASD and ID, researchers often use indirect measures of behavior such as "distance to the avoided stimulus" or "number of steps completed within a hierarchy" to measure fear or avoidance responses rather than measuring direct behaviors that indicate anxiety (Rapp, Vollmer, and Hovanetz, 2005).

PHYSIOLOGICAL MEASURES

The use of informant rating scales, clinical interviews, and behavioral observations is standard practice in clinical assessment. However, there are advancing efforts to translate physiological measures, which represent a variety of indices that reflect bodily and neural responses related to anxiety, in clinical research (De Los Reyes and Aldao, 2015). Though such measures are not yet diagnostic or in wide use in clinical practice, they can add valuable information as well as metrics of change inaccessible to self-report due to concerns about insight or verbal abilities.

Cortisol is a hormone that is responsible for regulating the human stress response (e.g., Stansbury and Gunnar, 2011). Cortisol is often assessed *via* salivary samples, and has been used to index the stress response in ASD, wherein individuals are exposed to situations thought to elicit stress or anxiety (e.g., Corbett et al., 2008). However, there is evidence to suggest that cortisol may be measuring generalized stress, rather than anxiety *per se*, in ASD (Lanni et al., 2012).

Heart rate, often measured by number of beats per minute *via* an electrocardiograph (ECG), is thought to index an individual's general state of arousal (Berntson et al., 1997). One examination found that individuals with ASD, compared to a TD group, had a higher heart rate in both low-anxiety and high-anxiety conditions (Kushki et al., 2013). However, a subsequent study found a blunted heart rate response following a stress test in anxious ASD youth, compared to the TD and non-anxious ASD groups, while reduced heart rate was related to higher levels of anxiety symptoms in the anxious ASD youth (Hollocks et al., 2014). Taken together, while ASD youth show increased heart rate to anxiety triggers, the relationship of heart rate to trait levels of anxiety in ASD is unclear.

The third measure is respiratory sinus arrhythmia (RSA), or vagal regulation of one's heart rate and sympathetic influences (Berntson et al., 1997). Like heart rate, RSA is measured using an ECG, as it is indexed *via* the *variability* in heart rate. Studies have found evidence for a decreased RSA in ASD, which is related to symptoms of anxiety (Bal et al., 2010; Guy et al., 2014), including during threatening situations (Van Hecke et al., 2009). These studies suggest increased levels of generalized arousal in ASD.

The fourth measure is the error-related negativity (ERN), an error-related potential (ERP) component, which is measured using an electro-encephalogram—an electrode array affixed to the head (see Olvet and Hajcak, 2009). The ERN is thought to represent monitoring of one's own performance; increased monitoring and corresponding ERN are associated with higher anxiety levels (see Olvet and Hajcak, 2009), a relationship which has been found in ASD (Henderson et al., 2015; for countervailing findings see Henderson et al., 2006). However, the inconsistent findings in this population suggest more research is needed to uncover the potentially unique patterns of self-monitoring seen in youth with ASD.

Presently, additional research is needed to more firmly establish how the aforementioned measures index the heterogeneous presentation of anxiety in ASD. Specifically, questions regarding clinical and incremental utility, feasibility, cost, and training will need to be explored. In the future, though, these measures may be integrated into clinical practice to improve assessment and diagnosis. However, it is important to note that measures of physiological arousal in individuals with ASD are not on their own diagnostic or indicative of anxiety, and could also be reflective of other physical or emotional states (e.g., anger). This is because the process of labeling one's state of affective arousal as "anxiety" or any other emotion is highly influenced by the situational context in which the arousal occurs (Bandura, 1988). For example, if one's heart were racing while exercising, the arousal would not likely be interpreted as anxiety, whereas if one's heart were racing while taking an exam, the arousal might be interpreted as anxiety because of the context in which the arousal occurs. Thus, information gained from physiological measures is most useful when interpreted in the context of a more comprehensive evaluation that incorporates multiple assessment methods from different informants (Moskowitz et al., 2013).

MULTIMETHOD ASSESSMENT OF ANXIETY IN YOUTH WITH ASD

Just as increased heart rate might indicate anxiety in one context but excitement or anger in another context, behaviors such as running away or crying might indicate anxiety in a child with ASD at certain times in certain contexts, but that same child might also run away or cry because he is tired, in pain, angry, sad, or because he *dislikes* an object, person, or situation (or simply prefers another situation). Indeed, Hagopian and Jennett (2014) differentiated between "simple avoidance" in which the individual with ASD avoids non-preferred stimuli or situations (e.g., wearing shoes, academic task) *versus* "anxious avoidance" in which the individual exhibits avoidant behavior accompanied by traditional symptoms of anxiety including facial expressions indicative of fear, increased physiological arousal and, if possible, self-reported anxiety. One way to differentiate between these two scenarios is to assess the context in which avoidant behavior and physiological arousal occur, as part of a multi-method assessment.

Given the difficulty of assessing anxiety in youth with ASD, particularly those who have ID or are minimally verbal, a multimethod assessment of the behavioral, physiological, and cognitive/affective/contextual components of anxiety is often warranted. To this end, Moskowitz et al. (2013) developed a multimethod assessment strategy to operationally define the construct of "anxiety" in children with ASD and ID. We measured the *affective/cognitive/contextual* component of anxiety using parent–report questionnaires and blind observers' Likert-type ratings, the *physiological* component of anxiety using heart rate (HR) and RSA, and the *behavioral* component of anxiety *via* direct observation (using idiosyncratic behavioral indicators of anxiety for each child). Regarding the affective/cognitive/contextual component, given the importance of identifying the context in which behaviors and physiological arousal occur, other-informant-report questionnaires such as the Stress Survey Schedule (SSS; Groden et al., 2011) can be used to identify situations that evoke anxiety in children with ASD, or one can simply ask parents and/or teachers (and even the child himself, if possible) which situations appear to evoke anxiety. In addition to relying on parent report, Moskowitz et al. (2013) also indexed the contextual or cognitive/affective component of anxiety (i.e., subjective fear or apprehension) by having blind observers rate the child's appearance of anxiety on a Likert-type scale (similar to Koegel et al., 2004). Regarding the physiological component, although increased heart rate or lower RSA in certain contexts can point to the presence of anxiety in those contexts, physiological indices are usually not realistic for parents, teachers, or providers to measure. In lieu of a device to measure physiology, it is still possible to assess observable symptoms that indicate physiological arousal, such as visible muscle tension, rapid breathing, sweating, flushed face, or trembling (Cautela, 1977). Although signs of physiological arousal appear difficult for caretakers to recognize in individuals with ASD and ID, increasing informants' awareness can help them to recognize signs such as tenseness and restlessness (Helverschou and Martinsen, 2011). Finally, regarding the behavioral component, to generate possible anxious behaviors, we initially created a comprehensive list of behavioral indicators of anxiety derived from a variety of sources, such as the Cues for Tension and Anxiety Survey Schedule (CTASS; Cautela, 1977), as well as from clinical observations of each child. Parents, teachers, staff members, or other caregivers identified behaviors the child typically displayed when anxious from this list of behavioral descriptors as well as identified other idiosyncratic behaviors that were not on the list but which the child displayed when anxious. Using this multimethod approach, we found that substantially more problem behaviors (as well as higher HR and lower RSA) occurred in High-Anxiety than in Low-Anxiety contexts (Moskowitz et al., 2013), suggesting that children with ASD may engage in problem behaviors to escape or reduce their anxiety. In sum, it is important to conduct a multimethod assessment incorporating multiple informants and direct observation when assessing for the presence of anxiety in children with ASD and ID because, although any behavior on its own does not necessarily indicate anxiety (e.g., someone may cry because he is feeling afraid, sad, angry, in pain, or ill), multiple sources of converging data may support that the behavior is a sign of anxiety.

CASE EXAMPLE

Jon was a 6-year-old boy of Jamaican descent, diagnosed with ASD and ID, who lived at home with his mother, father, and two younger brothers. Jon's level of adaptive functioning was in the low range, and he communicated through the use of 1–2-word phrases, primarily using language for making requests, negating, and scripted speech. Jon met criteria for Specific Phobia of birthday parties (classified as "Other Type") when his mother was interviewed using the ADIS-IV-C/P; she endorsed that he was more afraid of birthday parties than other kids his age, that he tries his hardest to avoid them or became extremely upset if he was forced to stay in the situation, and that his level of distress and avoidance interfered with both family and classroom activities. His fear of birthday parties had persisted for several years and there were never times when he was able to be around people singing "happy birthday!" in the presence of a birthday cake and remain in the situation calmly.

Affective/Cognitive/Contextual Component of Anxiety

To identify the context that was most likely to be associated with anxiety, Jon's parents were given the Stress Survey Schedule (SSS); they wrote in "birthday parties" when asked if there were any other stressors that were not listed, rating it as a "5" (with 1 being no anxiety to 5 being severe anxiety). Interviews based on the Functional Assessment Interview (FAI; O'Neill et al., 1997) were conducted with Jon's parents to identify, in greater detail, the specific events or situations that predicted the occurrence of anxiety. During the interview, Jon's parents identified birthday parties as the context that was most likely to evoke anxiety for Jon. As soon as children in class or family members at home or people in community settings starting sitting happy birthday while presenting a cake with lit candles, Jon immediately bolted out of the room or cowered in a corner if he could not leave the room, while crying and exhibiting other anxious behaviors. This context was confirmed as the most likely to evoke anxiety by Jon's teacher as well as by the clinician's direct observations. To further support the affective component of anxiety (as Jon himself could not self-report cognitions or emotions), on a scale of 0 (no anxiety) to 3 (high anxiety), Jon's appearance of anxiety was rated by blind observers as an average of 2.75 for each of the happy birthday contexts compared to a 0 for each of the low-anxiety contexts (Moskowitz et al., 2013).

Physiological Component of Anxiety

Jon wore the Alive heart rate monitor, a portable, wireless device with electrode transmitters that adhered to his chest and a receiver that was placed in a small fanny pack worn around his waist. We found that Jon exhibited significantly higher heart rate in the high-anxiety context (happy birthday) than in the low-anxiety context, and lower RSA in the high- than low-anxiety context (with the difference in RSA between the high- and low-anxiety context approaching significance) (Moskowitz et al., 2013).

Behavioral Component of Anxiety

Jon behaved differently in response to situations he simply disliked *versus* anxiety-provoking situations. He often verbally objected to things he did not like (such as if he were served pasta with tomato sauce instead of plain pasta, he would say "No!" and push it away) and he yelled or tantrummed when he was denied access to something such as his favorite video, but this was very different from the crying and fearful facial expression that occurred in response to birthday parties. The main way in which we discriminated between fear/anxiety versus dislike was by defining anxious behaviors and problem behaviors separately. Using a comprehensive list of behavioral descriptors compiled from existing measures (e.g., CTASS) as well as novel, idiosyncratic behaviors that were identified by Jon's mother, father, and teacher, we identified several "anxious behaviors" for Jon: clinging onto his mother, crying/tearfulness, freezing (lack of movement except for respiration), cowering (e.g., turning into corner), anxious vocalizations (e.g., whimpering, moaning, or idiosyncratic throat noises), and a fearful/anxious facial expression consisting of eyes wide open or eyes rapidly darting back and forth, eyebrows sloping down in an inverted V-shape, and frowning (turning down of the mouth). Problem behaviors identified for Jon were yelling or screaming, elopement (running away; leaving the room or attempting to leave the room), pushing another person, and pulling his mother's hair. Although Jon exhibited both anxious behavior and problem behavior in the context of happy birthday (given that his anxious behavior often escalated into problem behavior), he exhibited only problem behaviors such as yelling—not anxious behaviors—in contexts that were merely disliked versus anxiety-provoking. This made it easier to recognize that his anxious behaviors in response to "happy birthday" were distinctly different than his other problematic behaviors, and to conceptualize this as anxiety-based.

CONCLUSION

Despite longstanding clinical accounts of anxiety in children with ASD (e.g., Kanner, 1943), affective states such as fear and anxiety were rarely discussed or acknowledged in this population until relatively recently. Although fear and anxiety are reported to be more common in youth with ASD than in TD youth (e.g., Kuusikko et al., 2008) and those with other DDs (e.g., Brereton et al., 2006), it is worth remembering that almost all of the measures used to assess anxiety in ASD—with the exception of the ADIS/ASA, ACI-PL, and ASC-ASD—were designed for individuals without ASD. The prevalence of anxiety in ASD may be misrepresented given these measurement limitations, the varied and overlapping presentation of anxiety and ASD symptoms, and an over-reliance in anxiety assessment on self-reported or verbally-mediated symptoms (e.g., worries) that are at odds with deficits in communication and socio-emotional insight characteristic of ASD. There is a need for self-report and other-informant-report questionnaires and interviews designed to address these challenges, particularly in youth with ASD who have comorbid ID and/or are minimally verbal. We advocate for a multi-method approach using a variety of tools (e.g., interviews, questionnaires, direct observation) as well as multiple informants—and interpreting behaviors and physiological arousal within a given context—to assess anxiety in individuals with ASD. We must continue to further examine the best ways to discriminate between anxiety and other affective states, particularly in those with ID or who are minimally verbal, so that parents, teachers and clinicians do not misattribute anxiety to anger, frustration, sadness, boredom, or excitement, or *vice versa*.

REFERENCES

Aman, M.G., Tasse, M.J., Rojahn, J., Hammer, D., 1996. The Nisonger CBRF: a child behavior rating form for children with developmental disabilities. Res. Dev. Disabil. 17, 41–57.

Angold, A., Prendergast, M., Cox, A., Harrington, R., Simonoff, E., Rutter, M., 1995. The child and adolescent psychiatric assessment (CAPA). Psychol. Med. 25, 739–753.

Bandura, A., 1988. Self-efficacy conception of anxiety. Anxiety, Stress, & Coping 1, 77–98.

Bal, E., Harden, E., Lamb, D., Van Hecke, A.V., Denver, J.W., Porges, S.W., 2010. Emotion recognition in children with autism spectrum disorders: relations to eye gaze and autonomic state. J. Autism Dev. Disord. 40 (3), 358–370.

Berntson, G.G., Bigger, J.T., Eckberg, D.L., Grossman, P., Kaufmann, P.G., Malik, M., et al., 1997. Heart rate variability: origins, methods, and interpretive caveats. Psychophysiology 34 (6), 623–648.

Birmaher, B., Khetarpal, S., Brent, D., Cully, M., Balach, L., Kaufman, J., et al., 1997. The Screen for Child Anxiety Related Emotional Disorders (SCARED): scale construction and psychometric characteristics. J. Am. Acad. Child Adolesc. Psychiatry 36 (4), 545–553.

Birmaher, B., Brent, D.A., Chiappetta, L., Bridge, J., Monga, S., Baugher, M., 1999. Psychometric Properties of the Screen for Child Anxiety Related Emotional Disorders (SCARED): a Replication Study. J. Am. Acad. Child Adolesc. Psychiatry 38 (10), 1230–1236.

Brereton, A.V., Tonge, B.J., Einfeld, S.L., 2006. Psychopathology in children and adolescents with autism compared to young people with Intellectual Disability. J. Autism. Dev. Disord. 36, 863–870.

Cautela, J.R., 1977. Behavior analysis forms for clinical intervention. Research Press Co, Champaign, IL.

CDC, 2014. Prevalence of autism spectrum disorders among children aged 8 years: autism and developmental disabilities monitoring network, 11 sites, United States, 2010. MMWR Surveillance Summaries 63 (2), 1–22.

Chorpita, B.F., Yim, L., Moffitt, C., Umemoto, L.A., Francis, S.E., 2000. Assessment of symptoms of DSM-IV anxiety and depression in children: a revised child anxiety and depression scale. Behav. Res. Therapy 38 (8), 835–855.

Corbett, B., Mendoza, S., Wegelin, J., Carmean, V., Levine, S., 2008. Variable diurnal rhythm cortisol and anticipatory stress in children with autism. J. Intell. Disabil. Res. 51 (9), 654.

Cordeiro, L., Ballinger, E., Hagerman, R., Hessl, D., 2011. Clinical assessment of DSM-IV anxiety disorders in fragile X syndrome: prevalence and characterization. Journal of Neurodevelopmental Disorders 3, 57–67.

Davis, T.E., Moree, B.N., Dempsey, T., Reuther, E.T., Fodstad, J.C., Hess, J.A., et al., 2011. The relationship between autism spectrum disorders and anxiety: the moderating effect of communication. Res. Autism Spect. Disord. 5 (1), 324–329.

De Los Reyes, A., Aldao, A., 2015. Introduction to the special issue: toward implementing physiological measures in clinical child and adolescent assessments. J. Clin. Child Adolesc. Psychol. 44 (2), 221–237.

de Bruin, E.I., Ferdinand, R.F., Meester, S., de Nijs, P.F.A., Verheij, F., 2007. High rates of psychiatric co-morbidity in PDD-NOS. J. Autism. Dev. Disord. 37, 877–886.

Egger, H.L., Ascher, B.H., Angold, A., 1999. The preschool age psychiatric assessment: Version 1.1. Center for Developmental Epidemiology, Department of Psychiatry and Behavioral Sciences, Duke University Medical Center, Durham, NC.

Esbensen, A.J., Rojahn, J., Aman, M.G., Ruedrich, S., 2003. The reliability and validity of an assessment instrument for anxiety, depression and mood among individuals with mental retardation. J. Autism. Dev. Disord. 33, 617—629.

Fristad, M.A., Teare, M., Weller, E.B., Weller, R.A., Salmon, P., 1998. Study III: Development and concurrent validity of the Children's Interview for Psychiatric Syndromes—parent version (P-ChIPS). J. Child. Adolesc. Psychopharmacol. 8 (4), 221—226.

Gadow, K.D., Sprafkin, J., 2002. Child Symptom Inventory-4 Screening and Norms Manual. Checkmate Plus, Stony Brook, NY.

Gjevik, E., Eldevik, S., Fjaeran-Granum, T., Sponheim, E., 2011. Kiddie-SADS reveals high rates of DSM-IV disorders in children and adolescents with autism spectrum disorders. J. Autism. Dev. Disord. 41 (6), 761—769.

Grondhuis, S.N., Aman, M.G., 2012. Assessment of anxiety in children and adolescents with autism spectrum disorders. Res. Autism Spect. Disord. 6 (4), 1345—1365.

Groden, J., Cautela, J., Prince, S., Berryman, J., 1994. The impact of stress and anxiety on individuals with autism and developmental disabilities. In: Schopler, E., Mesibov, G.B. (Eds.), Behavioral issues in autism. Plenum Press, New York, pp. 178—190.

Guy, L., Souders, M., Bradstreet, L., Delussey, C., Herrington, J.D., 2014. Brief report: emotion regulation and respiratory sinus arrhythmia in Autism Spectrum Disorder. J Autism Dev Disord. 44 (10), 2614—2620.

Hagopian, L.P., Jennet, H.K., 2008. Behavioral assessment and treatment of anxiety in individuals with intellectual disabilities. J. Dev. Phys. Disabil. 20, 467—483.

Hallett, V., Ronald, A., Colvert, E., Ames, C., Woodhouse, E., Lietz, S., et al., 2013. Exploring anxiety symptoms in a large-scale twin study of children with autism spectrum disorders, their co-twins and controls. J. Child Psychol. Psychiatry Allied Disciplines 54 (11), 1176—1185.

Helverschou, S., Martinsen, H., 2011. Anxiety in people diagnosed with autism and intellectual disability: Recognition and phenomenology. Res. Autism. Spectr. Discord. 5 (1), 377—387.

Henderson, H., Schwartz, C., Mundy, P., Burnette, C., Sutton, S., Zahka, N., et al., 2006. Response monitoring, the error-related negativity, and differences in social behavior in autism. Brain Cogn. 61, 96—109.

Henderson, H.A., Ono, K.E., McMahon, C.M., Schwartz, C.B., Usher, L.V., Mundy, P.C., 2015. The costs and benefits of self-monitoring for higher functioning children and adolescents with autism. J. Autism Dev. Disord.1—12.

Hollocks, M.J., Howlin, P., Papadopoulos, A.S., Khondoker, M., Simonoff, E., 2014. Differences in HPA-axis and heart rate responsiveness to psychosocial stress in children with autism spectrum disorders with and without co-morbid anxiety. Psychoneuroendocrinology 46, 32—45.

Johnco, C.J., De Nadai, A.S., Lewin, A.B., Ehrenreich-May, J., Wood, J.J., Storch, E.A., 2015. Defining treatment response and symptom remission for anxiety disorders in pediatric autism spectrum disorders using the Pediatric Anxiety Rating Scale. J. Autism. Dev. Disord. 45 (10), 3232—3242.

Kanner, L., 1943. Autistic disturbances of affective contact. Nervous Child 2, 217—250.

Kaat, A.J., Lecavalier, L., 2015. Reliability and validity of parent- and child-rated anxiety measures in Autism Spectrum Disorder. J. Autism Dev. Disord. 45 (10), 3219—3231.

Kaboski, J.R., Diehl, J.J., Beriont, J., Crowell, C.R., Villano, M., Wier, K., et al., 2015. Brief report: a pilot summer robotics camp to reduce social anxiety and improve social/vocational skills in adolescents with ASD. J. Autism Dev. Disord 45 (12), 3862—3869.

Kaufman, J., Birmaher, B., Brent, D., Rao, U., Flynn, C., Moreci, P., et al., 1997. Schedule for affective disorders and schizophrenia for school-age children—present and lifetime version (K-SADSPL): Initial reliability and validity data. J. Am. Acad. Child. Adolesc. Psychiatry. 36, 980−988.

Kerns, C.M., Kendall, P.C., 2012. Anxiety in autism spectrum disorders: Core or comorbid psychopathology? Clinical Psychology: Science and Practice 12, 323−347.

Kerns, C.M., Kendall, P.C., Berry, L., Souders, M.C., Franklin, M.E., Schultz, R.T., et al., 2014. Traditional and atypical presentations of anxiety in youth with autism spectrum disorder. J. Autism. Dev. Disord. 44 (11), 2851−2861.

Kerns, C.M., Maddox, B.B., Kendall, P.C., Rump, K., Berry, L., Schultz, R.T., et al., 2015. Brief measures of anxiety in non-treatment-seeking youth with autism spectrum disorder. Autism. 969−979.

Kerns, C.M., Rump, K., Worley, J., Kratz, H., McVey, A., Herrington, J., et al., 2016. The differential diagnosis of anxiety disorders in cognitively-able youth with autism. Cogn. Behav. Practice 23, 530−547. Available from: http://dx.doi.org/10.1016/j.cbpra.2015.11.004.

Kerns, C.M., Renno, P., Kendall. P.C., Wood, J.J., & Storch, E.A. (in press). Anxiety Disorders Interview Schedule−Autism Addendum: Reliability and Validity in Children with Autism Spectrum Disorder. *Journal of Clinical Child and Adolescent Psychology.*

Koegel, R.L., Openden, D., Koegel, L.K., 2004. A systematic desensitization paradigm to treat hypersensitivity to auditory stimuli in children with autism in family contexts. Res. Practice Persons Severe Disabil. 29, 122−134.

Kuusikko, S., Pollock-Wurman, R., Jussila, K., Carter, A.S., Mattila, M.L., Ebeling, H., et al., 2008. Social anxiety in high-functioning children and adolescents with autism and Asperger syndrome. J. Autism Dev. Disord. 38, 1697−1709.

Kushki, A., Drumm, E., Pla Mobarak, M., Tanel, N., Dupuis, A., Chau, T., et al., 2013. Investigating the autonomic nervous system response to anxiety in children with autism spectrum disorders. PLoS ONE 8 (4).

La Greca, A.M., Lopez, N., 1998. Social anxiety among adolescents: linkages with peer relations and friendships. J. Abnormal Child Psychol. 26 (2), 83−94.

La Greca, A.M., Stone, W.L., 1993. Social anxiety scale for children-revised: factor structure and concurrent validity. J. Clin. Child Psychol. 22 (1), 17−27.

Lanni, K.E., Schupp, C.W., Simon, D., Corbett, B.A., 2012. Verbal ability, social stress, and anxiety in children with Autistic Disorder. Autism 16 (2), 123−138.

Lecavalier, L., Wood, J.J., Halladay, A.K., Jones, N.E., Aman, M.G., Cook, E.H., et al., 2014. Measuring anxiety as a treatment endpoint in youth with autism spectrum disorder. J. Autism Dev. Disord. 44, 1128−1143.

Lerner, M.D., Calhoun, C.D., Mikami, A.Y., De Los Reyes, A., 2012. Understanding parent−child social informant discrepancy in youth with high functioning autism spectrum disorders. J. Autism Dev. Disord. 42, 2680−2692.

Leyfer, O.T., Folstein, S.E., Bacalman, S., Davis, N.O., Dinh, E., Morgan, J., et al., 2006. Comorbid psychiatric disorders in children with autism: Interview development and rates of disorders. J. Autism. Dev. Disord. 36 (7), 849−861.

March, J.S., Parker, J.D., Sullivan, K., Stallings, P., Conners, C.K., 1997. The Multidimensional Anxiety Scale for Children (MASC): factor structure, reliability, and validity. J. Am. Acad. Child Adolesc. Psychiatry 36 (4), 554−565.

Matson, J.L., Gonzalez, M., 2007. Autism Spectrum Disorder − Comorbid for Children. Disability Consultants, LLC, Baton Rouge, LA.

Matson, J.L., Wilkins, J., Sevin, J.A., Knight, C., Boisjoi, J.A., Sharp, B., 2009. Reliability and item content of the Baby and Infant Screen for Children with aUtIsm Traits (BISCUIT): Parts 1−3. Res. Autism. Spectr. Discord. 3, 336−344.

Mattila, M.L., Hurtig, T., Haapsamo, H., Jussila, K., Kuusikko-Gauffin, S., Kielinen, M., et al., 2010. Comorbid psychiatric disorders associated with Asperger syndrome/high-functioning autism: A community- and clinic-based study. J. Autism. Dev. Disord. 40, 1080–1093.

Mazefsky, C.A., Kao, J., Oswald, D.P., 2011. Preliminary evidence suggesting caution in the use of psychiatric self-report measures with adolescents with high-functioning autism spectrum disorders. Res. Autism Spect. Disord. 5 (1), 164–174.

Mazefsky, C.A., Oswald, D.P., Day, T.N., Eack, S.M., Minshew, N.J., Lainhart, J.E., 2012. ASD, a psychiatric disorder, or both? Psychiatric diagnoses in adolescents with high-functioning ASD. Journal of Clinical Child & Adolescent Psychology 41 (4), 516–523.

McDougle, C.J., Scahill, L., Aman, M.G., McCracken, J.T., Tierney, E., Davies, M., et al., 2005. Risperidone for the core symptom domains of autism: Results from the study by the autism network of the research units on pediatric psychopharmacology. Am. J. Psychiatry. 162, 1142–1148.

Moskowitz, L.J., Mulder, E., Walsh, C.E., McLaughlin, D., Zarcone, J.R., Proudfit, G., et al., 2013. A multimethod assessment of anxiety and problem behavior in children with autism spectrum disorders and intellectual disability. American Journal on Intellectual and Developmental Disabilities 118 (6), 419–434.

Olvet, D.M., Hajcak, G., 2009. The stability of error-related brain activity with increasing trials. Psychophysiology 46, 957–961.

O'Neill, R.E., Horner, R.H., Albin, R.W., Storey, K., Newton, J.S., Sprague, J.R., 1997. Functional assessment and program development for problem behavior. Brooks/Cole, Pacific Grove, CA.

Rapp, J.T., Vollmer, T.R., Hovanetz, A., 2005. Evaluation and treatment of swimming pool avoidance exhibited by an adolescent girl with autism. Behav. Ther. 36, 101–105.

Renno, P., Wood, J.J., 2013. Discriminant and convergent validity of the anxiety construct in children with autism spectrum disorders. J. Autism. Dev. Disord. 43 (9), 2135–2146.

Reardon, T.C., Gray, K.M., Melvin, G.A., 2015. Anxiety disorders in children and adolescents with intellectual disability: Prevalence and assessment. Res. Dev. Disabil. 36, 175–190.

Reaven, J.A., Blakeley-Smith, A., Nichols, S., Dasari, M., Flanigan, E., Hepburn, S., 2009. Cognitive-behavioral group treatment for anxiety symptoms in children with high-functioning autism spectrum disorders: a pilot study. Focus Autism Other Dev. Disabil. 24 (1), 27–37.

Reynolds, C.R., Richmond, B.O., 1978. What I think and feel: a revised measure of children's manifest anxiety. J Abnorm Child Psychol 6 (2), 271–280.

Research Units for Pediatric Psychopharmacology (RUPP) Anxiety Study Group, 2002. The Pediatric Anxiety Rating Scale (PARS): Development and psychometric properties. Journal of the American Academy of Child & Adolescent Psychiatry 41, 1061–1069.

Rieske, R.D., Matson, J.L., Davis 3rd, T.E., Konst, M.J., Williams, L.W., Whiting, S.E., 2013. Examination and validation of a measure of anxiety specific to children with autism spectrum disorders. Dev. Neurorehabil. 16 (1), 9–16.

Rosen, T.E., Connell, J.E., Kerns, C.M., 2016. A review of behavioral interventions for anxiety-related behaviors in lower-functioning individuals with autism. Behavioral Interventions 31, 120–143.

Rodgers, J., Wigham, S., McConachie, H., Freeson, M., Honey, E., Parr, J.R., 2016. Development of the anxiety scale for children with autism spectrum disorder (ASC-ASD). Autism Res. Available from: http://dx.doi.org/10.1002/aur.1603.

Scahill, L., McDougle, C.J., Williams, S.K., Dimitropoulos, A., Aman, M.G., McCracken, J.T., et al., 2006. Children's Yale-Brown Obsessive Compulsive Scale modified for pervasive developmental disorders. Journal of the American Academy of Child & Adolescent Psychiatry 45 (9), 1114–1123.

Shaffer, D., Fisher, P., Lucas, C.P., Dulcan, M.K., Schwab-Stone, M.E., 2000. NIMH Diagnostic Interview Schedule for Children Version IV (NIMH DISC-IV): description, differences from previous versions, and reliability of some common diagnoses. Journal of the American Academy of Child & Adolescent Psychiatry 39 (1), 28–38.

Silverman, W.K., Albano, A.M., 1996. Anxiety Disorders Interview Schedule for DSM-IV.: Parent interview schedule, Vol. 1. Oxford University Press.

Simonoff, E., Pickles, A., Charman, T., Chandler, S., Loucas, T., Baird, G., 2008. Psychiatric disorders in children with autism spectrum disorders: Prevalence, comorbidity, and associated factors in a population-derived sample. J. Am. Acad. Child. Adolesc. Psychiatry. 47, 921–929.

Spence, S., 1998. A measure of anxiety symptoms among children. Behav. Res. Therapy 36, 545–566.

Spence, S.H., 1995. Social Skills Training, Enhancing Social Competence with Children and Adolescents: Research and Technical Support. NFER-Nelson Publishing Company Ltd, Windsor.

Spielberger, C.D., 1973. Manual for the State-Trait Anxiety Inventory for Children. Consulting Psychologists Press, Palo Alto, CA.

Stansbury, K., Gunnar, M.R., 2011. Activity and emotion. Emotion 59 (2), 108–134.

Sterling, L., Renno, P., Storch, E.A., Ehrenreich-May, J., Lewin, A.B., Arnold, E., et al., 2015. Validity of the Revised Children's Anxiety and Depression Scale for youth with autism spectrum disorders. Autism 19 (1), 113–117.

Stern, J.A., Gadgil, M.S., Blakeley-Smith, A., Reaven, J.A., Hepburn, S.L., 2014. Psychometric properties of the SCARED in youth with autism spectrum disorder. Res. Autism Spect. Disord. 8 (9), 1225–1234.

Storch, E.A., Wood, J.J., Ehrenreich-May, J., Jones, A.M., Park, J.M., Lewin, A.B., et al., 2012. Convergent and discriminant validity and reliability of the pediatric anxiety rating scale in youth with autism spectrum disorders. J. Autism Dev. Disord. 42 (11), 2374–2382.

Sukhodolsky, D.G., Scahill, L., Gadow, K.D., Arnold, L.E., Aman, M.G., McDougle, C.J., et al., 2008. Parent-rated anxiety symptoms in children with pervasive developmental disorders: frequency and association with core autism symptoms and cognitive functioning. J. Abnormal Child Psychol. 36 (1), 117–128.

Ung, D., Arnold, E.B., De Nadai, A.S., Lewin, A.B., Phares, V., Murphy, T.K., et al., 2014. Inter-rater reliability of the Anxiety Disorders Interview Schedule for DSM-IV in high-functioning youth with autism spectrum disorder. J. Dev. Phys. Disabil. 26, 53–65.

van Steensel Francisca, J.A., Bogels, S.M., Perrin, S., 2011. Anxiety disorders in children and adolescents with autistic spectrum disorders: A meta-analysis. Clin. Child. Fam. Psychol. Rev. 14 (3), 302–317.

Van Hecke, A.V., Lebow, J., Bal, E., Lamb, D., Harden, E., Kramer, A., et al., 2009. Electroencephalogram and heart rate regulation to familiar and unfamiliar people in children with autism spectrum disorders. Child Dev. 80 (4), 1118–1133.

White, S.W., Schry, A.R., Maddox, B.B., 2012. Brief report: the assessment of anxiety in high-functioning adolescents with autism spectrum disorder. J. Autism Dev. Disord. 42 (6), 1138–1145.

White, S.W., Oswald, D., Ollendick, T., Scahill, L., 2009. Anxiety in children and adolescents with autism spectrum disorders. Clin. Psychol. Rev. 29 (3), 216–229.

White, S.W., Lerner, M.D., McLeod, B.D., Wood, J.J., Ginsburg, G.S., Kerns, C., et al., 2015. Anxiety in youth with and without Autism Spectrum Disorder: examination of factorial equivalence. Behav. Therapy 46 (1), 40–53.

Witwer, A.N., Lecavalier, L., Norris, M., 2012. Reliability and validity of the Children's interview for psychiatric syndromes-parent version in autism spectrum disorders. J. Autism. Dev. Disord. 42 (9), 1949–1958.

Wood, J.J., Gadow, K.D., 2010. Exploring the nature and function of anxiety in youth with autism spectrum disorders. Clin. Psychol. Sci. Practice 17 (4), 281–292.

Wood, J.J., Drahota, A., Sze, K., Har, K., Chiu, A., Langer, D.A., 2009. Cognitive behavioral therapy for anxiety in children with autism spectrum disorders: a randomized, controlled trial. J. Child Psychol. Psychiatry Allied Disciplines 50 (3), 224–234.

Zainal, H., Magiati, I., Tan, J.W.L., Sung, M., Fung, D.S., Howlin, P., 2014. A preliminary investigation of the Spence Children's Anxiety Parent Scale as a screening tool for anxiety in young people with autism spectrum disorders. J. Autism. Dev. Disord. 44 (8), 1982–1994.

CHAPTER 6

Cognitive-Behavioral Principles and Their Applications Within Autism Spectrum Disorder

Paige M. Ryan, Maysa M. Kaskas and Thompson E. Davis
Louisiana State University, Baton Rouge, LA, United States

Autism Spectrum Disorder (ASD) is characterized as deficits in social communication and reciprocity, and distinctive repetitive behaviors that begin in the early years of life; these deficits cause pervasive impairment in domains of functioning. Although anxiety is not listed as a specific criterion for those with ASD, it has been found to be one of the most common comorbidities (de Bruin et al., 2007) and it has been difficult to tease apart from ASD symptoms (Kerns and Kendall, 2012). The rate of anxiety for those with ASD is even higher than that of the general population, ranging from 11% to 84%, with the average around 50% (White et al., 2009). A comparison of parent-reported anxiety in children with ASD and clinically anxious neurotypical children found that parents from the ASD group reported their children to have higher anxiety severity, more specific phobias, and lower overall quality of life (van Steensel et al., 2012).

Adolescents and school-aged children have the highest prevalence of anxiety (with 40% falling in the clinical range and 26% in the subclinical range). Additionally, higher IQ and lower ASD severity have been associated with higher levels of anxiety in preschool and school-aged children (Vasa et al., 2013). Reduced executive functioning, but not social cognitive ability, has also been associated with higher anxiety in those with ASD (Hollocks et al., 2014). Given the severity of symptoms and the frequent co-occurrence of ASD and anxiety, it is not surprising that a number of treatments have been developed to ease symptoms.

Treatments for children with comorbid anxiety and ASD include psychosocial and pharmacological treatments. Pharmacological treatments (e.g., Selective Serotonin Reuptake Inhibitors, or SSRIs) have commonly been used for the treatment of anxiety, occasionally with augmented components

Anxiety in Children and Adolescents with Autism Spectrum Disorder.
DOI: http://dx.doi.org/10.1016/B978-0-12-805122-1.00006-5
© 2017 Elsevier Inc.
All rights reserved.

(e.g., behavioral activation; Vasa et al., 2014). However, the efficacy of such interventions for anxiety is unclear and/or undocumented, and many report an increased risk of adverse side effects with these treatments in individuals with ASD, especially behavioral activation (Ji and Findling, 2015). At the same time, work has been underway to transport and modify neurotypical treatments for anxiety to children with ASD (Davis, 2012). Cognitive-behavioral therapy (CBT) has been established as an empirically-supported treatment for typically developing children with anxiety (Davis, 2009; Davis and Ollendick, 2005; Davis et al. 2011b; Kendall et al., 1997, 2008; Walkup et al, 2008). Knowledge of the efficacy of CBT for anxiety in ASD is modest but seems promising (White et al., 2013); however, several modifications may be necessary to accommodate for the specific characteristics in children with ASD, which will be our main focus.

CBT FOR ANXIETY IN TYPICALLY DEVELOPING CHILDREN

CBT is probably the most effective evidence-based treatment for those with anxiety disorders (Read et al., 2013). CBT typically involves various components that address three areas: distorted cognitions, dysfunctional behaviors (e.g., avoidance), and identification of emotions and physiological symptoms (Chorpita, 2007; Davis and Ollendick, 2005; Kendall, 1992, 1993; Friedberg and McClure, 2015). To address these problematic areas, a stepwise format for CBT has been formulated for neurotypical children. Read et al. (2013) include the following steps in their analysis of CBT: psychoeducation, relaxation training/somatic management, cognitive restructuring, problem solving, exposure tasks, and booster sessions/relapse prevention. The authors mention that additional steps may be necessary based on the client's specific needs. For example, Kendall (1993) mentions that additional strategies may be necessary when cognitive deficiencies (i.e., the lack of information processing when it would be beneficial as compared to cognitive distortions, which are biases in information processing) are present. Laying out these specific techniques for neurotypical children in the following sections will provide a clearer path from which to examine possible strategies for modification for children with ASD.

PSYCHOEDUCATION

In many CBT manuals, the clinician begins by informing the client about anxiety and describes the model that maintains the occurrence of anxiety.

For children, it is often helpful for the family to be involved in this step. The client can then better understand the environmental triggers, physiological responses, and factors that maintain their problems with anxiety. Furthermore, the client learns to no longer associate anxiety with something that is defective within them, but rather a normal, adaptive response that happens to everyone. Adaptations for young children may include using more concrete language, picture cards, and culturally appropriate metaphors (e.g., fire alarms, brain hiccups). Lastly, additional practice with the important skills of identifying and understanding emotions and establishing connections between thoughts, feelings, and actions can be beneficial for treatment progression, particularly for young children and those with impaired cognitive abilities (Read et al., 2013).

RELAXATION AND SOMATIC MANAGEMENT

This stage of treatment often encompasses both breathing exercises and muscle relaxation. The client learns to tense and relax specific muscle groups successively; this promotes awareness of tension that is caused by anxiety and relaxation as a solution for this tension. Deep diaphragmatic breathing is emphasized as well to counteract the quick and shallow breaths that occur with anxious physiological arousal (Read et al., 2013).

COGNITIVE RESTRUCTURING

By this stage, the therapist has usually already addressed the important link between thoughts, feelings, and actions, thus, the client understands that tackling biased "self-talk" (i.e., self-referential thoughts) is one way to address anxiety. The client first begins with identifying thoughts that may contribute to his/her anxious feelings and arousal. Next, the client begins to identify and categorize patterns in his/her biased thinking. The client can then challenge these errors with more accurate, probable, and adaptive responses. This step usually helps the client to reduce feelings of anxiety (Read et al., 2013).

PROBLEM SOLVING

Many individuals with anxiety may view their distress as uncontrollable and catastrophic in nature. However, this step specifically targets this distortion, as the client is told to view anxiety as a problem that can be solved. The therapist and the client act as a team to brainstorm ideas on decreasing the client's level of distress. The therapist should continuously encourage the client to come up with many alternatives to solve the problem and systematically "test" their viability in order to achieve the best outcome (Friedberg and McClure, 2015). Children might perceive the problem-solving phase as overwhelming and difficult to understand. In this case, the therapist should use concrete examples (e.g., looking for a lost toy) to more appropriately explain the steps of problem solving (Read et al., 2013).

EXPOSURE

Exposure is an essential component in the treatment of anxiety and is used in approximately 80% of all anxiety treatment models (CBT and other models; Chorpita and Daleiden, 2009). Behavioral avoidance is extremely common, and likely impairing, in those with anxiety disorders (Chorpita and Daleiden, 2009). Exposure is a systematic hierarchical presentation of fearful stimuli that, while mildly distressing, provides the client the opportunity to cope with the feared situation without the ability to avoid or escape. First, the hierarchy is built by the client's self-reported ratings of feared situations, from the least feared to the most catastrophic (and likely most impairing) fear. For younger children, the parents' ratings of the child's fears are typically included in building the hierarchy. During the actual exposure, the client practices and tests his/her coping skills learned in previous sessions. Furthermore, clients are taught to distinguish between their catastrophic perceptions of fear and the facts about the actual threat. In experiencing the exposure, clients learn that their beliefs about the outcome of the situation do not match the actual outcome of the exposure, discovering that they are able to successfully manage their fear and cope with the outcome. The goal is for clients to feel that they are able to successfully deal with distressing or threatening situations (Chorpita and Daleiden, 2009; Read et al., 2013).

Exposures can either be directly experienced in session (in vivo) or imagined (imaginal; in vitro). Imaginal exposures can be used when the situation is difficult to practically simulate in a session (e.g., getting smallpox). The therapist and the client work together to imagine a very vivid, detailed scene of the feared environment or stimulus, possibly while listening to an anxiety-inducing audio tape and/or viewing a group of pictures. Throughout the exposure, the client's level of distress is measured on a scale of subjective units of distress (SUDS), with 0 representing a state of total relaxation and a rating of 100 being the most fear the person can imagine. For children, a simpler scale of varying degrees of smiling/frowning faces or a numerical scale from 0 to 10 or 0 to 8 (per the Anxiety Disorders Interview Schedule Child/Parent; ADIS-IV-C/P) can be used to evaluate subjective anxiety (Friedberg and McClure, 2015).

Exposures are often repeated to allow the client to build a history of adaptive coping; this allows the client to habituate more quickly to successive exposures. Progress monitoring sheets can be used to track exposures and improve the client's sense of autonomy and self-efficacy. Exposure tasks can be practiced in multiple settings to encourage generalization of learning and coping. Additionally, exposures typically look different based on the client's particular fears and symptoms (Peterman et al, 2015).

TREATMENT OF ANXIOUS CHILDREN WITH ASD

ASD represents a cluster of varied characteristics that require careful assessment and treatment considerations. Communication disorders, intellectual disabilities, stereotypy, and mental health comorbidities are common in ASD (Myers and Johnson, 2007). These comorbid concerns may inhibit the individual's ability to independently complete self-report measures during assessment and understand some of the specific components of CBT during treatment (e.g., cognitive restructuring process). Therefore, modification of the traditional CBT process may be needed to maximize treatment efficacy for anxious children with ASD. Along these lines, commonly used treatments of anxiety for children with ASD include psychosocial interventions, medication, CBT modification (e.g., Coping Cat; Kendall and Hedtke, 2006a,b), and behavioral interventions (e.g., reinforcement for completion of exposure).

Psychosocial interventions usually include social skills training for children with distinct skill deficits (Schohl et al., 2014). Pharmacological interventions typically involve medication management strategies and occasionally other components (e.g., behavioral activation). This combination of approaches can be loosely defined as "treatment as usual" (TAU). Additionally, various studies have applied behavioral techniques (e.g., exposure plus reinforcement) for the treatment of anxiety in the ASD population (Chok et al., 2010; Love et al, 1990; Rapp et al., 2005; Schmidt et al.,2013). In a recent study, Storch et al. (2013) compared

TAU (defined as receiving pharmacological and medication management interventions, school counseling, special education services, and social skills training) to a modified version of CBT for anxious youth with ASD. The authors found that a personalized CBT intervention significantly reduced both anxiety symptoms and impairment with generally large effects observed across clinician–rated anxiety outcomes.

MODIFYING CBT FOR CHILDREN WITH ASD

An increasingly common option for anxiety treatment for children with ASD is modifying traditional CBT to fit the unique needs of these youth. Adapting CBT to improve outcomes for children with ASD may involve including more social skills and emotion recognition modules, incorporating more parental involvement in treatment (e.g., reviewing session content and homework assignments with parents), incorporating technology to guide clients through coping strategies, increasing use of visual aids (e.g., worksheets, cue cards), and modifying the pacing of treatment (e.g., scheduling more frequent sessions, spending more time reviewing material, including more exposure tasks; Scattone and Mong, 2013). Some characteristics inherent to youth with ASD (e.g., perseveration, restricted interests) can be leveraged to enhance treatment fidelity and outcomes. For example, the restricted interests of youth with ASD can be used both as a reward for session engagement and participation and also as a mechanism to explain the importance of strategies; e.g., a client's favorite movie character may be used consistently throughout the sessions to demonstrate skills, model appropriate cognitions, and reinforce brave behaviors (Danial and Wood, 2013).

One example of a modified CBT program for youth with comorbid ASD and anxiety is the modified Coping Cat program, a 16-week program which includes the following modifications for children with ASD: more time spent reviewing for skill generalization, additional visual materials (e.g., cue cards, schedules, scales), more concrete language, and increasing behavioral components (e.g., relaxation training, role playing). Furthermore, for children with motor skill difficulties, writing assignments were completed with the help of the therapist or a computer. Large effect sizes were reported for children participating in the modified Coping Cat treatment as compared to waitlist controls; importantly, these gains were maintained at two-month follow-up (McNally Keehn et al., 2013).

ESTIMATED EFFICACY OF CBT FOR CHILDREN WITH ASD

Though additional research is warranted, there is initial evidence to support the efficacy of CBT for children with ASD. Sukhodolsky et al. (2013) completed a review of the literature on CBT for children with ASD: although all reporters produced relatively large effect sizes, clinician- and parent-reported improvements in anxiety were slightly larger than child-rated improvements ($d = 1.19$ for clinician-rated improvements, $d = 1.2$ for parent-rated improvements, and $d = 0.68$ for self-reported improvements). Support for CBT applied to youth with ASD and anxiety has also been found across age groups, from preschoolers to adults. Although only a case study, improvements in a preschooler (age 4 years) with comorbid ASD and anxiety were reported and the gains were maintained at a four-month follow-up (Nadeau et al., 2015). Ehrenreich-May et al. (2014) evaluated CBT for adolescents with ASD and found a reduction of clinician-rated and parent-rated anxiety severity. Furthermore, level of impairment and behavioral problems were significantly reduced at post-treatment and maintained at a one-month follow up. Support has also been provided for CBT with adults with ASD and psychiatric comorbidity, including anxiety (Spain et al., 2015).

There is promising evidence for the efficacy of CBT in youth with ASD beyond improvements in anxiety symptomology. Drahota et al. (2011) noted that children with ASD often have difficulty in mastering and consistently applying basic daily living skills, resulting in impairments in functioning and greater dependence on caregivers to accomplish simple tasks. After a 16-week CBT program, participants' overall anxiety level and anxiety sensitivity significantly decreased. Interestingly, the children's total and personal daily living skills also improved, and their parents reported more independence and less need for involvement in their child's daily routine. These findings suggest broad utility for CBT in youth with ASD, as improvements were demonstrated across domains (e.g., anxiety, social skills, adaptive functioning).

High rates of comorbid OCD have been associated with ASD. Russell et al. (2013) investigated the outcome of children receiving CBT versus another active treatment (i.e., anxiety management) for OCD symptoms. Findings suggested that children who received CBT were more responsive to treatment, had slightly better outcomes at the end of treatment, and higher self-reported improvement scores. Last, given that high family accommodation of OCD symptomology has been associated with poorer outcomes, parent-training modifications of CBT for OCD in ASD may facilitate the best outcomes (see Davis et al., 2014 for more disorder-specific recommendations).

Current Research Limitations and Areas for Improvement

The data to date are promising, but, as Danial and Wood (2013) noted, there are some important considerations. For example, many treatment studies evaluating youth with comorbid anxiety and ASD have small sample sizes and rely heavily on parent report. Few studies have investigated associated characteristics for individuals with ASD that may complicate therapy progress (e.g., repetitive behaviors, sensory issues, comorbid disruptive behaviors) as well as characteristics that may increase probability of treatment response (e.g., advanced memory). Also, much of the literature examining the efficacy of CBT with persons with ASD and anxiety fails to assess the level of cognitive change (e.g., theory of mind skills) in addition to the amount of behavioral change (e.g., approach/avoidance in feared situations). More work is needed to examine the course of anxiety in those who also have comorbid ASD (e.g., Davis et al., 2011a). Needed are studies that help to dismantle CBT components to determine which of the varied components of modified CBT is most responsible for treatment outcomes. Additional empirical study is warranted to answer these and related questions that will optimize the efficacy of CBT for anxious youth with ASD.

SUGGESTIONS FOR SPECIFIC MODIFICATIONS OF CBT FOR CHILDREN WITH ASD

Careful assessment of the client before beginning therapy is vital in determining any special considerations and individualized components that may be necessary for successful implementation (Moree and Davis, 2010). For example, clinicians should assess for any sensory issues that may impede treatment (e.g., oversensitivity to material types, bright lights, loud noises) and pay attention to the need for the environment to be arranged so that the client feels comfortable and safe. Additional considerations may include using concrete visual displays and literal language (e.g., limiting use of metaphors or finding one that works and sticking with it) to improve understanding of new concepts for children with ASD, particularly for those with intellectual disability. Social skills training may be necessary for socially anxious individuals to remediate impairing skills deficits (e.g., emotional awareness, perspective taking) that often accompany ASD (White et al., 2010). Therapeutic approaches are best when tailored to the child's interests in order to increase motivation and rapport (Moree and Davis, 2010). For children with limited communication or intellectual abilities, structured preference assessments can determine potent reinforcers for completion of tasks related to treatment (e.g., exposure tasks, between-session activities; Hagopian et al., 2004). Clinicians report that children with ASD may require a slower pace throughout CBT, which may be attributed to rigidity, general executive dysfunction, or comorbid intellectual disability (Danial and Wood, 2013).

Clinicians may consider using the acronym "PRECISE" as a mnemonic device to recall the modifications needed to effectively conduct CBT with individuals with ASD (Davis et al., 2014). The "P" stands for a collaborative **p**artnership between the client and therapist that capitalizes on the client's strengths and assists with any difficulties. The collaborative partnership which emphasizes client strengths is particularly important in individuals with ASD, who might have difficulty connecting with others. The "R" stands for **r**ight developmental level (e.g., using visual cues, involving the parents along a continuum; Lang et al., 2010). The "E'" stands for **e**mpathy, and the "C" stands for **c**reative implementation (e.g., incorporating special or restricted interests). The "I" stands for **i**nvestigative approach (e.g., the use of behavioral experiments rather than verbal cognitive restructuring) and the "S" stands for **s**elf-discovery. Finally, the last "E" stands for **e**njoyable, which is particularly important for children in order to ensure their cooperation with treatment (Davis et al., 2014).

Due to the amount of time children with ASD spend with their caregivers, involving parents and aides in treatment can be important to a successful treatment response. Caregivers are valued sources of information, who can inform the clinician about the nature of the client's anxiety (e.g., antecedents, consequences, maintaining factors). Additionally, training the caregivers to conduct between-session activities and exposure tasks may be beneficial in treatment (Davis et al., 2014). For example, Storch et al. (2013) conducted a randomized 16-week trial of CBT, which was modified specifically for children with high-functioning ASD by increasing parental participation. The authors found that parental involvement was important for the completion of exposure tasks at home, which resulted in large treatment success effect sizes. Similarly, anxious youth with higher parent-rated autism spectrum symptoms have been found to respond better to family CBT compared to individual CBT

(Puleo and Kendall, 2011), again with family CBT having more at-home exposure tasks. It may be important for parents to complete training for problem behaviors (e.g., how to give consistent rewards and consequences, differential reinforcement) before beginning treatment for anxiety as such work may increase adherence to treatment by addressing problem behaviors which may serve to maintain the child's anxiety (e.g., facilitating avoidance) or interfere with treatment progress (e.g., refusal to participate; Davis et al., 2014). Finally, some degree of persistent impairment across the lifespan is typical for most individuals with an ASD diagnosis; involving parents in anxiety treatment is ideal for maintaining gains and consistent with the degree of parental involvement across development (Reaven and Blakeley-Smith, 2013).

Lickel et al. (2012) discussed how the assessment of the client's skill deficits can influence the treatment plan. For example, children with ASD tend to have difficulty with emotional regulation, perspective taking, and self-reflection. CBT for children with these difficulties could include additional components to teach affect discrimination and emotional awareness (Davis et al., 2014). Traditional CBT approaches include tasks such as detective thinking and identifying cognitive distortions; these tasks rely on the skill of cognitive control, the ability to manage internal reactions to distressing stimuli. Cognitive control may be a difficult skill for children with ASD to master. In modifying CBT for youth with ASD, these strategies could be made more concrete (e.g., using worksheets to write down all evidence for and against a thought). Children with ASD may also have difficulty in generating their own coping thoughts. If this is the case, it is recommended that therapists give the client a selection of coping thoughts that may be individualized according to their specific interests (Gross and Thompson, 2007).

According to Rieffe et al. (2011), individuals with ASD may struggle with rumination due to their problems with attentional networks and emotional awareness. For these children with deficits in emotional awareness or with alexithymia (inability to recognize emotions), more time should be spent on modules related to emotion identification and recognition prior to beginning CBT (Moree and Davis, 2010). Furthermore, individuals with ASD may benefit from learning how to address the experience of emotion and to express emotions in socially appropriate ways. Relaxation training and deep breathing are options for emotional regulation that are often part of CBT. A functional behavioral assessment helps to determine the function of specific therapy interfering behaviors (e.g., stereotypy, avoidance), and can thus be useful to address them appropriately (e.g., not allowing the client to escape, receive attention).

ADDITIONAL OPTIONS FOR TREATMENT

Modifying Exposure

When working with anxious youth, with or without ASD, mental health professionals are often encouraged to "think exposure" (Kendall et al., 2005; Peterman et al., 2015). One issue that frequently arises in anxiety treatment with children with ASD is how, when needed, to modify exposure. For example, in neurotypical individuals with specific phobias there is a growing body of evidence supporting the efficacy of a single exposure-based multi-hour treatment session (Choy et al., 2007; Davis et al., 2012). Davis et al. (2007) examined the potential utility of One-Session Treatment (OST), which combines graduated in vivo exposure with psychoeducation, modeling, reinforcement (e.g., verbal praise, pats on the back, access to preferred items), and cognitive challenges. The OST procedure was unmodified and administered for a verbal child with comorbid specific phobias (heights and water), developmental delays, and problematic behaviors, including self-injury, aggression, and disruption. A functional analysis of the child's problematic behavior indicated that the behaviors were primarily maintained by attention, suggesting the particular efficacy of verbal reinforcement delivered during the massed exposure. The child no longer met criteria for height phobia and water phobia at post-treatment (two months and four months). This case study suggests the possibility that exposure can be conducted unmodified in those who are not typically-developing children and adults; however, more than likely some degree of accommodation and modification will be necessary when conducting exposure tasks with children with ASD and anxiety.

An important part of treating anxiety is the fear hierarchy—individualized and disorder-specific—and interviews from caregivers can provide information about various fears to build a complete fear hierarchy. Studies have shown that video modeling (e.g., for exposure tasks) may be useful for individuals with ASD who prefer attending to videos more than human models (Davis et al., 2014). Some individuals with ASD may benefit from continuous access to preferred items during exposure, which may help to divert the attention away from the feared stimulus and weaken the association between the stimulus and the fearful response (Luscre and Center, 1996), or more than likely have a desensitizing rather than distracting effect (Davis, 2009).

GROUP THERAPY

CBT may be implemented in a small-group format and studies have found support for the efficacy of group CBT for children with comorbid ASD and anxiety. Reaven et al. (2012) conducted a 12-week randomized trial with 50 youth with high-functioning ASD and anxiety. These children were assigned to either a TAU group (which consisted of either medication to treat anxious symptomology, social skills interventions, school-based anti-bullying programs, individual coping or emotional regulation skills training sessions, or family-focused behavioral interventions) or a CBT intervention designed specifically for youth with ASD. The Facing Your Fears (FYF) intervention involved typical CBT components (e.g., relaxation, deep breathing, graduated exposure, strategies to promote emotion regulation, use of cognitive control) as well as ASD-specific modifications (e.g., increased reinforcement for behavior in group, visual cues such as multiple choice lists, hands-on activities, video modeling). The program also included a separate parent component and curriculum, which involved psychoeducation, coaching skills (e.g., supporting child brave behaviors, participation), and information about how to best parent a child with comorbid anxiety and ASD. Parents in the FYF program discussed the reciprocal relations between parental psychopathology (e.g., anxiety), parenting style (e.g., adaptive versus excessive protection), and the maintenance of anxiety symptoms in children. As children with ASD are prone to challenges with social skills and adaptive communication, "excessively protective" parenting styles are common in caregivers of youth with ASD. Caregivers who fall in the excessively protective category tend to allow their children to avoid anxiety-provoking or uncertain situations, therefore limiting their children's opportunities to practice adaptive coping skills and contributing to the maintenance of symptoms of anxiety. Participants in the FYF program exhibited significant reductions in anxiety (as compared to the TAU condition), suggesting that the group format may be an effective modification of CBT for youth with ASD (Reaven et al., 2012). However, no studies were found which directly compared the efficacy of group CBT to individual CBT. Additionally, due to the heterogeneity of symptoms associated with ASD, group interventions may not be appropriate for every child with comorbid ASD and anxiety.

FUTURE DIRECTIONS AND APPLICATIONS

Anxiety disorders can be extremely impairing, particularly in persons with pre-existing challenges (e.g., youth with ASD). van Steensel et al. (2013) compared the societal costs of children with high-functioning ASD and comorbid anxiety disorder(s) to typically-developing control children and neurotypical children with anxiety disorder(s), finding that costs in the comorbid group were 27 times higher than the comparison group and four times higher than the neurotypical anxiety disordered group. The authors concluded that these costs can be significantly decreased with efficacious therapies for anxiety in individuals with ASD. There is increasingly promising evidence for the application of CBT, an evidence-based treatment for many mental health problems in typically-developing individuals of all ages (Sukhodolsky et al., 2013).

Nearly all CBT principles and procedures can be used with individuals with ASD, especially if individualized. ASD severity may be the strongest moderator of response to treatment in individuals with ASD (even above children's language or overall cognitive abilities). Accordingly, it is important to conduct a thorough intake assessing level of functioning and symptom severity prior to treatment onset (Storch et al., 2015). This assessment can help to determine which modifications may improve likelihood of treatment adherence and success. These modifications typically include greater parent/caregiver involvement, social skills training, coping skills training, more time spent reviewing for skill generalization, additional visual materials (e.g., cue cards, schedules, scales), more concrete language, and increasing behavioral components (e.g., relaxation training, role playing; Scattone and Mong, 2013). However, it is important to apply CBT flexibly for all children with ASD, as one should expect treatment to progress at a slower pace than it would for neurotypical individuals (Storch et al., 2015).

Some youth with ASD may have more difficulty than others in adjusting to treatment. Teaching coping skills may aid progress; these skills may help individuals with ASD cope with discomfort during changes in routine, social interactions, and other fears or worries. Additionally, many children in therapy, who are often involuntarily taken by their parents, often lack motivation for treatment. Therapists can build both rapport and motivation for change by asking the child about the kinds of things they value, what they would like to improve, and how the therapist can help improve quality of life. Difficulties completing homework assignments can also interfere with treatment progress. Children with ASD may have executive functioning deficits which causes disorganization and forgetfulness with assignments. These individuals may benefit from additional support; e.g., homework assignments can be divided into small chunks, instructions can be simplified, additional practice can be built into sessions, and written and visual reminders to complete homework may be provided (Storch et al., 2015).

REFERENCES

Chok, J.T., Demanche, J.D., Kennedy, A.K., Studer, L., 2010. Utilizing physiological measures to facilitate phobia treatment with individuals with autism and intellectual disability: a case study. Behav. Intervent. 25 (4), 325–337.

Chorpita, B.F., 2007. Modular Cognitive-Behavioral Therapy for Childhood Anxiety Disorders. Guilford Press, New York, NY.

Chorpita, B.F., Daleiden, E.L., 2009. Mapping evidence-based treatments for children and adolescents: application of the distillation and matching model to 615 treatments. J. Counsell. Clin. Psychol. 77 (3), 566–579.

Choy, Y., Fyer, A.J., Lipsitz, J.D., 2007. Treatment of specific phobia in adults. Clin. Psychol. Rev. 27 (3), 266–286.

Danial, J.T., Wood, J.J., 2013. Cognitive behavioral therapy for children with autism: review and considerations for future research. J. Dev. Behav. Pediatrics 34 (9), 702–715.

Davis III, T.E., 2009. PTSD, anxiety, and phobia. Treating Childhood Psychopathology and Developmental Disabilities. Springer, New York, NY, pp. 183–220.

Davis III, T.E., 2012. Where to from here for ASD and anxiety? Lessons learned from child anxiety and the issue of DSM-5. Clin. Psychol. Sci. Pract. 19, 358–363.

Davis III, T.E., Ollendick, T.H., 2005. Empirically supported treatments for specific phobia in children: do efficacious treatments address the components of a phobic response? Clin. Psychol. Sci. Pract. 12 (2), 144–160.

Davis III, T.E., Kurtz, P., Gardner, A., Carman, N., 2007. Cognitive-behavioral treatment for specific phobias with a child demonstrating severe problem behavior and developmental delays. Res. Dev. Disabil. 28, 546–558.

Davis III, T.E., Hess, J.A., Moree, B.N., Fodstad, J.C., Dempsey, T., Jenkins, W., et al., 2011a. Anxiety symptoms across the lifespan in people with autistic disorder. Res. Autism Spectrum Disord. 5, 112–118.

Davis III, T.E., May, A.C., Whiting, S.E., 2011b. Evidence-based treatment of anxiety and phobia in children and adolescents: current status and effects on the emotional response. Clin. Psychol. Rev. 31, 592–602.

Davis III, T.E., Jenkins, W., Rudy, B., 2012. Empirical status of One-Session Treatment. In: Davis, T.E., Ollendick, T.H., Öst, L.-G. (Eds.), Intensive One-Session Treatment of Specific Phobias. Springer Science and Business Media, New York, pp. 209–226.

Davis III, T.E., White, S.W., Ollendick, T.H., 2014. Handbook of Autism and Anxiety. Springer, New York, NY.

de Bruin, E.I., Ferdinand, R.F., Meester, S., de Nijs, P.F., Verheij, F., 2007. High rates of psychiatric co-morbidity in PDD-NOS. J. Autism Dev. Disord. 37 (5), 877–886.

Drahota, A., Wood, J.J., Sze, K.M., Van Dyke, M., 2011. Effects of cognitive behavioral therapy on daily living skills in children with high-functioning autism and concurrent anxiety disorders. J. Autism Dev. Disord. 41 (3), 257–265.

Ehrenreich-May, J., Storch, E.A., Queen, A.H., Rodriguez, J.H., Ghilain, C.S., Alessandri, M., et al., 2014. An open trial of cognitive-behavioral therapy for anxiety disorders in adolescents with autism spectrum disorders. Focus Autism Other Dev. Disabil. 29 (3), 145–155.

Friedberg, R.D., McClure, J.M., 2015. Clinical Practice of Cognitive Therapy with Children and Adolescents: The Nuts and Bolts, second ed. Guilford Publications, New York, NY.

Gross, J.J., Thompson, R.A., 2007. Emotion regulation: conceptual foundations. In: Gross, J.J. (Ed.), Handbook of Emotion Regulation. Guilford Press, New York, NY, pp. 3–26.

Hagopian, L.P., Long, E.S., Rush, K.S., 2004. Preference assessment procedures for individuals with developmental disabilities. Behav. Modif. 28, 668–677.

Hollocks, M.J., Jones, C.G., Pickles, A., Baird, G., Happé, F., Charman, T., et al., 2014. The association between social cognition and executive functioning and symptoms of anxiety and depression in adolescents with autism spectrum disorders. Autism Res. 7 (2), 216–228.

Ji, N.Y., Findling, R.L., 2015. An update on pharmacotherapy for autism spectrum disorder in children and adolescents. Curr. Opin. Psychiatry 28 (2), 91–101.

Kendall, P.C., 1992. The Coping Cat Workbook. Workbook Publishing, Ardmore, PA.

Kendall, P.C., 1993. Cognitive-behavioral therapies with youth: guiding theory, current status, and emerging developments. J. Consult. Clin. Psychol. 61 (2), 235–247.

Kendall, P.C.,, Hedtke, K., 2006a. Coping Cat Workbook, second ed. Workbook Publishing, Ardmore, PA.

Kendall, P.C.,, Hedtke, K., 2006b. Cognitive-Behavioral Therapy for Anxious Children: Therapist Manual, third ed. Workbook Publishing, Ardmore, PA.

Kendall, P., Flannery-Schroeder, E., Panichelli-Mindel, S., Southam-Gerow, M., Henin, A., Warman, M., 1997. Therapy for youths with anxiety disorders: a second randomized clinical trial. J. Consult. Clin. Psychol. 65, 366–380.

Kendall, P.C., Robin, J., Hedtke, K., Suveg, C., Flannery-Schroeder, E., Gosch, E., 2005. Considering CBT with anxious youth? Think exposures. Cogn. Behav. Pract. 12, 136–148.

Kendall, P.C., Hudson, J., Gosch, E., Flannery-Schroeder, E., Suveg, C., 2008. Cognitive-behavioral therapy for anxiety disordered youth: a randomized clinical trial evaluating child and family modalities. J. Consult. Clin. Psychol. 76, 282–297.

Kerns, C.M., Kendall, P.C., 2012. The presentation and classification of anxiety in autism spectrum disorder. Clin. Psychol. Sci. Pract. 19, 323–347.

Lang, R., Regester, A., Lauderdale, S., Ashbaugh, K., Haring, A., 2010. Treatment of anxiety in autism spectrum disorders using cognitive behavior therapy: a systematic review. Dev. Neurorehabil. 13 (1), 53–63.

Lickel, A., MacLean, W.E., Blakeley-Smith, A., Hepburn, S., 2012. Assessment of the prerequisite skills for cognitive behavioral therapy in children with and without autism spectrum disorders. J. Autism Dev. Disord. 42 (6), 992–1000.

Love, S.R., Matson, J.L., West, D., 1990. Mothers as effective therapists for autistic children's phobias. J. Appl. Behav. Anal. 23, 379–385.

Luscre, D.M., Center, D.B., 1996. Procedures for reducing dental fear in children with autism. J. Autism Dev. Disord. 26, 547–556.

McNally Keehn, R.H., Lincoln, A.J., Brown, M.Z., Chavira, D.A., 2013. The Coping Cat program for children with anxiety and autism spectrum disorder: a pilot randomized controlled trial. J. Autism Dev. Disord. 43 (1), 57−67.

Moree, B.N., Davis, T.E., 2010. Cognitive-behavioral therapy for anxiety in children diagnosed with autism spectrum disorders: modification trends. Res. Autism Spectrum Disord. 4 (3), 346−354.

Myers, S.M., Johnson, C.P., 2007. Management of children with autism spectrum disorders. Pediatrics 120 (5), 1162−1182.

Nadeau, J.M., Arnold, E.B., Selles, R.R., Storch, E.A., Lewin, A.B., 2015. A cognitive-behavioral approach for anxiety in a preschool-aged child with autism spectrum disorder. Clin. Case Studies 14 (1), 47−60.

Peterman, J., Read, K., Wei, C., Kendall, P.C., 2015. The art of exposure: putting science into practice. Cogn. Behav. Pract. 22, 379−392.

Puleo, C.M., Kendall, P.C., 2011. Anxiety disorders in typically developing youth: autism spectrum symptoms as a predictor of cognitive-behavioral treatment. J. Autism Dev. Disord. 41, 275−286.

Rapp, J.T., Vollmer, T.R., Hovanetz, A.N., 2005. Evaluation and treatment of swimming pool avoidance exhibited by an adolescent girl with autism. Behav. Ther. 36, 101−105.

Read, K.L., Puleo, C.M., Wei, C., Cummings, C.M., Kendall, P.C., 2013. Cognitive-behavioral treatment for pediatric anxiety disorders. Pediatric Anxiety Disorders. Springer, New York, NY, pp. 269−287.

Reaven, J., Blakeley-Smith, A., 2013. Parental involvement in treating anxiety in youth with high-functioning ASD. In: Scarpa, A., Williams White, S., Attwood, T., Scarpa, A., Williams White, S., Attwood, T. (Eds.), CBT for Children and Adolescents with High-Functioning Autism Spectrum Disorders. Guilford Press, New York, NY, pp. 97−122.

Reaven, J., Blakeley-Smith, A., Culhane-Shelburne, K., Hepburn, S., 2012. Group cognitive behavior therapy for children with high-functioning autism spectrum disorders and anxiety: a randomized trial. J. Child Psychol. Psychiatry 53 (4), 410−419.

Rieffe, C., Oosterveld, P., Tewogt, M.M., Mootz, S., van Leeuwen, E., Stockmann, L., 2011. Emotion regulation and internalizing symptoms in children with autism spectrum disorders. Autism 15 (6), 655−670.

Russell, A.J., Jassi, A., Fullana, M.A., Mack, H., Johnston, K., Heyman, I., et al., 2013. Cognitive behavior therapy for comorbid obsessive-compulsive disorder in high-functioning autism spectrum disorders: a randomized controlled trial. Depress. Anxiety 30 (8), 697−708.

Scattone, D., Mong, M., 2013. Cognitive behavior therapy in the treatment of anxiety for adolescents and adults with autism spectrum disorders. Psychol. Schools 50 (9), 923−935.

Schmidt, J.D., Luiselli, J.K., Rue, H., Whalley, K., 2013. Graduated exposure and positive reinforcement to overcome setting and activity avoidance in an adolescent with autism. Behav. Modif. 37, 128−142.

Schohl, K.A., Van Hecke, A.V., Carson, A.M., Dolan, B., Karst, J., Stevens, S., 2014. A replication and extension of the PEERS intervention: Examining effects on social skills and social anxiety in adolescents with autism spectrum disorders. J. Autism Dev. Disord. 44 (3), 532−545.

Spain, D., Sin, J., Chalder, T., Murphy, D., Happé, F., 2015. Cognitive behaviour therapy for adults with autism spectrum disorders and psychiatric co-morbidity: a review. Res. Autism Spect. Disord.9151−9162.

Storch, E.A., Arnold, E.B., Lewin, A.B., Nadeau, J.M., Jones, A.M., De Nadai, A.S., et al., 2013. The effect of cognitive-behavioral therapy versus treatment as usual for anxiety in children with autism spectrum disorders: a randomized, controlled trial. J. Am. Acad. Child Adolesc. Psychiatry 52 (2), 132−142.

Storch, E.A., Sachs, R., Gaus, V., Hoffman, J.H., Kerns, C.M., Lerner, M. (2015). Addressing real and imagined constraints in utilizing CBT for autistic spectrum disorder: best practices regarding applicability of CBT to ASD. Clinical round table conducted at the meeting of the Association for Behavioral and Cognitive Therapies, Chicago, IL.

Sukhodolsky, D.G., Bloch, M.H., Panza, K.E., Reichow, B., 2013. Cognitive-behavioral therapy for anxiety in children with high-functioning autism: a meta-analysis. Pediatrics 132 (5), e1341−e1350.

van Steensel, F.J., Bögels, S.M., Dirksen, C.D., 2012. Anxiety and quality of life: clinically anxious children with and without autism spectrum disorders compared. J. Clin. Child Adolesc. Psychol. 41 (6), 731−738.

van Steensel, F.J., Dirksen, C.D., Bögels, S.M., 2013. A cost of illness study of children with high-functioning autism spectrum disorders and comorbid anxiety disorders as compared to clinically anxious and typically developing children. J. Autism Dev. Disord. 43 (12), 2878−2890.

Vasa, R.A., Kalb, L., Mazurek, M., Kanne, S., Freedman, B., Keefer, A., et al., 2013. Age-related differences in the prevalence and correlates of anxiety in youth with autism spectrum disorders. Res. Autism Spectrum Disord. 7 (11), 1358−1369.

Vasa, R.A., Carroll, L.M., Nozzolillo, A.A., Mahajan, R., Mazurek, M.O., Bennett, A.E., et al., 2014. A systematic review of treatments for anxiety in youth with autism spectrum disorders. J. Autism Dev. Disord. 44 (12), 3215−3229.

Walkup, J., Albano, A.M., Piacentini, J., Birmaher, B., Compton, S., Sherrill, J., et al., 2008. Cognitive behavioral therapy, sertraline, or a combination in childhood anxiety. New Engl. J. Med. 359, 2753−2766.

White, S.W., Oswald, D., Ollendick, T., Scahill, L., 2009. Anxiety in children and adolescents with autism spectrum disorders. Clin. Psychol. Rev. 29 (3), 216−229.

White, S.W., Albano, A.M., Johnson, C.R., Kasari, C., Ollendick, T., Klin, A., et al., 2010. Development of a cognitive-behavioral intervention program to treat anxiety and social deficits in teens with high-functioning autism. Clin. Child Family Psychol. Rev. 13 (1), 77−90.

White, S.W., Scahill, L., Ollendick, T.H., 2013. Multimodal treatment for anxiety and social skills difficulties in adolescents on the autism spectrum. In: Scarpa, A., Williams White, S., Attwood, T., Scarpa, A., Williams White, S., Attwood, T. (Eds.), CBT for Children and Adolescents with High-Functioning Autism Spectrum Disorders. Guilford Press, New York, NY, pp. 123−146.

CHAPTER 7

Individual CBT for Anxiety and Related Symptoms in Children With Autism Spectrum Disorders

Jeffrey J. Wood, Sami Klebanoff, Patricia Renno, Cori Fujii and John Danial
University of California, Los Angeles, CA, United States

In addition to the significantly impairing effects of core Autism Spectrum Disorder (ASD) symptoms, individuals with ASD commonly struggle with emotion dysregulation. In many individuals with ASD, poor emotion regulation manifests as an internalizing disorder (i.e., anxiety, depression, obsessive compulsive disorder) or an externalizing disorder (i.e., disruptive behavior disorders; e.g., Wood and Gadow, 2010; Gerstein et al., 2011). Gerstein et al. (2011) and Baker et al. (2003) estimate that developmental delays may place children at three times the risk for developing behavior problems as typically developing children. While it has been difficult to accurately diagnose co-occurring anxiety in youth with ASD, anxiety appears to be extremely common in children and adolescents with ASD, with estimates ranging from 7% to 57% depending on the specific type of anxiety being examined (Wood and Gadow, 2010).

Cognitive behavioral therapy (CBT) is an established treatment approach for anxiety and emotion dysregulation in both typically developing adults and children (e.g., In-Albon and Schneider, 2007; Ishikawa et al., 2007). It is increasingly being used to target co-occurring disorders related to emotion dysregulation (i.e., anxiety, OCD, depression, disruptive behavior) in verbal youth with ASD. CBT is based on the assumptions that cognition impacts behavior, cognition can be changed, and that changes in cognition can alter behavior (Dobson and Dozois, 2001). CBT is also derived from the memory retrieval competition model (Brewin, 2006), which dictates that in order to challenge

Anxiety in Children and Adolescents with Autism Spectrum Disorder.
DOI: http://dx.doi.org/10.1016/B978-0-12-805122-1.00007-7
© 2017 Elsevier Inc.
All rights reserved.

maladaptive thought and behavior patterns, competing retrievable memories of adaptive patterns of thought and behavior must be developed. Techniques such as cognitive restructuring, in which negative maladaptive thoughts are challenged by positive adaptive thoughts, facilitate the formation of adaptive retrievable memories that can be used to better cope with challenging real-life situations.

Because CBT is a frontline treatment for emotion dysregulation disorders and these disorders are very common in youth with ASD, numerous studies have begun to examine the use of CBT programs adapted for youth with ASD. While the use of CBT in treating children and adolescents with ASD has increased, the quality of the extant studies is mixed. In this chapter, we review the evidence base in the extant studies examining individual CBT as an evidence-based treatment (EBT) for children with ASD, emphasizing anxiety since that target area has been the greatest emphasis of the current set of studies. However, it is impossible to meaningfully separate anxiety from other areas of mental health and psychosocial functioning in children with ASD (e.g., Wood and Gadow, 2010) given the overlapping underlying causes (e.g., common genes, stress associated with having ASD, executive dysfunction) and interdependency of symptom areas (e.g., poor social skills related to ASD can reduce social confidence and increase self-consciousness, the fight-or-flight component of anxiety can heighten aggression and defiance). Thus, this review addresses individual CBT for children and youth with ASD including any target areas addressed within studies using adequate methodology (defined below).

While substantial progress has been made in identifying EBTs for preschool children with ASD, less attention has been paid to the identification of EBTs for school-aged youth (6- to 18-year-olds) with ASD. Many youth with ASD continue to experience significant impairment in areas such as social communication and emotion regulation into the elementary and secondary school years (Macintosh and Dissanayake, 2006). Furthermore, roughly 10−30% of youth with ASD show behavioral deterioration during adolescence (Gillberg and Schaumann, 1982; Rutter, 1970). Some have suggested that for adolescents with high-functioning autism, growing awareness of their social difficulties and differences can lead to psychosocial stress (Carrington et al., 2003; Loveland and Tunali-Kotoski, 2005; Shea and Mesibov, 2005), which may translate into the development of concurrent internalizing disorders (Wood and Gadow, 2010).

USE OF UNPROVEN TREATMENTS BY PARENTS AND PROFESSIONALS

The wide-ranging impairments experienced by school-aged youth with ASD have led to a proliferation of interventions aimed at core autism symptoms as well as commonly co-occurring symptoms and disorders. Parents and professionals are largely unaware of which treatments are evidence-based and are thus left with little direction as to which interventions to select (Christon et al., 2015; Goin-Kochel et al., 2007). Among 6- to 10-year-old with high-functioning ASD, the average child uses about seven current services (e.g., therapies, medications), with around 50% using behavioral interventions at a given time, 50% also using other skills-based interventions (e.g., social skills), and another 50% using psychiatric medication (Green et al., 2006; Thomas et al., 2007). Families frequently utilize interventions, such as complementary and alternative medicine (CAM) treatments, that have very little or no empirical support (Christon et al., 2010). In a sample of 248 families, 70% had tried at least one CAM treatment and 50% were currently using a CAM treatment (Christon et al., 2010). The most frequently used alternative treatments were special diets (29%), vitamins (27%), animal therapy (24%), auditory integration training (16%), music therapy (16%), and chelation (11%; Christon et al., 2010). In addition, a large percentage of children with ASD receive speech and language therapy (88%) and occupational therapy (78%; McLennan et al., 2008). It is unclear whether children are benefitting from these treatments.

As a result of the long-standing tradition in the field of utilizing controversial and unproven treatments, numerous calls have been made for use of EBTs (e.g., Lord et al., 2006; National Research Council, 2001; Simpson, 2005). However, the autism community has yet to arrive at a generally agreed upon classification system for determining which interventions are efficacious (Simpson, 2005; US Department of Education, 2003). This would be an important first step in long-term efforts to achieve clarity regarding which treatments qualify as evidence-based to improve awareness of comparative treatment options for individuals with ASD.

Extant definitions of treatment efficacy are significantly less stringent in the ASD field than those currently used in related mental health fields, rendering them less meaningful and less able to discriminate between treatments. In the general arena of clinical psychology, well-accepted efficacy criteria recently updated by Southam-Gerow and Prinstein (2014) are widely used to review treatment approaches for various disorders. This classification system is distinguished by its specificity and use of stringent methodological criteria. In the following section, we will apply Southam-Gerow and Prinstein's (2014) rigorous classification system to individual CBT treatments for school-aged youth with ASD.

SUMMARY OF EBT CLASSIFICATION SYSTEM

Within Southam-Gerow and Prinstein's (2014) classification system, interventions are evaluated based on five methods criteria and then classified into one of five levels of efficacy. A treatment study is considered of good quality if it: (1) involves a randomized controlled trial (RCT) design; (2) utilizes a treatment manual; (3) clearly specifies its target population and inclusion criteria; (4) uses reliable and valid outcome measures assessing the intervention targets; and (5) uses appropriate statistical analyses and a sample size large enough to detect possible intervention effects. An intervention is considered "well-established" once it has been shown to be either significantly superior to an active control group or not significantly different from another well-established intervention in at least two studies conducted by at least two independent research groups in at least two research settings. Well-established treatments must also meet all five methods criteria. "Probably efficacious" treatments must meet all five methods criteria and be found to be superior to a wait list control group in at least two studies or meet well-established criteria in at least one study. A treatment qualifies as "possibly efficacious" if it has been found to be superior to wait-list control in at least one RCT or if it has demonstrated efficacy in at least one study meeting methods criteria 2, 3, 4, and 5. A treatment is considered "experimental" if it has not been tested in a RCT or if its efficacy has been demonstrated in at least one study not meeting "possibly efficacious" criteria. "Treatments of questionable efficacy" have been examined in quality clinical studies and found to have no discernable treatment effect or to be inferior to either active control or wait-list control groups.

METHOD

In order to identify well-established, probably and possibly efficacious individual CBT treatments for school-aged youth with ASD, we conducted a three-step procedure. We chose to review only psychosocial CBT treatments for ASD, excluding pharmacological and physical health-related interventions. Children enter first grade at roughly age 6 and graduate secondary school at roughly 18 years of age. Therefore, school-aged is defined as ages 6−18.

Step 1: Keyword search. We conducted a search of relevant electronic databases (PsycINFO, PsycARTICLES, and ERIC). We used keywords "autism," OR "Asperger's," OR "Asperger's syndrome" OR "Asperger syndrome" OR "pervasive developmental disorder" OR AND "cognitive behavioral therapy," OR "CBT," OR "cognitive therapy." We then reviewed the bibliographies of articles found in this initial search for additional studies to review.

Step 2: Inclusion criteria. Studies pertaining to pharmacological and physical health-related interventions, case studies and studies only reported in book chapters rather than peer-reviewed journals were excluded. Studies including participants ages 6−18 were then included for subsequent review.

Step 3: EBT classification. We determined the number of methods criteria met by each study. We grouped studies by symptoms targeted (e.g., anxiety, core ASD). After determining the number and methodological quality of studies within each intervention category, we determined the level of efficacy for the intervention categories.

RESULTS

CBT for Anxiety and Core Autism Symptoms

CBT for Anxiety in ASD

CBT, an efficacious treatment for numerous child and adult disorders, is currently being used to treat a variety of symptoms associated with ASD. Because anxiety disorders are frequently comorbid in individuals with ASD (Wood and Gadow, 2010), CBT has been adapted for use with youth with ASD. CBT for children with autism and concurrent anxiety commonly consists of basic CBT elements, such as replacing irrational thoughts with rational, adaptive beliefs, and graded exposures to feared situations, alongside various adaptations for children with ASD (e.g., incorporating perseverative interests and visual representations of concepts; Danial and Wood, 2013).

In one waitlist-control RCT, an efficacious CBT program for typically developing youth with anxiety, the Coping Cat program, was modified for use with youth ($N = 22$; ages 8−14 years) with ASD and anxiety randomly assigned to treatment or waitlist (McNally Keehn et al., 2013). Treatment consisted of 16 weekly 90 minute one-on-one sessions. The major components of the Coping Cat manual are coping techniques, emotion recognition and understanding, cognitive restructuring, self-evaluation, and self-reinforcement. The modified version of the program involved use of participants' special interest to foster engagement, session content, and homework review at the end of sessions, longer sessions (from 60 to 90 minutes), use of visual aids, breaks, as well as technique and reward individualization. In the waitlist group, all participants continued to meet criteria for their primary anxiety disorder on the Anxiety Disorders Interview Schedule-Parent version (ADIS-P; Silverman and Albano, 1996), while in the treatment group 58% no longer met criteria for their primary anxiety disorder. The principal investigator was the therapist for all cases in the study, which raises questions about whether less experienced therapists would be able to successfully deliver the protocol. Regarding weaknesses, the study utilized a small sample size and one experienced therapist.

A 16-session family-based CBT program, Behavioral Interventions for Anxiety in Children with Autism (BIACA), was developed for children with ASD and clinical anxiety, drawing upon successful elements of both programs for ASD (e.g., pivotal response treatment: Koegel et al., 2005) and anxiety CBT programs for children. In the initial study examining the BIACA program, children ages 7−11 years ($N = 40$) were randomly assigned to an immediate treatment group or a waitlist control group (Wood et al., 2009). On average, the participants met criteria for four anxiety disorders on the ADIS-IV-C/P at baseline. At posttreatment, over half the children in the treatment group did not meet criteria for an anxiety disorder and parents reported significant reductions in anxiety. Both of these outcome variables showed a significant treatment effect for BIACA compared to waitlist. There were no significant reductions in anxiety at posttreatment according to child report. However, the children in the study reported low overall anxiety levels at baseline and the study used measures that have not been validated for use in children with ASD.

In a second study conducted by the same research group (Fujii et al., 2013), 16 additional sessions were added to the protocol in order to enhance the generalizability of the skills learned to real-life settings. Participants ($N = 16$, ages 7−11) were randomly assigned to a 32 week treatment condition or a 16-week treatment-as-usual (TAU) condition. The initial 16 weeks were similar to the original BIACA protocol and focused on decreasing anxiety. The second half of the treatment empha-sized developing the skills and relationships that would facilitate coping with anxiety in real-life situations. Parents, therapists, and school profes-sionals were trained to be social coaches, helping the participants apply their skills in everyday contexts, such as parks or the schoolyard. Due to numerous missed sessions, four participants were not included in the analyses. At posttreatment, five of the seven children in the BIACA group did not meet criteria for their primary anxiety disorders on the ADIS-IV-C/P, while all participants in TAU continued to meet criteria for an anxiety disorder, a statistically significant difference. While the outcome is promising, the study is limited by its small sample size and the greater number of sessions received by the CBT group.

An independent research group also found BIACA to be efficacious in a recent randomized controlled trial (Storch et al., 2013). Participants ($N = 45$, ages 7–11) were randomly assigned to receive BIACA for 16 weeks or TAU for 16 weeks. The same BIACA manual was implemented in 60–90 minute weekly sessions, as in prior BIACA trials. At posttreat-ment, the participants who received BIACA demonstrated significantly greater reductions in anxiety than those who received TAU.

Two recent randomized controlled trials by two independent research groups examined the efficacy of BIACA in treating anxiety in early ado-lescents with ASD. In one study, participants ($N = 33$, ages 11–15) were randomized to either an immediate treatment or waitlist group (Wood et al., 2015). The treatment was similar in length (i.e., 16 weekly 90 minute sessions) to that of previous studies. Developmental modifica-tions were made to the BIACA manual, such as fostering independence and age-appropriate social skills. The BIACA group experienced signifi-cantly greater reductions in anxiety severity than the waitlist group on the Pediatric Anxiety Rating Scale (PARS; Research Units on Pediatric Psychopharmacology Anxiety Study Group, 2002). A significantly greater percentage of the BIACA group qualified as treatment responders (79%) than the waitlist group (28%) on the Clinical Global Impressions-Improvement (CGI-I) scale. Parent report measures also demonstrated decreases in autism symptom severity in the BIACA group. However, no significant differences between groups were found for anxiety disorder diagnoses on the ADIS-IV-C/P.

Another randomized controlled trial conducted by an independent research group examined the efficacy of BIACA for early adolescents with ASD and anxiety (Storch et al., 2015). In this RCT, participants

($N = 31$, ages 11—16) were randomly assigned to either a 16 week BIACA group or a 16 week TAU group. Participants received the same developmentally modified version of BIACA implemented in Wood and colleagues' (2015) study. At posttreatment, the BIACA group experienced significantly greater improvements than the TAU group on all clinician-rated anxiety measures (i.e., the PARS, ADIS-IV-C/P, CGI-I) and the measure of autism symptom severity (i.e., the Social Responsiveness Scale). Improvements were maintained at 1-month follow-up for the CBT group.

Since BIACA has demonstrated efficacy in four RCTs from two different research groups (Storch et al., 2013, 2015; Wood et al., 2009, 2015), it meets criteria for probable efficacy and, to the extent that a TAU comparison group is considered an active treatment, also meets criteria as a well-established treatment.

White and colleagues (2013) combined one-on-one therapy, group therapy, and parent education to target both anxiety and social skills in adolescents with ASD. In this randomized controlled trial, participants ($N = 30$, ages 12—17) were assigned to either CBT or a waitlist control group. Participants received up to 13 one-on-one therapy sessions, seven group therapy sessions, and a parent education component during each individual and group session. Sessions targeted social skills using techniques, such as social reinforcement and modeling. The treatment also targeted anxiety with established techniques, such as cognitive restructuring and exposure. Parents were instructed to promote generalization by practicing exposure tasks in real-life settings. While results showed significant differences between the CBT and control groups on social skills outcomes, there were no significant differences between groups on the anxiety outcome measures. These results suggest that while this particular protocol may be helpful in developing social skills in adolescents with ASD, it may not be an effective treatment for anxiety in this population.

Clinical Features of CBT for Anxiety in Children with ASD

As an efficacious individual CBT treatment for the ASD population, the clinical features of BIACA are described forthwith. BIACA was adapted from the Building Confidence CBT program (Wood et al., 2008), which was developed for general childhood anxiety problems. Both parent and child attend 16 weekly sessions lasting approximately 90 minutes each. The therapist typically spends 30 minutes with the child and 60 minutes with the parent/family. Similar to other childhood anxiety CBT programs, the BIACA manual includes psychoeducation, coping skills training (e.g., emotion recognition, cognitive restructuring), and in vivo exposure (facing feared situations gradually and repeatedly until habituation to the situation occurs). Usually after the first couple sessions, when adequate background information has been gathered and rapport established, the therapist creates a fear hierarchy with the child and/or parent, in which they rate how fearful the child is in certain situations. This hierarchy serves as a guide for the remainder of the treatment sessions. Starting with the least distressing situations, children gradually work their way up the fear hierarchy through in vivo exposures in session with the therapist and practice tasks at home. Children are rewarded for their efforts in session and at home with reward charts and point systems. The BIACA manual includes several parent-training components throughout the course of the treatment, in which parents learn parenting techniques to help their child when he or she is feeling anxious (e.g., using positive reinforcement, reflecting emotions, extinction).

There were numerous enhancements to the original Building Confidence manual to simultaneously address common deficits associated with ASD in conjunction with treating anxiety symptoms. These additions were designed to treat poor social skills, adaptive skills deficits, circumscribed interests and stereotypies, poor attention and motivation, and common comorbidities in ASD (e.g., disruptive behavior disorders). In particular, new modules were added to address difficulties children with ASD have in forming and maintaining peer relationships. These modules focus on teaching key skills needed to make and keep friends, such as being a good play date host. In session, the child and therapist discuss "social rules" to follow during play dates (e.g., letting the friend choose the activity, giving compliments) and key "super friend" behaviors are illustrated through cartoons and role-playing (cf. Frankel and Myatt, 2003). The complimentary parent module reviews tips for ensuring successful play dates (e.g., keeping them short, having the children decide on an activity to do beforehand), as well as, sources of potential friends for their child (e.g., extracurricular activities, clubs). Additionally, in these modules, children are given social coaching by the therapist, parents, and school staff on appropriate ways to play and converse with their peers in different situations. Therapists, parents, and school staff provide social coaching immediately before the social activity as a priming tool to maximize success in the interaction (Koegel et al., 2005). These skills are practiced at the park, on play dates, and at school and are reinforced with a comprehensive reward system that typically includes daily privileges and longer term rewards. Another module that targets social isolation at school focuses on implementing a peer buddy system and mentoring program at school. For this module, the child with ASD can benefit from serving as both the mentee and mentor and it is intended to enhance social acceptance and perspective taking skills (cf. Fulk and King, 2001; King-Sears, 2001; Maheady et al., 2001; Rogers, 2000). Typically, the therapist meets with the school one to two times to teach the intervention techniques to the school staff (e.g., aides, teachers).

The manual also includes modules aimed at increasing the child's adaptive skills by building independent daily self-help skills (e.g., dressing, showering). Typically two to three skills are identified and broken down into steps to work on at home. In session, the therapist focuses on providing motivation for the child (e.g., "you're going to be so grown-up!") and emphasizes to the parent the importance of developing these daily living skills for future independent living. Additionally, children's circumscribed interests and sterotypies are incorporated throughout treatment. To establish rapport and maximize attention and motivation in session, special interests are employed to teach therapeutic concepts (e.g., emotion regulation) by using the characters in the examples. Special interests are also used as reinforcers to increase motivation and participation during the session. Stereotypies and special interests that are interfering with the child's success socially (e.g., will only talk about a special interest with peers, engages in hand flapping during recess) are addressed later in treatment through a suppression approach. The therapist works with the child and parent to increase the amount of time per day in which the child refrains from discussing this topic or engaging in the stereotypy (cf. Sze and Wood, 2007). To provide a rationale for the child, the therapist discusses with the child social expectations by illustrating other children's perspectives through cartoons and role-plays (e.g., these behaviors are fine in private but tend to confuse peers and get in the way of friendship).

There are also modules in the BIACA program that address behavior problems associated with comorbid disruptive behavior disorders by including behavioral goals (e.g., following directions, keeping hands, and feet to self) on the child's weekly homework chart and providing the parent with strategies for dealing with difficult behaviors (e.g., planned ignoring). These items are also incorporated into the child's reward system. For example, a child may earn a point for speaking calmly and respectfully each day. School personnel can also be recruited to keep track of daily target behaviors at school through a "school-home" note from which the child also earns points and privileges.

The BIACA manual's modular format allows therapists to choose modules on a session-by-session basis depending on the child's most pressing needs and treatment trajectory. Typically, modules focusing on teaching coping skills are delivered early in the intervention with in vivo exposure modules conducted for the remainder of the treatment sessions. The modules addressing ASD-related deficits can be interspersed through-out the treatment, as needed. Usually, adaptive skill deficits and behavior problems are addressed early in treatment, with social skill modules deliv-ered later in treatment (see Sze and Wood, 2007). The manual is flexible and the modular format allows the treatment to be individualized depending on the needs of the child. Despite this flexibility, at least three sessions are spent on basic coping skills and eight on in vivo exposure to ensure adequate doses of CBT for anxiety across cases.

Clinical Examples of CBT for Anxiety in ASD

In the following section, we will provide two brief clinical exemplars of CBT for anxiety in ASD. These case examples illustrate ways in which CBT for anxiety has been adapted for children with ASD using the BIACA protocol, as well as key techniques employed. Key details of the cases have been changed to protect confidentiality.

Case example 1: Jordan. Jordan was a 9-year-old boy who met criteria for ASD as well as social phobia, obsessive compulsive disorder, general-ized anxiety disorder, and concurrent ADHD-combined type at intake. Jordan presented as overly shy and would often fail to speak with unknown individuals until he became comfortable with them. Jordan was often anxious in social situations involving peers, stating that he was worried that others would not think he was "cool." He frequently avoided parties and get-togethers with peers from school due to his fear that the other children would not like him and would think he was weird. Jordan spent half of his school day in a special day class and was excessively worried that other kids would find out that he was in that class and negatively evaluate him. As a result, Jordan would often isolate himself during periods of free play, choosing to sit alone in the library. While in the special day class Jordan would often participate, however in his mainstream classes he would never participate unless compelled by the teacher. Two main goals for Jordan were to increase his participation in his mainstream class as well as to increase his peer interactions during unstructured free-time.

During therapy sessions, Jordan was encouraged, through a structured rewards program, to gradually increase his interactions with new same-aged children, with a similar program focused on increasing interactions with his peers implemented within his classroom by his primary teacher. In addition, Jordan was taught in sessions what it meant to be a "friend" and was encouraged to spend time with his peers both in and out of school. Jordan's mother encouraged Jordan to go on play dates and hosted several at her home to promote his use of appropriate social skills learned during therapy sessions. Jordan's teacher was also instrumental in encouraging these behaviors during the school day. With the establishment of a rewards system for all attempts Jordan took during free-time to interact with peers, and additional points earned for participating in class, Jordan was able to slowly increase both of these targeted behaviors. By the end of treatment he was able to approach and interact with unknown peers and sustain interactions with even small groups of children, something that would have paralyzed him with anxiety at the beginning of treatment.

Case example 2: Beth. Beth was a seven-year-old girl diagnosed with ASD as well as generalized anxiety disorder, social phobia, and separation anxiety disorder. A primary area of concern for Beth and her family was her heightened anxiety in social situations with peers and unfamiliar adults. She was concerned about being negatively judged by other people. She worried about joining conversations with peers, anticipating that peers would ignore her or she would embarrass herself. She tended to avoid interacting with peers and directed most of her social overtures to one close friend at school.

A main goal for treatment was to address Beth's social phobia and concurrently enhance her social-communication skills. Beth's relationship with her one friend was high in conflict and they isolated themselves from other peers. Despite only positive interactions with other peers (although infrequent), Beth would avoid these interactions due to fear of rejection. In session Beth was taught to change her negative cognitions about approaching and interacting with peers, by instead focusing on the positive interactions she had previously had with her peers. She was also encouraged in session and school to gradually increase her interactions with peers, with a structured rewards program in place for all attempts made to interact with peers both in and outside of school. In addition, concepts about friendship such as the meaning of being a good friend and the qualities Beth preferred in friends were discussed. Further, play dates with other peers in her class were set up to expand Beth's friendships. Beth learned and practiced play date hosting skills to promote successful get-togethers. As play dates with a variety of girls from her class occurred, Beth became increasingly aware of the poor quality of her friendship with her "close" friend. Eventually, she used this realization and her success in the play dates to develop closer friendships with other girls in her class, increasing her network of friends to play with at school. By the end of treatment Beth was consistently playing with other peers for the majority of time at school and would often engage in play dates with these new friends.

CBT for Core ASD Symptoms

Growing evidence supports the use of individual CBT to address core social functioning deficits in children and adolescents with ASD (e.g., Storch et al., 2013, 2015; Wood et al., 2009, 2015). While CBT for core autism symptoms has been delivered in varying dosages and formats (i.e., one-on-one and group), interventions frequently involve emotion recognition, cognitive restructuring related to social competencies, and in vivo exposure (Danial and Wood, 2013). Several open trials, RCTs, and multiple-baseline design group intervention studies examining CBT for core autism symptoms demonstrate significant improvements in domains such as pro-social behavior, social problem solving, and peer engagement. In two RCTs targeting both anxiety and core autism symptoms (Storch et al., 2013; Wood et al., 2009), individualized CBT including parent and school involvement produced gains in parent-reported autism symptoms that were maintained at 3-month follow-up in one study. In another RCT targeting both anxiety and social skills in adolescents with ASD, youth social skills improved significantly, while anxiety did not (White et al., 2013). Improvements in social awareness, cognition, and communication were also found in a recent RCT comparing CBT with treatment as usual for adolescents with ASD (Storch et al., 2015; also see Wood et al., 2015). The above examples of CBT for anxiety also illustrate how CBT is applied to autism symptoms such as isolation and social skill challenges, and how closely anxiety and social challenges may be interrelated in this population.

Overall, preliminary findings suggest that one-on-one individualized formats may be capable of producing more generalizable, lasting changes than group formats, although further study in this area is warranted (cf. Danial and Wood, 2013). Individualized CBT has been shown to improve core autism symptoms in two RCTs comparing CBT to wait-list control and in two RCTs comparing CBT to treatment as usual; therefore, CBT for core autism symptoms in youth with ASD meets criteria for probable efficacy.

CBT for Externalizing Behavior in Children With ASD

Stepping Stones Triple P—Positive Parenting Program (SSTP) is a specialized form of CBT for parents of children ages 2—16 years with a variety of disabilities that targets child internalizing and externalizing problems by altering parenting style and improving parent mental health (Sanders et al., 2002). It utilizes a tiered, public health approach in which parents begin with less intensive versions of the intervention and move on to more intensive intervention if their needs are not met. The intervention approach consists of five levels: level 1 is delivered *via* media; level 2 consists of a few group seminars; level 3 is brief and individually delivered; level 4 is a longer course of 10 individual, group, or self-directed sessions; level 5 involves additional modules targeting specific problems (e.g., partner conflict). In a RCT comparing level 3 SSTP to a care as usual control condition, families of children with ASD ages 2—9 in the SSTP group demonstrated improvements in parent-reported child behavior problems, parenting style, parent confidence, parent stress, parent relationship conflict, and parent relationship satisfaction, which were largely maintained at 6-month follow-up (Tellegen and Sanders, 2014). However, significant improvements were not found on observational measures of child behavioral problems and parent aversive behavior (Tellegen and Sanders, 2014). While level 3 SSTP may meet possibly efficacious criteria, further research examining other levels of SSTP and using observational measures will help to determine the efficacy of this approach for families of school-aged youth with ASD.

DISCUSSION

The results of this review provide support for classifying individual CBT as a probably efficacious treatment for anxiety and core autism symptoms in youth with ASD. Individual CBT demonstrates promise as a treatment for externalizing behavior in youth with ASD. Studies from more than one research group comparing CBT for disruptive behaviors in youth with ASD to active control groups will be needed in order to further establish its efficacy (see Table 7.1).

While many of the studies reviewed were high quality randomized controlled trials, they were limited by several factors. Several studies used

Table 7.1 RCTs of probably efficacious EBTs for school-aged youth with ASD

Study authors & year	Symptoms targeted	Design	Age range	Outcome measures
McNally Keehn et al. (2013)	Anxiety	RCT (wait-list control)	8–14	ADIS-IV-C/P; SCAS-C/P
Storch et al. (2013)	Anxiety + core ASD	RCT (TAU control)	7–11	PARS, ADIS-IV-C/P, CGI-S, CGI-I; CBCL; CIS-P; MASC-P; SRS; RCMAS
Storch et al. (2015)	Anxiety + core ASD	RCT (active control)	11–16	PARS, ADIS-IV-C/P, CGI-S, CGI-I; CBCL; CIS-P; MASC-P; SRS; RCADS
White et al. (2013)	Anxiety + core ASD	RCT (wait-list control)	12–17	SRS; CASI-Anx; PARS; CGI-I; DD-CGAS
Wood, Drahota, Sze, Van Dyke et al. (2009)	Core ASD	RCT (wait-list control)	7–11	SRS
Wood et al. (2009)	Anxiety + core ASD	RCT (wait-list control)	7–11	ADIS-IV-C/P; CGI-I; MASC-C; MASC-P
Wood et al. (2015)	Anxiety + core ASD	RCT (wait-list control)	11–15	ADIS-IV-C/P; CGI-I; MASC-P; PARS; RCADS; SRS
Tellegen and Sanders (2014)	Behavior Problems	RCT (TAU control)	2–9	ECBI; PS; PTC; DASS-21; PSS; FOS; PPC; RQI; GAS

Note: RCT, randomized controlled trial; EBT, evidence-based treatment; TAU, treatment as usual; CBT, cognitive-behavioral therapy; SST, social skills training.

small sample sizes that limit their generalizability. A strength of many of the studies was that they used the ADIS-IV-C/P, a reliable and valid outcome measure administered by independent evaluators blind to treatment condition. However, while the ADIS-IV-C/P is administered by independent evaluators, it does rely on parent report. Future studies would benefit from the use of multiple reporters as well as observational measures.

A few of the reviewed studies also relied on a high degree of involvement from the principal investigator. It is unclear if therapists with less expertise, training, and experience would be able to implement these complex interventions. Ultimately, if individual CBT is found to be a well-established treatment in university settings, the next step will be to test its effectiveness in community settings. Future studies including less involvement from principal investigators and expert clinicians would help to shed light on the transportability of CBT for anxiety in ASD to community settings.

While extant research on CBT for anxiety in youth with ASD has made important strides in providing evidence for individual CBT as an EBT for ASD, further research is needed before CBT can be categorized as a well-established treatment. Larger randomized controlled trials using active control groups beyond treatment as usual, with broader measurement batteries, are the next logical step in this line of research. According to Southam-Gerow and Prinstein's (2014) criteria, CBT would need to outperform either an active control group or another well-established treatment in at least two studies conducted by two independent research groups.

Individual CBT has demonstrated promise in treating anxiety, core ASD symptoms, and externalizing behavior in high-functioning, verbal school-aged children and adolescents with ASD. However, the efficacy of individual CBT for minimally verbal youth with ASD has yet to be tested. A few studies have examined the efficacy of CBT for adolescents with ASD, but none have tested the efficacy of CBT in treating co-occurring disorders and core ASD symptoms in adults with ASD. Future research on CBT for these understudied subpopulations within ASD is warranted.

CBT is a treatment with a long-standing history of success in treating a wide range of emotion dysregulation disorders in typically developing children and adults. The results of this review suggest that individual CBT may be an efficacious treatment for a range of target symptoms in youth with ASD. There is ample reason to proceed with larger scale trials to examine individual CBT for youth with ASD. In the meantime, clinicians have a basis for selecting CBT as a sensible treatment option for higher functioning clients with ASD.

REFERENCES

Baker, B.L., McIntyre, L.L., Blacher, J., Crnic, K., Edelbrock, C., Low, C., 2003. Preschool children with and without developmental delay: behaviour problems and parenting stress over time. J. Intell. Disabil. Res. 47 (4–5), 217–230.

Brewin, C.R., 2006. Understanding cognitive behaviour therapy: a retrieval competition account. Behav. Res. Ther. 44 (6), 765–784.

Carrington, S., Templeton, E., Papinczak, T., 2003. Adolescents with Asperger Syndrome and Perceptions of Friendship. Focus Autism Other Dev. Disabil. 18 (4), 211−218.

Christon, L.M., Mackintosh, V.H., Myers, B.J., 2010. Use of complementary and alternative medicine (CAM) treatments by parents of children with autism spectrum disorders. Res. Autism Spectrum Disord. 4 (2), 249−259.

Christon, L.M., Arnold, C.C., Myers, B.J., 2015. Professionals' reported provision and recommendation of psychosocial interventions for youth with Autism Spectrum Disorder. Behav. Ther. 46 (1), 68−82.

Danial, J.T., Wood, J.J., 2013. Cognitive behavioral therapy for children with autism: review and considerations for future research. J. Dev. Behav. Pediatrics 34 (9), 702−715.

Dobson, K.S., Dozois, D.J., 2001. Historical and philosophical bases of the cognitive-behavioral therapies. In: Dobson,, K.S. (Ed.), Handbook of Cognitive-Behavioral Therapies, second ed Guilford Press, New York, NY.

Frankel, F., Myatt, R., 2003. Children's Friendship Training. New York: Brunner-Routledge. (pp. xii, 198).

Fujii, C., Renno, P., McLeod, B.D., Lin, C.E., Decker, K., Zielinski, K., et al., 2013. Intensive cognitive behavioral therapy for anxiety disorders in school-aged children with autism: a preliminary comparison with treatment-as-usual. School Mental Health 5 (1), 25−37.

Fulk, B.M., King, K., 2001. Classwide peer tutoring at work. Teach. Except. Child. 34 (2), 48−52.

Gerstein, E.D., Arbona, A.Py, Crnic, K.A., Ryu, E., Baker, B.L., Blacher, J., 2011. Developmental risk and young children's regulatory strategies: predicting behavior problems at age five. J. Abnormal Child Psychol. 39 (3), 351−364.

Gillberg, D.C., Schaumann, H., 1982. Infantile autism and puberty. J. Autism Dev. Disord. 11 (4), 365−371.

Goin-Kochel, R.P., Myers, B.J., Mackintosh, V.H., 2007. Parental reports on the use of treatments and therapies for children with autism spectrum disorders. Res. Autism Spectrum Disord. 1 (3), 195−209.

Green, V.A., Pituch, K.A., Itchon, J., Choi, A., O'Reilly, M., Sigafoos, J., 2006. Internet survey of treatments used by parents of children with autism. Res. Dev. Disabil. 27 (1), 70−84.

In-Albon, T., Schneider, S., 2007. Psychotherapy of childhood anxiety disorders: a meta-analysis. Psychother. Psychosomat. 76 (1), 15−24.

Ishikawa, S., Okajima, I., Matsuoka, H., Sakano, Y., 2007. Cognitive behavioural therapy for anxiety disorders in children and adolescents: a meta-analysis. Child Adolesc Mental Health 12 (4), 164−172.

King-Sears, M.E., 2001. Institutionalizing peer-mediated instruction and interventions in schools beyond "Train and Hope". Remedial Special Educ. 22 (2), 89−101.

Koegel, R.L., Werner, G.A., Vismara, L.A., Koegel, L.K., 2005. The effectiveness of contextually supported play date interactions between children with autism and typically developing peers. Res. Pract. Persons Severe Disabil. 30 (2), 93−102.

Lord, C., Wagner, A., Rogers, S., Szatmari, P., Aman, M., Charman, T., et al., 2006. Challenges in evaluating psychosocial interventions for autistic spectrum disorders. J. Autism Dev. Disord. 35 (6), 695−708.

Loveland, K.A., Tunali-Kotoski, B., 2005. The school-age child with an autistic spectrum disorder. In: Volkmar, F.R., Paul, R., Klin, A., Cohen, D. (Eds.), Handbook of Autism and Pervasive Developmental Disorders. John Wiley & Sons, Inc., pp. 247−287.

Macintosh, K., Dissanayake, C., 2006. Social skills and problem behaviours in school aged children with high-functioning autism and Asperger's disorder. J. Autism Dev. Disord. 36 (8), 1065−1076.

Maheady, L., Harper, G.F., Mallette, B., 2001. Peer-mediated instruction and interventions and students with mild disabilities. Remedial Special Education 22 (1), 4—14.

McLennan, J.D., Huculak, S., Sheehan, D., 2008. Brief report: pilot investigation of service receipt by young children with autistic spectrum disorders. J. Autism Dev. Disord. 38 (6), 1192—1196.

McNally Keehn, R.H., Lincoln, A.J., Brown, M.Z., Chavira, D.A., 2013. The coping cat program for children with anxiety and autism spectrum disorder: a pilot randomized controlled trial. J. Autism Dev. Disord. 43 (1), 57—67.

National Research Council, 2001. Educating Children with Autism. National Academy Press, Washington, DC.

Research Units on Pediatric Psychopharmacology Anxiety Study Group, 2002. The pediatric anxiety rating scale (PARS): development and psychometric properties. J. Am. Acad. Child Adolesc. Psychiatry 41 (9), 1061—1069.

Rogers, S.J., 2000. Interventions that facilitate socialization in children with autism. J. Autism Dev. Disord. 30 (5), 399—409.

Rutter, M., 1970. Autistic children: infancy to adulthood. Semin. Psychiatry 2 (4), 435—450.

Sanders, M.R., Turner, K.M.T., Markie-Dadds, C., 2002. The development and dissemination of the triple P—positive parenting program: a multilevel, evidence-based system of parenting and family support. Prevent. Sci. 3 (3), 173—189.

Shea, V., Mesibov, G.B., 2005. Adolescents and adults with autism. In: Volkmar, F.R., Paul, R., Klin, A., Cohen, D. (Eds.), Handbook of Autism and Pervasive Developmental Disorders. John Wiley & Sons, Inc., pp. 288—311.

Silverman, W.K., Albano, A.M., 1996. The Anxiety Disorders Interview Schedule for Children (ADIS-C/P). Psychological Corporation, San Antonio, TX.

Simpson, R.L., 2005. Evidence-based practices and students with autism spectrum disorders. Focus Autism Other Dev. Disabil. 20 (3), 140—149.

Southam-Gerow, M.A., Prinstein, M.J., 2014. Evidence base updates: the evolution of the evaluation of psychological treatments for children and adolescents. J. Clin. Child Adolesc. Psychol. 43 (1), 1—6.

Storch, E.A., Arnold, E.B., Lewin, A.B., Nadeau, J.M., Jones, A.M., Nadai, D., et al., 2013. The effect of cognitive-behavioral therapy versus treatment as usual for anxiety in children with autism spectrum disorders: a randomized, controlled trial. J. Am. Acad. Child Adolesc. Psychiatry 52 (2), 132—142, e2.

Storch, E.A., Lewin, A.B., Collier, A.B., Arnold, E., De Nadai, A.S., Dane, B.F., et al., 2015. A randomized controlled trial of cognitive-behavioral therapy versus treatment as usual for adolescents with autism spectrum disorders and comorbid anxiety. Depress. Anxiety 32 (3), 174—181.

Sze, K., Wood, J., 2007. Cognitive behavioral treatment of comorbid anxiety disorders and social difficulties in children with high-functioning autism: a case report. J. Contemp. Psychother. 37 (3), 133—143.

Tellegen, C.L., Sanders, M.R., 2014. A randomized controlled trial evaluating a brief parenting program with children with autism spectrum disorders. J. Consult. Clin. Psychol. 82 (6), 1193—1200.

Thomas, K.C., Ellis, A.R., McLaurin, C., Daniels, J., Morrissey, J.P., 2007. Access to care for autism-related services. J. Autism Dev. Disord. 37 (10), 1902—1912.

US Department of Education, 2003. Identifying and Implementing Educational Practices Supported by Rigorous Evidence: A User Friendly Guide. Author, Washington, DC.

White, S.W., Ollendick, T., Albano, A.M., Oswald, D., Johnson, C., Southam-Gerow, M.A., et al., 2013. Randomized controlled trial: multimodal anxiety and social skill intervention for adolescents with autism spectrum disorder. J. Autism Dev. Disord. 43 (2), 382—394.

Wood, J.J., Gadow, K.D., 2010. Exploring the nature and function of anxiety in youth with autism spectrum disorders. Clin. Psychol. Sci. Practice 17 (4), 281–292.

Wood, J.J., McLeod, B.D., Hiruma, L.S., Phan, A.Q., 2008. Child Anxiety Disorders: A Family-based Treatment Manual for Practitioners, Vol. xiii. W W Norton & Co, New York, NY, US.

Wood, J.J., Drahota, A., Sze, K., Har, K., Chiu, A., Langer, D.A., 2009. Cognitive behavioral therapy for anxiety in children with autism spectrum disorders: a randomized, controlled trial. J. Child Psychol. Psychiatry 50 (3), 224–234.

Wood, J.J., Ehrenreich-May, J., Alessandri, M., Fujii, C., Renno, P., Laugeson, E., et al., 2015. Cognitive behavioral therapy for early adolescents with autism spectrum disorders and clinical anxiety: a randomized, controlled trial. Behav. Ther. 46 (1), 7–19.

CHAPTER 8

Group Cognitive Behavior Therapy for Children and Adolescents With Anxiety and Autism Spectrum Disorders

Judy Reaven and Kirsten Willar
University of Colorado Anschutz Medical Campus School of Medicine, Aurora, CO, United States;
Children's Hospital Colorado, Aurora, CO, United States

INTRODUCTION

The origins of group therapy can be traced to when Joseph Pratt convened patients with tuberculosis in small groups with the purpose of providing education about their disease process (Pratt, 1945). The unexpected psychological benefits of working with individuals with similar life circumstances in small groups were soon realized and others began to apply group work to individuals with other medical conditions. At around the same time, Jacob Moreno began to explore the potential benefits of working with female prostitutes in what later became known as "self-help" groups. He reported that the process of each woman taking turns to share her stories and experiences in the presence of the group yielded profound benefits. The group therapy format was described as not only helping to create a supportive and cohesive community among the participants, but also increasing self-awareness and providing opportunities to learn adaptive strategies for coping and problem solving (Moreno, 1946; Christner et al., 2007).

The group treatment format for children has been influenced by Adler, Bender, and Slavson among others (Bender, 1937; Dreikurs and Corsini, 1954) who observed that working with children together with their peers permitted them to be challenged in ways that were very different than when they were seen in individual therapy. Providing children with the opportunity to observe the impact of their behavior on others in a safe and supportive environment was thought to promote insight and awareness of behavior, which clinicians believed was necessary to impact change.

Anxiety in Children and Adolescents with Autism Spectrum Disorder.
DOI: http://dx.doi.org/10.1016/B978-0-12-805122-1.00008-9
© 2017 Elsevier Inc.
All rights reserved.
143

Over the past decades, group therapy has been used for many different psychological symptoms. It can be argued that certain mental health difficulties may specifically lend themselves to group treatment, such as improving social skills and interaction abilities, and building empathy (Kronenberger and Meyer, 2001). More recently, group treatments, frequently from a cognitive behavior therapy (CBT) perspective, have addressed aggression, anger, depression, and anxiety in typically developing children and adolescents (e.g., Flannery-Schroeder and Kendall, 2000; Lochman and Wells, 2003). Group therapies may be especially appealing as they can address long wait lists and maximize resources. Caring communities are created, the potential for hope and change is instilled, and behavior is "normalized." Many group members feel less isolated as they begin to recognize the universality of their experiences (Yalom and Leszcz, 2005). Furthermore, participation in group therapy can motivate less interested participants, promote interpersonal skill development, provide opportunity for peer modeling, and offer a safe space for practice of new skills within a naturalistic environment (Flannery-Schroeder and Kendall, 2000; Kronenberger and Meyer, 2001; Reaven et al., 2009). In spite of these benefits, group therapy is not without its disadvantages. Individualized attention is limited, inappropriate behaviors may be displayed and modeled by group members and inaccurate information and perspectives can be perpetuated by well-meaning group members.

This chapter reviews group CBT approaches to treat anxiety disorders in children and adolescents with Autism Spectrum Disorders (ASD). The review begins with a description of the initial efforts to use the group therapy format and techniques with children and teens with ASD, beginning with social skills interventions. An exploration of existing group CBT treatments for anxiety in youth with ASD is followed by an in-depth review of advantages and potential disadvantages of conducting group therapies for these youth. Practical suggestions for delivering group CBT interventions are provided to help practitioners make informed decisions about whether a group therapy approach is appropriate for the clients they work with *and* whether group therapies can be effectively delivered in their practice or setting. Specific examples from one group treatment program, Facing Your Fears: Group Therapy for Managing Anxiety in Children with High-Functioning Autism Spectrum Disorders (FYF; Reaven et al., 2011) are detailed. Finally, recommendations for future clinical and research efforts are offered.

GROUP TREATMENT FOR YOUTH WITH
ASD—INITIAL FOCUS

Not surprisingly, the group format for treatments of youth with ASD has largely focused on addressing social skill deficits (Reichow and Volkmar, 2010; Reichow et al., 2012). Although there are multiple methods to improve social skill development, including naturalistic and peer-mediated approaches among others (Kasari et al., 2012), clinic-based social skills training (SST) groups are common and have been used extensively with high-functioning school-aged children and adolescents with ASD (Bellini et al., 2007; Rao et al., 2008). SST entails direct instruction that facilitates the acquisition or performance of social skills and teaches group members ways to interact with others. Targeted skills for youth with ASD may include teaching conversational skills, increasing social motivation, expanding and developing friendship networks, emotion recognition and regulation, and social problem solving (Frankel et al., 2010). Group SSTs typically meet weekly for 12–20 consecutive weeks (Reichow et al., 2012).

A variety of strategies have been used to teach social interaction skills, as there is no single agreed upon approach for teaching social skills to children with ASD (Cappadocia and Weiss, 2011). According to a review of various group SST programs, treatment methods based upon applied behavior analysis, naturalistic techniques, peer-mediated training, visual supports, and video modeling were all found to be effective treatment strategies for teaching social skills (Reichow and Volkmar, 2010). Behavioral rehearsal, role-play demonstrations, performance feedback, homework assignments, and parent involvement can promote continued practice and generalization of skills (Laugeson and Park, 2014; Rao et al., 2008; Otero et al., 2015).

Over the past decade, there has been a dramatic increase in the amount of research on SSTs for individuals with ASD, including a focus on different aspects of social competence (Reichow and Volkmar, 2010; Cotugno, 2009). Overall, the evidence supports that group SSTs can greatly improve social abilities in youth with ASD (Reichow et al., 2012; Cappadocia and Weiss, 2011). That said, SSTs come with their own set of inherent limitations: for example, many group SSTs occur outside of natural contexts, potentially making it more difficult for participants to generalize and maintain the skills over time (Kasari et al., 2012). Peer-mediated approaches may be more ecologically valid than clinic-based

SSTs for improving social outcomes in youth with ASD, although more research is needed (Kasari et al., 2012). Furthermore, the majority of social skills groups that have been developed to date have served only a subset of individuals on the autism spectrum. The applicability and effectiveness of SSTs with individuals with ASD who are more cognitively impacted needs to be studied (Reichow and Volkmar, 2010).

Although social skills can be taught to youth with ASD in both group and individual contexts, there are no head-to-head randomized clinical trials comparing one modality to the other. Many would argue that the use of group treatment is more beneficial in the teaching of social skills to children with ASD because the group format allows for the instruction and practice of newly learned skills in an interactive manner that approximates a naturalistic setting (Barry et al., 2003; Kroeger et al., 2007). Additionally, a group setting can create opportunities for structured interactions with peer support and feedback, and allows participants to practice social skills in a protected and predictable environment (Burgess and Turkstra, 2006).

DETERMINING TREATMENT FOCUS—SOCIAL SKILLS OR ANXIETY-BASED INTERVENTIONS?

As previously indicated, most group treatments for youth with ASD have been social skills based and these SSTs have been exclusively focused on building social competence in youth with autism. However, unaddressed anxiety problems can undermine the benefits of intervention. For example, youth with high levels of anxiety may be less able to make use of social skills training and avoid opportunities to practice newly learned social skills (White et al., 2013). To address both sets of challenges, the Multimodal Anxiety and Social Skills Intervention (MASSI) was developed to focus on treatment of both anxiety symptoms and social skills. Preliminary findings have been positive for adolescents with ASD who participated in the treatment, as improvement in social impairment and anxiety were noted (White et al., 2013). Treatments that target the acquisition and improvement in social skills may position youth with ASD to engage in graded social exposures, a core component of anxiety interventions. Conducting graded exposure practice for social goals (e.g., engaging in conversation with peers) without the requisite skills necessary for social interaction may be frustrating and potentially unsuccessful.

It has yet to be determined whether one treatment (e.g., anxiety or social skills) should be prioritized over the other, or whether a combination of treatment approaches is more beneficial for youth with ASD. On the one hand, many youth with anxiety and ASD may not need explicit social skills training as brief social coaching immediately prior to social interaction may be adequate (Wood et al., 2009). Furthermore, young children with ASD commonly present with less socially focused anxiety symptoms such as specific phobias and separation fears (van Steensel et al., 2011), perhaps making it less necessary that direct social skills instruction be included as part of the intervention for these children. Youth with ASD and social anxiety may be a different story, as these youth may require the inclusion of both social skills and anxiety based strategies as part of their treatment program.

Because youth with ASD can present with such a broad range of anxiety symptoms (van Steensel et al., 2011), more research is needed to determine the core treatment components for these youth. Ultimately an over-focus on determining treatment approach for youth with ASD and anxiety may be "much ado about nothing" because group treatments, whether they are anxiety or social skills focused, are in fact, exposures (Flanner-Schroeder and Kendall, 2000). There is already substantial overlap in group SST programs and anxiety-based programs for youth with ASD, especially when anxiety symptoms are socially-focused. For example, although the FYF program is designed to address the anxious symptoms of youth with ASD, the FYF manual specifically highlights the "social skills" that naturally occur within the group setting (e.g., listening to others, talking in front of a group, and increasing emotional expression). During each FYF session, group facilitators encourage child participants to develop these "social skills" even as they identify anxiety-provoking situations, develop coping strategies and begin to face fears.

GROUP THERAPY FOR ANXIETY IN YOUTH WITH ASD

The past decade has been witness to a burgeoning interest in the assessment and treatment of co-occurring mental health symptoms in youth with ASD (Reaven and Wainer, 2015). Perhaps because prevalence studies have indicated that anxiety disorders occur at very high rates in children and adolescents with ASD (van Steensel et al., 2011), much attention has been devoted to the development of psychosocial treatment programs to address anxious symptoms. Both individual (e.g., McNally Keehn et al., 2013;

Wood et al., 2009) and group treatment programs (e.g., Chalfant et al., 2007; McConachie et al., 2014; Sung et al., 2011) have been developed, almost exclusively from a CBT perspective. Regardless of modality, the majority of these programs contain the core elements of CBT for anxiety treatment, including a cognitive component, somatic management, and graded exposure (Kendall, 1994). Similarly, all treatment programs, whether delivered in an individual or group context, modified their programs to meet the specific social, communication, and learning needs of youth with ASD. Adaptations that cut across treatment programs included the development of disorder specific hierarchies, use of concrete visual supports, incorporation of child-specific interests, and parent involvement (Moree and Davis, 2010).

At least five randomized controlled trials (RCT) have used a group CBT approach to manage the anxiety symptoms in youth with ASD (Chalfant et al., 2007; McConachie et al., 2014; Reaven et al., 2012a; Sofronoff et al., 2005; Sung et al., 2011). As indicated earlier, one program used a combination of individual and group treatment to address both the anxiety symptoms as well as social challenges in teens with ASD (White et al., 2013). Youth participants in these studies were both male and female, considered to be "high functioning" (IQs greater than 70), and ranged in age from 8 to 17 years. Each treatment program was careful to create groups that were well matched by age (younger/older cohorts) as well as by gender. Group size varied across treatment programs, although most interventions for youth with ASD and anxiety indicate that 3–5 children (and their parents) comprise a "group," along with two to four group facilitators (Chalfant et al., 2007; McConachie et al., 2014; Reaven et al., 2011; Sofronoff et al., 2005; Sung et al., 2011). For the most part, the group treatments targeted generalized anxiety, social anxiety, separation anxiety, and specific phobia symptoms (Chalfant et al., 2007; Reaven et al., 2012a). Parent involvement varied across studies, ranging from limited parent involvement (Sung et al., 2011), to concurrent parent/child groups (e.g., Chalfant et al., 2007; Sofronoff et al., 2005), to fully integrated parent participation via parent/child dyadic work and large group activities (parents and children altogether), in addition to concurrent parent/child groups) (Reaven et al., 2012a).

Session length and, thus, subsequent intervention dosage ranged from a low of 6 sessions (Sofronoff et al., 2005) to a high of 20 sessions (White et al., 2013). For the most part, psychologists or trainees in psychology delivered the treatment. Core CBT components established for typically developing youth with anxiety disorders are included in the group treatments, with the exception of two treatment programs that did not include graded exposure, but focused primarily on building strategies for managing anxiety symptoms (McConachie et al., 2014; Sofronoff et al., 2005). To enhance the accessibility of core CBT content for youth with ASD, some researchers made adaptations and modifications to existing protocols (e.g., McNally Keehn et al., 2013—Coping Cat; Kendall and Hedtke, 2006a; Kendall and Hedtke, 2006b; Chalfant et al., 2007—Cool Kids; Barrett et al., 2003; and Wood et al., 2009—Building Confidence; Wood and McLeod, 2008). Others developed treatment programs specifically for individuals with ASD (e.g., McConachie et al., 2014—Exploring Feelings; Attwood, 2004; Reaven et al., 2012a—Facing Your Fears; Reaven et al., 2011).

Results from efficacy studies indicated that across treatment programs significant improvements in anxiety symptoms were apparent following participation in intervention, according to parent reported measures of youth anxiety (e.g., Anxiety Disorders Interview Schedule-Child/Parent-IV, Parent version-ADIS-IV-C/P; Silverman and Albano, 1996; Screen for Child Anxiety and Related Emotional Disorders, Parent version-SCARED; Birmaher et al., 1999). Because each study measured youth treatment outcome somewhat differently, it is difficult to directly compare outcomes across programs. For example, one study documented significant loss (71%) of the principal anxiety diagnosis post-treatment (Chalfant et al., 2007), while other studies measured more general decreases in anxiety post-treatment (e.g., Sofronoff et al., 2005). Our own RCT yielded significant decreases in Clinician Severity Ratings (CSRs) (per the ADIS-IV-C/P) for the four main anxiety diagnoses (Social Anxiety, Separation Anxiety, Specific Phobia, and Generalized Anxiety) and total number of anxiety diagnoses for participants assigned to the FYF treatment, compared with participants assigned to Treatment as Usual (TAU). In addition, participants in FYF also demonstrated significant and clinically meaningful improvements in global ratings of anxiety symptoms (according to clinician ratings) compared with TAU (Reaven et al., 2012a). Finally, in a sample of 70 children ages 9–16 years old, with ASD and anxiety, Sung et al. (2011) found significant decreases in anxiety symptoms for all participants, regardless of whether they were randomized to CBT treatment or to a social recreation comparison group. Participants in both groups demonstrated significant reductions in anxiety according to child self-report as well as clinician report of anxiety. The authors indicated that although there was sufficient power to detect a statistically significant difference between groups, they raised the possibility that the current sample size may have been insufficient to detect a difference in symptoms given that the comparison was between two active treatments. Further, the authors also hypothesized that the significant decreases in anxiety across both groups may have been due to the commonalities between the two conditions, i.e., the structured group setting, presence of consistent therapists, social exposure, and use of ASD strategies.

Although there have been no head–to–head comparisons of individual CBT versus group CBT for youth with ASD, research exploring individual and group treatment modalities in general pediatric samples has indicated that group treatments can be at least as effective as individual approaches (Manassis et al., 2002). Direct comparisons of individual versus group CBT treatment have included anxious youth between the ages of 8 and 14 years, and for the most part, there were few substantial differences in outcome. Results across programs reveal that both children and parents report significant decreases in anxiety post-treatment, regardless of modality (Manassis et al., 2002; Flannery-Schroeder and Kendall, 2000). Interestingly, highly socially anxious children reported greater improvements in symptoms when assigned to individual CBT compared with group CBT. Anxious youth in individual CBT also experienced significant improvement on measures of anxious distress, and as a whole, were better at recalling the content of what they learned in group, compared to youth participants in group CBT (Manassis et al., 2002; Flannery-Schroeder and Kendall, 2000). Thus, individual CBT may be a preferable modality for some anxious youth, as group treatment may be viewed as overwhelming with less opportunity for individualized attention. More research is needed to determine the advantages and disadvantages of group versus individual CBT approaches for anxious youth with ASD, with a focus on "fit" between youth characteristics and treatment modality as an area for additional study.

CHALLENGES/RECOMMENDATIONS FOR CONDUCTING GROUP THERAPY WITH YOUTH WITH ASD AND ANXIETY

Many of the challenges detailed in this section represent universal challenges, and are not unique to any one group CBT program for youth with ASD. However, given the scope of this chapter, recommendations offered in this section are primarily informed by the FYF program for anxiety in youth with ASD.

Logistical considerations: In comparison with individual treatment, conducting group therapy can be an exercise in intense coordination, as many variables need to be juggled to maximize successful recruitment of even a single group. Family and clinician schedules need to be synchronized such that all participants are available on the same day during the week, and on average, for a minimum of 12–16 consecutive weeks of intervention (e.g., Reaven et al., 2011; Storch et al., 2013; Sung et al., 2011). In addition, identifying 2–4 "qualified" clinicians with coordinated schedules can also be challenging. Although the majority of studies conducted thus far have utilized advanced students and degreed-professionals in mental health-related professions, there is a lack of established guidelines for *who* can facilitate these group treatments. Even if agencies determined that mental health clinicians were essential to the delivery of group CBT, many clinical settings do not have the resources to provide 2–4 experienced clinicians, limiting the feasibility of offering group therapy in some environments (Reaven et al., 2014).

Recommendations: When scheduling groups, it may be most helpful to map group schedules onto school calendars. When group therapy sessions extend beyond school semesters (e.g., spring semester through summer) there may be a higher risk of participant drop-out. For families who desire summer groups, containing the group treatment to the summer months may be preferable to increase attendance. Explicitly outlining expectations for attendance at the outset is important (e.g., requirement to attend a minimum of 85% of sessions) and can maximize attendance. In addition, enlisting trainees to participate as co-therapists may be one way to select group facilitators. Although it is recommended that at least 1–2 experienced mental health professionals be part of the treatment team, it may be less critical that *all* facilitators have a mental health background. Rather, clinicians who possess strong group management skills may be more important to consider than clinician background or discipline, given the high potential for behavioral challenges to occur in a group setting. However, research is needed to determine the facilitator background, experience, and training necessary to deliver group treatment programs to fidelity.

Recruitment challenges: The heterogeneity of ASD coupled with the diverse and even atypical presentation of anxiety symptoms in youth with ASD (Kerns et al., 2014) can make selection of a cohesive group of youth (and their families) a daunting task. The cognitive, social, and linguistic characteristics of youth with ASD vary tremendously (Kerns and Kendall, 2012). Differences in social ability, relative comfort in a group setting, processing speed, self-regulatory skill, and expressive language ability (particularly emotional expression) are only a handful of the disparities that may exist among group members. Other essential variables to consider may include age, gender, race and ethnicity, and socioeconomic status. Determining which of the aforementioned variables are most critical to consider (and match) in recruitment selection is nearly impossible. In addition, little empirical investigation has occurred to provide guidelines for decision-making regarding group composition.

Not all children with ASD and anxiety may be appropriate for a group CBT treatment. Some youth may have extreme difficulty separating from their parents for any length of time, display significant aggressive or disruptive behaviors, chronically resist treatment, and/or have other mental health conditions. If a child presents with any of these difficulties they may not be "group ready" and could benefit from an alternative treatment focus or modality (Reaven et al., 2011).

Further complicating recruitment is the ambivalence that some families experience when considering participation in group treatment. For example, confidentiality may be of particular concern in a group context as children and their parents may be worried that their privacy may be potentially violated by other group members. Additionally, parents may express concern that their children will "catch" the fears, worries or inappropriate behaviors of the other group members. Parents may compare their child to the other children in the group, and express embarrassment in the child's conduct, particularly when non-compliant, dysregulated, or inappropriate behaviors are displayed. Additionally, parents may worry that their child is too "high-functioning" for the group, or conversely, too impacted by ASD symptoms to participate effectively in group treatment. Of course, parents themselves may also experience varying levels of comfort in group participation, further impacting group selection and retention.

Finally, the identification and assessment of co-occurring mental health symptoms, including clinical anxiety symptoms in youth with ASD can be difficult (Reaven and Wainer, 2015). Misdiagnoses and/or failure to provide an accurate diagnosis may prevent access to appropriate treatment for youth with ASD. Confusion can result when children are selected for group participation, but do not have clinical anxiety symptoms. The mismatch between the child's behavioral presentation and the intended behavioral targets of the treatment program can lead to feelings of frustration for parents and children.

Recommendations: Clear inclusion/exclusion criteria for group participation can be helpful to recruitment. Results from several treatment studies (e.g., Reaven et al., 2009; Reaven et al., 2012a) have yielded following inclusion criteria that may be helpful when recruiting for a clinical group using FYF (Reaven et al., 2011): (1) youth with ASD between the ages of 8–14, creating aged based groups (e.g., 8–11 yrs.; 11–14 yrs.), have been the most successful. Although the majority of treatment groups will likely be comprised of boys, when girls meet the inclusion criteria for group participation it may be important to recruit at least two girls at a time to decrease the potential for social isolation; (2) cognitive ability at least in the low average/average range, with verbal IQ at approximately 80 or above[1]; (3) documented diagnosis of ASD according to parent report[2]; (4) clinical anxiety symptoms on an objective measure of anxiety such as the SCARED (Birmaher et al., 1999); and (5) ability to separate from the parent for 30 minutes or more. Children with ASD and anxiety who have other diagnoses (e.g., ADHD) are appropriate for group, although anxiety should be the primary problem, relative to other co-occurring symptoms. Youth with severe behavioral disturbance (e.g., aggression, self-injurious behavior), severe mood disorder, or active psychotic symptoms are not appropriate for FYF, and should be referred to an appropriate treatment provider. If group facilitators are uncertain as to whether a child is "group ready," a trial period of three treatment sessions can be proposed to allow for an extended assessment period. If within the trial period the child is not able to participate without marked distress that cannot be abated by the facilitators, the lead clinician may decide to end the child's participation in group and recommend that the family participate in an individual modality (Reaven et al., 2011).

Educating parents that anxiety symptoms typically include irrational and excessive fear, worry, or avoidant behaviors that are persistent and interfere with day-to-day functioning can be helpful in appropriately

---

[1] Verbal IQ criterion is intended as a general guideline only. Some verbally fluent youth have responded well to the FYF treatment, even when the verbal IQ score was lower than recommended criterion.

[2] Our research studies have required a well-characterized sample of youth with ASD, including the administration of autism specific measures such as the ADOS-2. The same diagnostic rigor is not required for clinical groups.

identifying symptoms. Parents are encouraged to look for moments of "anxious avoidance" or the combination of anxiety symptoms (e.g., increased physiological arousal, self-report anxiety) paired with avoidant behavior (Hagopian and Jennett, 2014) as an additional way to assess anxiety. While it may be tempting to label a range of problem behaviors as examples of anxious symptoms, careful assessment is important. For instance, there may be various explanations as to why a child refuses to complete homework that has nothing to do with anxiety. Challenges with the planning, initiation or organization of doing homework, mismatch of academic expectations compared with the child's learning ability, or difficulties transitioning from preferred to non-preferred activities may be just a handful of the problems that may account for a child's reluctance to complete homework. Evaluating the correct contributor(s) to the challenging behaviors is essential to identifying a suitable treatment approach (see Chapter 5 "Assessment of Anxiety in Youth With ASD" for more information).

When parents express concerns about their child's inappropriate displays of behavior, talking directly with parents can be quite helpful. Normalizing the behavior (e.g., "many children have difficulties with group participation, especially at first") can allay many of the parents' fears about the appropriateness of group for their child. When parents directly ask if their child will "catch" the fears of others, we indicate that although children have "tried on" the fears of others for short periods, we have not experienced any situations where a group participant has permanently "caught" the fears of other group members. Further, emphasizing the benefits of group therapy for youth with ASD, including the opportunity to observe peers being brave and "facing fears," can also be extremely beneficial.

Finally, directly addressing the importance of confidentiality with all group members is critical. Talking with all participants about what it means to keep information "private" is essential so that the children and their parents feel safe sharing information. Employing the "Las Vegas" rule can be helpful to share with group members—"what happens in group, stays in group."

Lack of individualization and flexibility in delivery of material: As has been well documented, children with ASD are exceedingly heterogeneous in their presentations of anxiety (Kerns et al., 2014; van Steensel et al., 2011). Severity of core deficits, intellectual functioning and language abilities are just some of the variables that influence an individual's presentation. Thus, a common disadvantage when working with youth with ASD in group therapy is the lack of individual attention that can be provided to each participant. The variability in cognitive functioning, severity and type of anxiety symptoms, and potential for behavioral challenges (see below) during a group therapy session may make it difficult to reliably execute lessons from a manual-based treatment program. For example, comprehension differences alone can thwart completion of a particular lesson as some group members may require additional instruction to complete even one task, while other members may be able to finish a series of activities independently. Thus, decisions about how long to spend on a particular activity, or whether to move on to the next activity even though some children may not have completed, or maybe even understood the lesson, are constant and frequently difficult to make.

Recommendations: As with other manual-based treatments, FYF emphasizes the importance of "flexibility within fidelity" (Kendall and Beidas, 2007). For example, throughout the FYF program, there are activities that have been designated as "optional." For example, "story time" can be included for younger children, whereas older youth may find the story content childish. Group leaders can make decisions about whether to include these optional activities based on the group composition and functioning. In addition, some activities are designed to be completed *either* independently *or* as small group activities; again, decisions that can be made based on facilitator discretion. For example, to teach the concepts of anxious self-talk and coping self-talk (Kendall, 1994), FYF uses the terms "active minds" and "helpful thoughts" (Garland and Clark, 1995; Reaven et al., 2011). In this activity, group members are presented with worksheets depicting a child who is faced with an anxiety provoking situation (e.g., seeing a snake at the zoo). Examples of "active minds" are shown in thought bubbles drawn above the child's head with statements such as "oh no, the snake will escape and come to my house." Rather than requiring the children to generate suggestions for "helpful thoughts" on an individual basis (which may be challenging for some youth with ASD), group facilitators can draw a picture of a child on a large poster board, adding blank thought bubbles above the child's head. The group then works together to generate "helpful thoughts" to manage the "active minds." Completing this activity as a group may enhance task comprehension in a way that completing it individually could not.

Another example of flexible delivery of the FYF intervention involves length of time spent on various activities. That is, some group activities can be shortened, particularly if they occur in large group settings when group members are more likely to become behaviorally dysregulated. For example, a "getting to know you" activity occurs in the first session, and is designed as a large group activity (parents, children and facilitators altogether). The activity encourages all child participants to identify different categories of "favorites" (e.g., foods, video games, and vacations) and gives children and adults the opportunity to respond to all of the categories. However, this can be a lengthy activity and potentially overwhelming for some youth. Group leaders can closely monitor participation and abbreviate the activity so that only the children provide responses, thus allowing the activity to end on a positive note.

Providing individual attention "bursts" (if the number of facilitators in group allows for this), to particular group members to support understanding of an activity, and in some cases to help with compliance may be helpful. For children who work quite slowly, it may be important to talk with the parent about completing some activities at home, although this has rarely been necessary in FYF. Children who work quickly may assist the facilitators or another peer with some activities, which in turn may promote social engagement. This strategy can be especially effective if there is a group comprised of both younger and older youth. Finally, carrying over an activity from one session to another is allowable in FYF. Even in sessions that are content heavy, delivering the information in a thorough manner is much more preferable to completing activities quickly and within designated sessions. On the other hand, some children with ASD may not fully comprehend the psychoeducation component of FYF. Similar to other CBT programs, graded exposure is viewed as a critical component (Peterman et al., 2015). Therefore, rather than spend extensive time teaching "tools" to manage anxiety, it may be more beneficial to move more quickly to the introduction of graded exposure strategies.

Managing behavioral challenges: One of the biggest challenges of conducting group treatment with youth with ASD is managing difficult behaviors. Challenging behavior can take many forms. In the FYF groups, we have worked with youth who are quick to "meltdown", refuse to participate, deny that anxiety is a problem, withdraw from social interaction, or become silly and dysregulated. Even encouraging children to regularly attend group can be a struggle for some families. Although challenging behaviors obviously can occur in both group and individual psychotherapeutic contexts, managing difficult behaviors in a group setting is much more problematic because of the extent to which these behaviors interfere with group process. Thus, finding ways to effectively manage these behaviors can promote group functioning and is crucial to the success of treatment.

Recommendations: A "meltdown" is perhaps one of the most difficult behaviors to manage in a group context. In the exact moment that the behavior is happening, it may be hard to do anything other than react (e.g., help the child to calm down, keep the child and other group members safe). Depending on the severity of the behavior, it may be necessary to temporarily remove the child from group and/or enlist parent support to help the child calm down.

Once the child has been taught some of the initial FYF content, it may be helpful to employ key aspects from the psychoeducation portion of FYF to manage "meltdowns." For example, similar to other CBT programs, FYF includes a segment on managing the body's reaction to worry and focuses on developing somatic management as well as emotion regulation skills. During this segment, the children first identify the vocabulary words they prefer to use to describe their upset, as well as identify words that they *do not* want others to use to describe their anxiety (e.g., "worry," "agitated," "afraid," "upset"). Group members are next taught to "externalize" their worry (March and Mulle, 1998). Here, the children are asked to imagine that their worry is an entity separate from themselves. The process of labeling and eventually creating a "worry bug" allows children, parents and group facilitators to work together to manage the child's worry through externalization. In other words, "the person is not the problem, but the problem is the problem" (Freedman and Combs, 1996, p. 47). Using phrases such as "that sounds like your worry bug," (without overuse) when the child is displaying excessive, unrealistic worry, and/or prior to a meltdown can potentially prevent power struggles between children and adults and creates opportunities for the child to feel supported.

Following externalization of worry, the children learn how to "measure" the intensity of worry/upset using a "stress-o-meter" (an 8-point scale with green, yellow, and red zones). Then, numerous strategies for calming down are generated and reviewed (e.g., deep breathing, take a break; encourage coping self-talk such as "the worry feelings will go away" or "this is just my worry bug"). Children are encouraged (and rewarded) for using these strategies when they find themselves in red or yellow zones, and are also rewarded for staying in green zones. Group members are encouraged to create a "plan to get to green" with their parents that details the range of coping strategies that the children can use both in group and at home when they experience significant worry or upset.

Once the stress-o-meter and other related concepts have been introduced, it can be quite helpful to use these tools to assist the children in labeling how they are feeling currently (if they are in the middle of a meltdown), as well as to remind them of strategies they can use to "get to green." The a priori development of the "plan to get to green" can be part of a longer term solution for managing meltdowns. Assisting parents in identifying specific Do's (e.g., stay calm; model strategies you want the child to do; keep everyone safe) and Don'ts (e.g., talk or try to problem-solve while the child is upset; teach a new strategy; say "just calm down") during a child's meltdown may be particularly useful. If the meltdowns or other displays of challenging behaviors persist, it may be helpful to conduct a modified functional assessment of behavior (FBA) to understand and identify the triggers for the inappropriate behavior so that additional antecedent strategies can be employed (Koegel et al., 1996).

Importantly, the range of strategies outlined above may also be used to address other forms of challenging behavior such as withdrawn or "shut down" behavior, and silly or dysregulated behaviors. Emotional dysregulation can take many forms; emphasizing somatic management and emotion regulation skills through labeling the experience, measuring intensity of emotions, and employing the "plan to get to green" may be effective in targeting the range of problematic behaviors that can occur in a group setting.

Noncompliance or refusals to participate in group activities occur, and although the aforementioned strategies may be helpful here too, it may also be important to implement additional strategies. Gathering additional information about *why* the refusals or non-compliant behaviors are occurring (via FBA) can also provide direction on the selection of various intervention strategies. As a rule, in the FYF program we do not *require* that children participate in group activities (particularly at first); rather, children are supported to be successful through participation in very small behavioral increments at a time. For example, many children decline to speak in group, especially during large group activities. We may start by encouraging a child to respond either verbally or nonverbally to direct yes or no questions as a way to foster small steps toward participation. If this approach does not work, we request that parents speak for their children (e.g., "let's have your mom share your work") until the child feels comfortable in group.[3] Because youth with ASD may be particularly sensitive to some aspects of a given activity such as deep breathing, offering an alternative to the activity may work for some group members (e.g., squeezing and relaxing muscles, chair push-ups). Rewarding (via token reward system or social praise) successive approximations and any efforts toward participation is essential. Scheduling a pleasurable activity following group may provide an additional incentive for attendance and participation. Finally, ignoring minor displays of undesirable behavior (provided it is not disruptive to group members), while simultaneously praising the other children for on-task behavior, may be an effective strategy. Explicitly stating that it is important for group members to disregard their peers' silly or inappropriate behaviors can also become a potential group rule, and referred to throughout intervention if needed.

It is not uncommon for children with ASD to begin group denying that they experience worry or anxiety. This stance can be disconcerting for families, as they often express concern that their children will not respond to treatment because they deny the presence of their own anxiety symptoms. These denials may occur for a number of reasons. For example, recognizing and accurately identifying anxiety for some children with ASD can be difficult, because of core difficulties with emotional understanding and expression. In other circumstances, children may be reluctant to admit that they have "problems." Emphasizing the universal and human experience of anxiety can be a helpful place to begin. It may also be important to establish how to talk about the worry. For example, if some youth have a strong reaction to the word "worry," then you may try using words that the child previously identified as preferable such as "upset," "nervous," or "irritated." In addition, when parents and youth disagree about the nature of the anxiety symptoms, do not require parents and children to reach consensus, but rather, take the stance of "agreeing to disagree." Over time, it has been our experience that most child participants do eventually become aware of their anxiety, employ coping strategies and begin facing fears.

Working with parents: Parents of children with ASD play a critical role in intervention programs, as they can help their children generalize newly learned skills from one setting to another (Reaven et al., 2011). In fact, when anxious youth with high rates of parent-reported ASD

---

[3] Youth with selective mutism are appropriate for FYF, but will likely require psychoeducation and a graded exposure hierarchy to address more thoroughly

symptoms, received family CBT as opposed to individual CBT, results indicated that parents were more involved with the homework (exposure) tasks, and the anxiety reduction outcomes were better (Puleo and Kendall, 2011). Because parents appear key to the success of treatment for youth with ASD, parents are an integral part of FYF and are required to attend every therapy session along with their child. Parents regularly interact with their children in large group contexts, as well as during parent/child dyadic work throughout treatment. There are also times during FYF, when the parents and children work in separate groups that meet concurrently. Disagreements can occur between parents and children during the program. For instance, conflict may be initially apparent when parents and children start to identify worries and fears. Difficulties may also arise when parents meet alone as a group. As with other group treatments, at times one or more individuals may dominate the discussion, making it hard for all of the parents to be heard. In addition, some parents may use the parent group as a venting session to air complaints about their child, school teams, or family members, potentially making the other parents feel uncomfortable. Some parents may be obliged to generate solutions for a parent's dilemma, which in turn may side track the discussion altogether.

Recommendations: One primary benefit of involving parents in the FYF program is that as parents get to know each other, they can become a source of support for each other. Parents have frequently commented on how helpful it is for them to meet other families who experience similar struggles to their own. In order to maximize the benefits of meeting with the parents separately, it is important to balance the delivery of the therapeutic content with opportunity for parents to more informally share concerns about their child. Beginning each parent group with a clear schedule of what topics will be covered in group can let parents know the session agenda. Empathizing with parents' struggles and explicitly stating that you will leave time at the end of group to discuss additional issues may be another way to balance content with group process. Some parents may require additional direct contact outside of group, particularly if there are specific concerns about a parent/child dyad that cannot be addressed in the group context (e.g., safety issues). Although we try to keep additional contacts to a minimum, sometimes connecting with parents outside of group is unavoidable. Finally, some parents may openly struggle with helping their children identify worries, use coping strategies and face fears. When this occurs, it can be most beneficial to invite other parents in group to help problem-solve and offer suggestions for change. Hearing from another parent can be much more powerful to group members, rather than relying solely on facilitator input.

Conducting exposure practice in a group context: The delivery of the psychoeducational content (e.g., identification of anxious symptoms and anxiety provoking stimuli, increased awareness of anxious and coping self-talk, strategies to improve somatic management and emotion regulation) of FYF is fairly straightforward. Even clinicians who deliver FYF after only reading the manual demonstrate very good treatment adherence to content (Reaven et al., manuscript in preparation).

Conducting exposure practice, on the other hand, can be quite challenging, even in an individual therapeutic context (Abramowitz, 2013). Encouraging four to five children with ASD to face their fears in a group setting can be an even more daunting task. For instance, children and their parents may disagree about which fear to target first. Children may choose fears that their parents do not view as "true" fears. This can be particularly unsettling to parents who commonly want their child to target fears that interfere with daily functioning. However, if parents are allowed to select fears on their child's behalf, they may underestimate the amount of anxiety or distress involved in facing the fear. As a result, the child may feel extremely reluctant to tackle the fear, and refuse to face the fear at home and/or in group. Even when a fear is identified and agreed upon by both parents and children, generating the steps in a stimulus hierarchy can also be quite challenging, particularly for generalized worries.

Recommendations: In the FYF program, we frequently support the child's selection of a fear, even if parents may disagree with this choice. Once the child gains confidence and experiences success in facing the initial fear, s/he will likely become much more willing to tackle more challenging fears in the future. As a fear is identified, a stimulus hierarchy needs to be created. To guide this process it is important to ask the child (and family) the following questions: (1) How does your fear of _____ interfere with your life? (2) What are you avoiding as a result of your fear of _____? (3) How will you know when you have conquered your fear of _____? Are there things that you would like to do, but cannot do because of your fear? These questions can lead to identification of a goal, an important first step in the creation of a fear hierarchy.

Once the hierarchy is created, the child can begin to face his/her fear. In the FYF program, after exposure is introduced (approximately half-way through the treatment), each subsequent session begins with parent/child dyadic work. To maximize exposure practice, parents and children are encouraged to identify at least the initial step on their hierarchy and begin facing fears right away in session. (If hierarchies are not fully completed, it may be more appropriate to complete the hierarchy when the parents meet together later in the session). Some fears may require some amount of planning, while other fears can easily be conducted in a clinic setting. For example, social fears such as talking to new people can be fairly easy to accomplish in session (e.g., encouraging children to approach office staff and ask pre-planned questions such as "do you know where the bathroom is?"). Other fears may require more planning; for instance, fear of fire alarms or tornados may require props to simulate these experiences. In these cases, it is important to identify the fears that children will be facing ahead of time, so that in the following sessions each exposure practice can be as meaningful as possible.

For children who are reluctant to begin facing fears, it may be important to pair them with another parent/child dyad, particularly if their fears are similar to other group members. For example, children who may be afraid of the dark can simultaneously enter dark rooms (side by side), creating the opportunity for the children to debrief together following the exposure. Supporting and praising each other as they face their fears together can be powerful by-product of group treatment for youth with ASD. Social learning occurs throughout group therapy, as one child watches another child face a fear, thus promoting brave behavior.

For the most part, exposure practice usually occurs in parent/child dyads, with initial support from one group facilitator. Parents initially observe the facilitator guiding their children to face fears. As the parents gain increased comfort with graded exposure, they are urged to lead the practice since they will be responsible for encouraging the child to face fears at home. All parent/child dyads are engaged in exposure practice at the same time. Assuming that there are more parent/child dyads than there are facilitators, it would be important for facilitators to "float" between pairings, helping children begin to face fears. After the children have had a chance to face their fears, they are encouraged to share their progress with the group. To capitalize on the group context, all efforts to be brave and face fears are rewarded with much praise and applause from group members.

Importantly, the degree of parental participation and guidance in exposure practice is notably different for adolescents with ASD and anxiety.

In the development of the adolescent version of FYF, we found that it was more developmentally appropriate to encourage exposure practice to occur during the separate teen group, rather than with teens and their parents in dyadic work (Reaven et al., 2012b). Exposures in the teen group can occur simultaneously, but more commonly, exposure practice tends to occur one by one, in front of the group, to provide the teens with the opportunity to support and encourage each other to face fears.

Positive, meaningful, and tangible rewards can also be used to encourage exposure practice. We have used "punch cards" as a way to document and reward individual exposure practice (one punch for every practice). Once a child has accumulated 5–10 "punches" on a card, he may turn the card in for small prizes. To enhance group cohesion and support, group members can identify an achievable goal of cumulative exposure practices (e.g., 150 exposure practices) that the group as a whole can accomplish by the end of the program. Facilitators can then document the number of practices (or punches) that each child has completed over the course of the week and help the group keep track of the progress from week to week. A special reward, such as a pizza party, can happen during graduation to reward the group for reaching their goal.

For some youth with ASD, we have found that particular fears may require an exposure hierarchy *and* identification of specific skills that need to be taught directly to the child. For example, if a child is facing his fear of having a conversation with a peer, group facilitators may need to teach the peer how to: select an appropriate peer, determine what questions to ask, decide what comments to make, and end the conversation appropriately. In many cases, skill building can be embedded within the exposure hierarchy.

Finally, although we teach "graded" exposure strategies during FYF, we also emphasize specific approaches from an "inhibitory learning" approach (Arch and Craske, 2011; Craske et al., 2014) to deepen exposure practice, which in turn may enhance learning and prevent relapse. For example, varying exposure steps and length, and eliminating safety signals (e.g., people, props, or lucky charms that one has to have to face fears) are encouraged. Although a core tenet of exposure therapy is that habituation to feared stimulus occurs, the length of time that it may take for this process to occur is unknown for children with ASD. Additionally, some children with ASD may not experience fear reduction at all, as they face fears. As such, progress and success are defined as whether the child was able to face his fear, rather than whether the fear or anxiety decreased over time. Thus, the extent to which habituation occurs is less the focus of exposure practice, but rather it is whether the child was able to "act with anxiety" that is the measure of success (Abramowitz, 2013).

SUMMARY

There are several group CBT treatments for anxiety in youth with ASD. Specific advantages and potential disadvantages of conducting group therapies for youth with ASD and anxiety have been presented, alongside practical suggestions and advice for delivering group CBT interventions. Given the challenges associated with working with individuals with autism and anxiety, it is hoped that the information provided has given practitioners a road map for how to effectively deliver group CBT to youth with ASD.

FUTURE DIRECTIONS

Although the handful of RCTs focused on group CBT treatment with ASD and anxiety have yielded positive outcomes, there are areas where additional research is needed. Head-to-head comparisons of individual treatment versus group treatment for youth with ASD should be conducted, as it is not yet known who is best suited for group or individual approaches. Also, assessments of the long-term maintenance of skills are needed. The lion's share of group treatment thus far has focused exclusively on improving social skills and/or anxiety. Given that individuals with ASD are at high risk for developing a multitude of co-occurring mental health conditions, it would be valuable for research to address these additional interfering symptoms.

The majority of group treatments developed for youth with ASD and anxiety, thus far, have occurred in tightly controlled settings. It is essential to begin to bridge the research to practice gap and facilitate the portability of group therapies beyond lab settings and into the hands of clinicians across settings (Reaven et al., 2014). Initial efforts to train clinicians unfamiliar with FYF have been quite promising, as new clinicians were able to deliver FYF with excellent fidelity, after participating in an interactive training workshop paired with ongoing consultation (Reaven et al., 2014). Preliminary findings from this small pilot study (N = 16) also indicated that meaningful reductions in anxiety symptoms were obtained following participation in FYF. Given the proliferation of manualized interventions, it may particularly important for future research to systematically compare the clinician training methods necessary (e.g., workshop plus ongoing consultation; workshop alone) to deliver evidence-based interventions for youth with ASD.

Finally, the extent to which group CBT interventions for youth with ASD must be delivered by clinicians with a mental health background and/or with CBT experience is unknown. Preliminary efforts to explore this issue with the FYF program have begun with a cross-cultural collaboration with schools in Southeast Asia (Drmic, Sharifah, and Reaven, manuscript in preparation). Preliminary results indicated that significant decreases in anxiety symptoms occurred for students ages 13—15 with ASD and anxiety (N = 30), following participation in a school-based version of FYF. Importantly, the intervention was delivered by educators, who were coached by mental health professionals. In many cases, the educators had limited CBT experience; thus, the positive findings obtained in this pilot study reflect the potential to serve youth with ASD in more naturalistic settings, and improve access to services for this high risk and underserved population.

ACKNOWLEDGMENTS

The authors are supported, in part, by the Health Resources and Services Administration (HRSA) under the Leadership Education in Neurodevelopmental Disabilities (LEND) GrantT73MC11044 and by the Administration on Intellectual and Developmental Disabilities.

(AIDD) under the University Center of Excellence in Developmental Disabilities (UCDEDD) Grant 90DD0632 of the U.S. Department of Health and Human Services (HHS). JR was also supported in part by the National Institutes of Health (NIH) Grant R33MH089291—03. This information or content and conclusions are those of the authors and should not be construed as the official position or policy of, nor should any endorsements be inferred by NIH, HRSA, HHS, or the US government. The authors extend a special thanks to Audrey Blakeley-Smith, Nora Klemencic, Gilah Haber, Victoria Kolakowski, Gail Stickney-Mills, Katherine Sidhom, and Gina Barona for reading through this chapter and providing thoughtful feedback.

REFERENCES

Abramowitz, J., 2013. Exposure Therapy for Anxiety: Principles and Practice. The Guilford Press, New York, NY.

Arch, J.J., Craske, M.G., 2011. Addressing relapse in cognitive behavioral therapy for panic disorder: methods for optimizing long-term treatment outcomes. Cogn. Behav. Pract. 18, 306—315.

Attwood, T., 2004. Exploring Feelings (Anxiety). Future Horizons, Arlington, TX.

Barrett, P.M., Sonderegger, R., Xenos, S., 2003. Using FRIENDS to combat anxiety and adjustment problems among young migrants to Australia: a national trial. Clin. Child Psychol. Psychiatry 8, 241–260. Available from: http://dx.doi.org/10.1177/1359104503008002008.

Barry, T.D., Klinger, L.G., Lee, J.M., Palardy, N., Gilmore, T., Bodin, S.D., 2003. Examining the effectiveness of an outpatient clinic-based social skills group for high-functioning children with autism. J. Autism Dev. Disord. 33, 489–507.

Bellini, S., Peters, J.K., Benner, L., Hope, 2007. A meta-analysis of school-based social skills interventions for children with autism spectrum disorders. Remedial Special Educ. 28, 153–162. Available from: http://dx.doi.org/10.1177/07419325070280030401.

Bender, L., 1937. Group activities on a children's ward as a method of psychotherapy. Am. J. Psychiatry 93, 151–173.

Birmaher, B., Brent, D.A., Chiappetta, L., Bridge, J., Monga, S., Baugher, M., 1999. Psychometric properties of the Screen for Child Anxiety Related Emotional Disorders (SCARED): a replication study. J. Am. Acad. Child Adolesc. Psychiatry 38 (10), 1230–1236. Available from: http://dx.doi.org/10.1097/00004583-199910000-00011.

Burgess, S., Turkstra, L., 2006. Social skills intervention for adolescents with autism spectrum disorders: a review of the experimental evidence. EBP Briefs 1 (4), 1–21.

Cappadocia, M.C., Weiss, J.A., 2011. Review of social skills training groups for youth with asperger syndrome and high functioning autism. Res. Autism Spect. Disord. 5 (1), 70–78. Available from: http://dx.doi.org/10.1016/j.rasd.2010.04.001.

Chalfant, A.M., Rapee, R., Carroll, L., 2007. Treating anxiety disorders in children with high functioning autism spectrum disorders: a controlled trial. J. Autism Dev. Disorders 37 (10), 1842–1857. Available from: http://dx.doi.org/10.1007/s10803-006-0318-4.

Christner, R., Stewart, J., Freeman, A., 2007. Handbook of Cognitive-Behavior Group Therapy With Children and Adolescents-Specific Settings and Presenting Problems. Routledge, New York, NY.

Cotugno, A., 2009. Social competence and social skills training and intervention for children with Autism Spectrum Disorders. J. Autism Dev. Disord. 39 (9), 1268–1277. Available from: http://dx.doi.org/10.1007/s10803-009-0741-4.

Craske, M.G., Treanor, M., Conway, C.C., Zbozinek, T., Vervliet, B., 2014. Maximizing exposure therapy: an inhibitory learning approach. Behav. Res. Therapy 58, 10–23. Available from: http://dx.doi.org/10.1016/j.brat.2014.04.006.

Dreikurs, R., Corsini, R., 1954. Twenty years of group psychotherapy; purposes, methods and mechanisms. Am. J. Psychiatry 110 (8), 567–575.

Flannery-Schroeder, E., Kendall, P., 2000. Group and individual cognitive-behavioral treatments for youth with anxiety disorders: a randomized clinical trial. Cogn. Ther. Res. 24 (3), 251–278.

Frankel, F., Myatt, R., Sugar, C., Whitham, C., Gorospe, C.M., Laugeson, E., 2010. A randomized controlled study of parent assisted children's friendship training with children having autism spectrum disorders. J. Autism Dev. Disord. 40, 827–842. Available from: http://dx.doi.org/10.1007/s10803-009-0932-z.

Freedman, J., Combs, G., 1996. Narrative Therapy. W.W. Norton & Company, New York, NY.

Garland, E., Clark, S., 1995. Taming Worry Dragons: A Manual for Children, Parents and Other Coaches. British Columbia's Children's Hospital, Vancouver, Canada.

Hagopian, L.P., Jennett, H.K., 2014. Behavioral assessment and treatment for anxiety for those with autism spectrum disorder. In: Davis III, T.E., White, S.W., Ollendick, T.H. (Eds.), Handbook of Autism and Anxiety. Springer, New York, NY, pp. 155–169.

Kasari, C., Rotheram-Fuller, E., Locke, J., Gulsrud, A., 2012. Making the connection: randomized controlled trial of social skills at school for children with autism spectrum disorders. J. Child Psychol. Psychiatry 53 (4), 431–439. Available from: http://dx.doi.org/10.1111/j.1469-7610.2011.02493.x.

Kendall, P.C., Beidas, R.S., 2007. Smoothing the trail for dissemination of evidence-based practices for youth: flexibility within fidelity. Prof. Psychol. Res. Pract. 38, 13–20.

Kendall, P.C., Hedtke, K., 2006a.). Coping Cat Workbook, 2nd ed. Workbook Publishing, Ardmore, PA.

Kendall, P.C., Hedtke, K., 2006b. Cognitive-Behavioral Therapy for Anxious Children: Therapist Manual, 3rd ed. Workbook Publishing, Ardmore, PA.

Kerns, K., Kendall, P., 2012. The presentation and classification of anxiety in autism spectrum disorder. Clin. Psychol. 19 (4), 323–347. Available from: http://dx.doi.org/10.1111/cpsp.12009.

Kerns, C.M., Kendall, P.C., Berry, L., Souders, M.C., Franklin, M.E., Schultz, R.T., et al., 2014. Traditional and atypical presentations of anxiety in youth with autism spectrum disorder. J. Autism Dev. Disord. 44 (11), 2851e2861. Available from: http://dx.doi.org/10.1007/s10803-014-2141-7.

Koegel, L., Koegel, R., Dunlap, G., 1996. Positive Behavioral Support: Including People with Difficult Behavior in the Community. Paul Brookes Publishing, Baltimore, MD.

Kroeger, K.A., Schultz, J.R., Newsom, C., 2007. A comparison of two group-delivered social skills programs for young children with autism. J. Autism Dev. Disorders 37, 808–817. Available from: http://dx.doi.org/10.1007/s10803-006-0207-x.

Kronenberger, W.G., Meyer, R.G., 2001. The Child Clinician's Handbook, 2nd ed. Allyn & Bacon, Needham Heights, MA.

Laugeson, E.A., Park, M.N., 2014. Using a CBT approach to teach social skills to adolescents with autism spectrum disorder and other social challenges: the PEERS method. J. Ration. Emotive Cogn. Behav. Therapy 32 (1), 84–97. Available from: http://dx.doi.org/10.1007/s10942-014-0181-8.

Lochman, J.E., Wells, K.C., 2003. The Coping Power program for preadolescent aggressive boys and their parents: effects at the one-year follow-up. J. Consult. Clin. Psychol. 72 (4), 571–578.

Manassis, K., Mendlowitz, S.L., Scapillato, D., Avery, D., Fiksenbaum, L., Freire, M., et al., 2002. Group and individual cognitive-behavioral therapy for childhood anxiety disorders. A randomized trial. J. Am. Acad. Child Adolesc. Psychiatry 41, 1423–1430. Available from: http://dx.doi.org/10.1097/01.CHI.0000024879.60748.5E.

McConachie, H., McLaughlin, E., Grahame, V., Taylor, H., Honey, E., Tavernor, L., et al., 2014. Group therapy for anxiety in children with autism spectrum disorder. Autism 18 (6), 723–732. Available from: http://dx.doi.org/10.1177/1362361313488839.

McNally Keehn, R.H., Lincoln, A.J., Brown, M.Z., Chavira, D.A., 2013. The Coping Cat program for children with anxiety and autism spectrum disorder: a pilot randomized controlled trial. J. Autism Dev. Disord. 43 (1), 57–67. Available from: http://dx.doi.org/10.1007/s10803-012-1541-9.

Moree, B.N., Davis, T.E., 2010. Cognitive-behavioral therapy for anxiety in children diagnosed with autism spectrum disorders: modification trends. Res. Autism Spect. Disord. 4 (3), 346–354. Available from: http://dx.doi.org/10.1016/j.rasd.2009.10.015.

Moreno, J.L., 1946. Psychodrama and group psychotherapy. Sociometry 9 (2/3), 249–253.

Otero, T., Schatz, R., Merrill, A., Bellini, S., 2015. Social skills training for youth with autism spectrum disorders: a follow-up. Child Adolesc. Psychiatric Clin. N. Am. 24 (1), 99–115.

Peterman, J., Read, K., Wei, C., Kendall, P.C., 2015. The art of exposure: putting science into practice. Cogn. Behav. Pract. 22, 379–392.

Pratt, J., 1945. The group method in the treatment of psychosomatic disorders. Sociometry 8, 85–93.

Puleo, C.M., Kendall, P.C., 2011. Anxiety disorders in typically developing youth: autism spectrum symptoms as a predictor of cognitive–behavioral treatment. J. Autism Dev. Disord. 41, 275–286.

Rao, P.A., Beidel, D.C., Murray, M.J., 2008. Social skills interventions for children with asperger's syndrome or high-functioning autism: a review and recommendations. J. Autism Dev. Disord. 38, 353–361. Available from: http://dx.doi.org/10.1007/s10803-007-0402-4.

Reaven, J., Wainer, A., 2015. Children and adolescents with ASD and co-occurring psychiatric conditions: current trends in intervention. Int. Rev. Res. Dev. Disabil. 49, 45–90. Available from: http://dx.doi.org/10.1016/bs.irrdd.2015.06.001.

Reaven, J., Blakeley-Smith, A., Nichols, S., Dasari, M., Flanigan, E., Hepburn, S., 2009. Cognitive-behavioral group treatment for anxiety symptoms in children with high-functioning autism spectrum disorders: a pilot study. Focus Autism Other Dev. Disabil. 24 (1), 27–37. Available from: http://dx.doi.org/10.1177/1088357608327666.

Reaven, J., Blakeley-Smith, A., Nichols, S., Hepburn, S., 2011. Facing Your Fears: Group Therapy for Managing Anxiety in Children With High-Functioning Autism Spectrum Disorders. Paul Brookes Publishing, Baltimore, MD.

Reaven, J., Blakeley-Smith, A., Culhane-Shelburne, K., Hepburn, S., 2012a. Group cognitive behavior therapy for children with high-functioning autism spectrum disorders and anxiety: a randomized trial. J. Child Psychol. Psychiatry 53 (4), 410–419.

Reaven, J., Blakeley-Smith, A., Leuthe, E., Moody, E., Hepburn, S., 2012b. Facing your fears in adolescence: cognitive-behavioral therapy for high-functioning autism spectrum disorders and anxiety. Autism Res. Treat. Available from: http://dx.doi.org/10.1155/2012/423905.

Reaven, J., Blakeley-Smith, A., Beattie, T., Sullivan, A., Moody, E., Stern, J., et al., 2014. Improving transportability of a cognitive-behavioral intervention for anxiety in youth with autism spectrum disorders: results from a US-Canada collaboration. Autism. Available from: http://dx.doi.org/10.1177/1362361313518124.

Reichow, B., Volkmar, F., 2010. Social skills interventions for individuals with autism: evaluation for evidence-based practices within a best evidence synthesis framework. J. Autism Dev. Disorders 40 (2), 149–166. Available from: http://dx.doi.org/10.1007/s10803-009-0842-0.

Reichow, B., Steiner, M., Volkmar, F., 2012. Social skills groups for people aged 6 to 21 with autism spectrum disorders (ASD). Campbell Syst. Rev.1–75. Available from: http://dx.doi.org/10.1002/14651858.

Silverman, W., Albano, A., 1996. Anxiety Disorders Interview Schedule for Children for DSM-IV: (Child and Parent Versions). Psychological Corporation, San Antonio, TX.

Sofronoff, K., Attwood, T., Hinton, S., 2005. A randomized controlled trial of a CBT intervention for anxiety in children with Asperger syndrome. J. Child Psychol. Psychiatry 46, 1152–1160. Available from: http://dx.doi.org/10.1111/j.1469-7610.2005.00411.x.

Storch, E.A., Arnold, E.B., Lewin, A.B., Nadeau, J.M., Jones, A.M., De Nadai, A.S., et al., 2013. The effect of cognitive-behavioral therapy versus treatment as usual for anxiety in children with autism spectrum disorders: a randomized, controlled trial. J. Am. Acad. Child Adolesc. Psychiatry 52 (2), 132–142. Available from: http://dx.doi.org/10.1016/j.jaac.2012.11.007.

Sung, M., Ooi, Y.P., Goh, T.J., Pathy, P., Fung, D.S.S., Ang, R.P., et al., 2011. Effects of cognitive-behavioral therapy on anxiety in children with autism spectrum disorders: a randomized controlled trial. Child Psychiatry Hum. Dev. 42 (6), 634–649. Available from: http://dx.doi.org/10.1007/s10578-011-0238-1.

van Steensel, F., Bogels, S., Perrin, S., 2011. Anxiety disorders in children and adolescents with autistic spectrum disorders: a meta-analysis. Clin. Child Fam. Psychol. Review 14, 302–317. Available from: http://dx.doi.org/10.1007/s10567-011-0097-0.

White, S., Ollendick, T., Albano, A., Oswald, D., Johnson, C., Southam-Gerow, M., et al., 2013. Randomized controlled trial: multimodal anxiety and social skill intervention for adolescents with Autism Spectrum Disorder. J. Autism Dev. Disord. 43 (2), 382–394. Available from: http://dx.doi.org/10.1007/s10803-012-1577-x.

Wood, J., Drahota, A., Sze, K., Har, K., Chiu, A., Langer, D., 2009. Cognitive behavioral therapy for anxiety in children with autism spectrum disorders: a randomized, controlled trial. J. Child Psychol. Psychiatry 50 (3), 224–234. Available from: http://dx.doi.org/10.1111/j.1469-7610.2008.01948.x.

Wood, J.J., McLeod, B.D., 2008. Child Anxiety Disorders: A Treatment Manual for Practitioners. Norton, New York, NY.

Yalom, I., Leszcz, M., 2005. The Theory and Practice of Group Psychotherapy, 5th Edition Basic Books, New York, NY.

CHAPTER 9

Behavioral Treatments for Anxiety in Adults With Autism Spectrum Disorder

Susan W. White[1], Caitlin M. Conner[2] and Brenna B. Maddox[3]
[1]Virginia Tech, Blacksburg, VA, United States
[2]University of Colorado School of Medicine, Aurora, CO, United States
[3]The Children's Hospital of Philadelphia, Philadelphia, PA, United States

INTRODUCTION

Although Autism Spectrum Disorder (ASD) is most often identified during early childhood, it is becoming increasingly apparent that recognition can be delayed and that initial diagnosis of ASD can occur during adulthood. As Lai and Baron-Cohen (2015) proposed, adult identification may be due to an increasing public awareness of ASD as well as a broadening of the diagnostic criteria to include higher functioning individuals who would likely not be seen as having sufficiently severe symptoms during childhood to warrant a diagnosis. Regardless of the underlying causes for the increased, and still increasing, number of adults with ASD and heightened recognition of the disorder in adulthood, it is abundantly clear that more research is needed to inform effective treatment of co-occurring mental health conditions in adults with ASD, including anxiety disorders. In this chapter, we describe the presentation and prevalence of anxiety disorders in adults with ASD and evidence-informed approaches to assess and treat anxiety in this population.

PREVALENCE AND CLINICAL PRESENTATION

It is only in recent years that researchers have begun to investigate adult outcomes among people diagnosed with ASD as children. Largely, the extant research has focused on stability of the ASD diagnosis and severity of ASD over time (Louwerse et al., 2015; Woolfenden et al., 2012) and quality of life in adulthood and variables associated with adult outcomes (Howlin, 2000). Recently, however, data on rates of psychiatric

Anxiety in Children and Adolescents with Autism Spectrum Disorder.
DOI: http://dx.doi.org/10.1016/B978-0-12-805122-1.00009-0
© 2017 Elsevier Inc.
All rights reserved.

comorbidity in adults with ASD have been reported (e.g., Lai and Baron-Cohen, 2015). Although this research is fairly young and epidemiological research is very limited, it is apparent that adults diagnosed with ASD have more co-occurring medical and mental health diagnoses than do adults without ASD. This finding has been reported in international samples and when psychopathology is viewed diagnostically as well as dimensionally.

For example, a large, case controlled study of health records has shown that rates of all the major mental health disorders, including anxiety disorders, are elevated among adults with ASD relative to age- and sex-matched nonASD adults (Croen et al., 2015). In addition, Bruggink and colleagues (2016) found that adults with ASD self-reported significantly more symptoms anxiety and depression, compared to an age- and gender-matched control sample of adults and Croen and colleagues (2015) found that more than half of their sample ($n = 1507$) of adults with ASD were diagnosed with at least one additional mental health condition. Anxiety disorders were more commonly diagnosed than any other mental health diagnosis. Almost one-third (29%) of the sample had anxiety disorder diagnoses (not including obsessive-compulsive disorder [OCD], which was an additional 8%). By comparison, among the age- and sex-matched controls (10 controls for every proband), 9% had an anxiety disorder. Hofvander and colleagues (2009) found that anxiety disorders were second only to mood disorders in terms of prevalence. Half of their clinical sample of 122 adults met criteria for at least one anxiety disorder, with generalized anxiety disorder (GAD) being the most frequently diagnosed anxiety disorder (15%), followed closely by social anxiety disorder (SAD; 13%).

In a follow-up study with adults who were diagnosed with ASD as children and who had at least average cognitive ability, 56% of the sample ($n = 58$, mean age = 44 years) experienced mental health problems in adulthood (Moss et al., 2015). Although specific disorders were not diagnosed, 10% of the sample surpassed the clinical cut-off on a self-reported anxiety scale (Beck Anxiety Inventory: BAI; Beck and Steer, 1990) and 29% surpassed the cut-off for OCD (based on Y-BOCS (Goodman et al., 1989) with items added from the Children's Yale-Brown Obsessive-Compulsive Scale-Pervasive Developmental Disorders: CY-BOCS-PDD; Scahill et al., 2006).

There is a slowly emerging picture of the onset and course of co-occurring anxiety problems in ASD among adults. Although problems with anxiety can emerge during adulthood, for the majority of adults with ASD, it is more likely that anxiety onset is during childhood. In a retrospective study of adults diagnosed with ASD without intellectual disability, Maddox and White (2015) found that, among adults with ASD and SAD, onset of impairing social anxiety was most often during middle school.

Cognitive and verbal ability may be predictive of problems with anxiety in this population. Gotham and colleagues (2015) found that verbal IQ was positively associated with anxiety among adults with ASD. ASD severity, gauged by self-report *via* the Autism Spectrum Quotient (AQ; Baron-Cohen et al., 2001), has also been found to be positively associated with social anxiety (Bejerot et al., 2014). There is evidence that anxiety is more problematic among women than men with ASD (Croen et al., 2015) and that anxiety symptoms worsen more sharply during adolescence and early adulthood for females with ASD, compared to males with ASD (Gotham et al., 2015). This gender difference has not been found consistently. Lugnegård and colleagues (2011) found no gender differences with respect to rates of psychiatric comorbidity in their high-functioning adult sample. The potentially moderating role of gender is consistent with prior research showing that in childhood, girls are at greater risk for anxiety and mood problems than boys with ASD (May et al., 2013; Solomon et al., 2012), but divergent from the comparable rates of anxiety disorders across the genders seen in treatment seeking children with anxiety who do not have ASD (Kendall et al., 2010).

In one of the only qualitative studies on the phenomenology of anxiety in ASD during adulthood, Trembath and colleagues (2012) conducted focus groups with 11 diagnosed adults. They found the primary sources of anxiety identified by these individuals to be related to the environment (e.g., crowds), social interaction, concern for others (e.g., broad societal issues), fearful anticipation, and disappointment. These anxiety triggers are similar to the findings of Gillott and Standen (2007) who, using a quantitative approach, found that anxiety was associated with having to cope with change, anticipation, personal contact, and sensory stimulation among adults with ASD.

Based on this fairly limited research base on anxiety in adults with ASD and extrapolating from the more mature research base with children and adolescents, we can surmise that anxiety, of all types, is common among adults with ASD. Adults with ASD experience more anxiety, based on self- and other-report, than do neurotypical adults and adults with other types of developmental disabilities. Additionally, anxiety may be more problematic, or at least more often recognized, among adults who do not have co-occurring intellectual disability. However, this conclusion is tentative as the majority of prior studies have been with higher functioning, cognitive unimpaired samples. It is possible that reliance on verbalization of internal symptoms and self-report diminishes our ability to accurately assess for anxiety in adults with ASD who are less verbal or cognitively impaired, thus inflating the actual effect of cognitive ability. The limited research with adult samples with ASD and intellectual disability, however, suggests that anxiety is more problematic for those who have co-occurring ASD than for adults with intellectual disability without ASD (Cervantes and Matson, 2015).

EVIDENCE-INFORMED ASSESSMENT OF ANXIETY IN ADULTS WITH ASD

Historically, the degree to which any anxiety disorder can truly be "comorbid" alongside ASD has been unclear. Specifically, given the high prevalence of anxiety in the context of ASD it has been debated whether anxiety *could* be diagnosed as a comorbid disorder, or whether anxiety was a phenomenological manifestation, more core to the ASD itself (Kerns and Kendall, 2012). Most experts now agree that anxiety disorders, as clinical conditions distinct from ASD in terms of etiology and treatment, can and do frequently co-occur with ASD and, as such, can be separable diagnosable disorders (e.g., Lai and Baron-Cohen, 2015). Although the mechanisms underlying co-occurrence of anxiety in ASD are not fully understood, Lai and Baron-Cohen (2015) suggest that two probable pathways are shared causative factors (e.g., amygdala hyper-reactivity) and anxiety resulting, directly or indirectly, from the ASD itself (e.g., social alienation, need for sameness).

How anxiety is assessed (e.g., observational tools, self-reports) and conceptualized (e.g., as a separable condition that is the same as anxiety in neurotypical individuals or something related to ASD) greatly affect how the manifest symptoms are "counted" or categorized diagnostically. Accurate diagnostic assessment of apparent anxiety problems in adults with ASD is often challenging. Primary reasons for this challenge include limited insight into and reliance on verbal reporting for internal symptoms of anxiety (e.g., worries, self-doubt, fear of negative evaluation), which affect self-reporting. Alexithymia, or the inability to identify and label one's own emotions, as well as impaired attention and executive function (e.g., inability to step back and contemplate what one is fearful about, outside of the moment or after the situation has passed) also contribute to this diagnostic quandary.

The research base on anxiety, and its treatment, in adults with ASD has primarily relied on measures developed for evaluating anxiety in typical, nonASD adults. Self-report measures, such as the BAI (Beck and Steer, 1990) and the Symptom Check List (SCL-90; Derogatis, 1977), have been used (e.g., Bruggink et al., 2016; Moss et al., 2015). Researchers (e.g., Maddox and White, 2015) have also used semi-structured diagnostic interviews, such as the Anxiety Disorders Interview Schedule for DSM-IV (ADIS-IV-C/P; Brown et al., 1994), with cognitively unimpaired adults. With respect to measurement of specific types of anxiety disorder symptoms, arguably the most research has occurred in the area of social anxiety. The Social Anxiety Scale (SAS; La Grecaand Lopez, 1998) has been used as both self- and parent-report (e.g., Swain et al., 2015). There has been very little development of tools for assessing anxiety specifically in adults with ASD. The Social Anxiety Scale for People with ASD (SASPA; Kreiser and White, 2011) is one exception. The SASPA is a self-report measure of social anxiety symptoms that are not confounded by core ASD symptoms, such as behavioral avoidance owing to lack of social interest. Unfortunately, there is very little rigorous evaluation of the sensitivity or validity of most of these measures, including the SASPA. Additionally, there is a dearth of measures that are appropriate for adults yet available as both caregiver- and self-report, which poses a considerable challenge for service providers attempting to assess adults with ASD who may also have cognitive limitations or be functionally delayed (e.g., living with parents, no employment). In this situation, the evaluator typically must decide between using a measure for children or adolescents, that might better lend itself to parental report (e.g., rely on behavioral indicators), or asking the caregiver to try to intuit about symptoms that are difficult for any third party to ascertain in a valid way (e.g., feelings of despair, negative interpretations).

Clinically, it can be helpful to set up situations, or presses, that are likely to trigger the symptoms of interest in order to assess them "in the moment." For instance, the clinician can observe how the client responds when a new student introduces herself (social stress) or when there is an unanticipated event, such as changing to a different, unfamiliar assessment room. Sequencing symptoms, and associated impairment, is also helpful. Although impairments in socialization and interpersonal communication must be present (even if not identified as such) early in childhood for diagnosis of ASD, new symptoms in this domain or their worsening during late adolescence or in adulthood may be suggestive of anxiety in addition to the ASD. Caution must be taken, however, as core and secondary symptoms of ASD often change over the course of development. For example, whereas behavioral avoidance of social situations tends to decline during adolescence among typically developing youth, behavioral avoidance as well as fear of negative evaluation has been found to be higher among adolescents with ASD relative to children (under 12 years) with ASD, based on cross-sectional data (Kuusikko et al., 2008). As such, a carefully illustrated timeline and an informed understanding of the heterotypic continuity within ASD can inform the clinician's differential diagnosis, as well as help the client with reporting on events and symptom onset.

The practice demand for empirically supported tools for the screening and diagnosis of anxiety disorders in people with ASD is great. Indeed, many adults are referred for additional diagnostic evaluation due to problems with mood and anxiety (e.g., Hofvander et al., 2009). Evidence-based assessment of co-occurring conditions, including anxiety disorders, in adult ASD warrants further study. As this research base develops, given the substantial phenotypic overlap between many of the anxiety disorders and ASD symptoms, we suggest a nuanced assessment that goes beyond symptom count, duration, distress, and interference when determining if an anxiety disorder in comorbidity presents in a client with ASD.

The conceptual overlap between anxiety disorders and ASD is perhaps best exemplified by considering SAD and ASD. Social awkwardness and difficulty in social interaction, which are hallmark features of ASD, are often considered in the evaluation of possible SAD. This type of social difficulty can be due to impaired ability to infer others' thoughts and feelings (theory of mind impairment), underdeveloped interaction skills, or awkward social behaviors (i.e., a fluency deficit). Social difficulty can also be due to anxiety and related social avoidance. In a person with ASD, all these factors may underlie the manifest social difficulty. In practice, when faced with a client who is socially avoidant and hyper-aroused in social interaction and performance situations, the clinician probes into the reasons for avoidance and variability in arousal. The client with ASD who does not have co-occurring SAD may, for instance, report feelings of discomfort when around others due to a variety of reasons (e.g., too loud, unsure of what to do or say socially), but deny any socio-evaluative fears or perhaps even thoughts about the repercussions of social missteps. If these factors are not evaluated, the SAD diagnosis may be misapplied. In this example, a consideration of the factors underlying the observed problem (e.g., social avoidance) will inform diagnosis and the treatment approach that is taken. In this case, for example, the clinician may target skill deficits primarily and general anxiety and sensory sensitivities adjunctively, but not engage in exposures targeting fear of social evaluation.

TARGETING KEY MECHANISMS

Determination of the processes that influence and give rise to co-occurring psychopathology can allow for the targeting of specific symptoms in treatment. Likewise, ascertainment of the mechanisms that mediate clinical changes (e.g., symptom reduction) as a result of effective treatment can facilitate treatment personalization (the choice of one treatment over another for a given client), improve treatment outcome, and augment adaptations to current and future treatments (Kazdin, 2007; Norcross and Wampold, 2011; Paul, 1967). Because the understanding of *how, why,* and *for whom* these treatments work is largely unknown, despite the number of empirically based treatments for anxiety in individuals with ASD (mostly for children and adolescents), study of the etiological and treatment mechanisms is an essential next step in our growing research base.

BASIC PROCESSES UNDERLYING ANXIETY IN ASD

Several commonly seen deficits among individuals with ASD could underlie anxiety symptoms. The social deficits required for a diagnosis of ASD have been postulated to contribute to increased anxiety, especially social anxiety symptoms, at least for a subset of individuals with insight into their social deficits (White et al., 2014). Additionally, social motivation, the extent to which a person is interested in interacting with others, could play a role in anxiety among individuals with ASD. Swain and colleagues (2015) found that greater social motivation was associated with higher social anxiety among 69 young adults with ASD, who participated in a social skills intervention, suggesting that the desire to interact may also increase anxiety for adults with ASD.

Alternatively, there may be core processes that contribute independently to both symptoms of ASD and symptoms of anxiety. For instance, alexithymia may contribute to or exacerbate social deficits, as well as lead to anxiety among individuals with ASD. Up to 50% of individuals with ASD have been observed to experience difficulty in identifying and describing their emotions (Lombardo et al., 2007). Difficulties in labeling others' emotional states likely contribute to theory of mind deficits, the ability to surmise another person's perspective and emotional state, which compromise social interaction and may lead to discomfort or anxiety (Mazefsky and Herrington, 2014). Indeed, adults with ASD have been found to misinterpret happy face stimuli as negative, potentially indicative of a bias that could lead to anxiety (Eack et al., 2015). These results are consistent with a previous meta-analysis of emotion recognition research in ASD across the lifespan, finding that individuals with ASD are significantly less able to recognize emotions other than happiness in face stimuli (Uljarevic and Hamilton, 2012). In addition, individuals with ASD have been shown to have difficulties with their own emotion expression (Trubanova, 2015), which can also diminish the ability to interact with others.

The second cluster of symptoms in the diagnostic criteria for ASD, repetitive and restricted behaviors or interests, contains several behaviors that overlap with anxiety symptomatology. Symptoms that may be present for a diagnosis of ASD include resistance to changes in routine and in one's environment, as well as sensory hypersensitivity or hyposensitivity (APA, 2013). These symptoms may lead individuals to experience their world as volatile and overwhelming, thus contributing to fear and anxiety (Mazefsky and Herrington, 2014). Similarly, intense focus or perseveration on specific topics of interest, although typically thought of as relating to topics that the individual enjoys, may signify an overall emotional and cognitive style characterized by difficulty shifting one's attention (Mazefsky and Herrington, 2014; White et al., 2014). This cognitive "stickiness" can easily be re-construed as rumination if focused upon negative thoughts or emotions, and has been hypothesized to account for increased negative affect and emotional lability for individuals with ASD (Keehn et al., 2013).

EMOTION REGULATION

Emotion regulation (ER) can be defined as one's attempts to monitor and modulate their emotional experience (Gross and Thompson, 2007).

Traditionally, research has categorized ER strategies as typically adaptive or maladaptive, although whether ER is adaptive for the individual is dependent upon context (Aldao and Nolen-Hoeksema, 2012). Among typically developing individuals, ER impairment or over-reliance on maladaptive ER strategies has been posited to be associated with many forms of psychopathology (Aldao et al., 2010; Gross, 2002). Similarly, ER deficits have been studied as a potential underlying factor for many of the associated behavioral problems seen in ASD, such as aggression, irritability, and anxiety (Mazefsky and White, 2014; Mazefsky et al., 2013; Samson et al., 2015; Weiss, 2014; White et al., 2014). White and colleagues (2014) proposed a model of how various social-cognitive, neurological, and physiological mechanisms contribute to ER impairments, thus leading to heightened levels of anxiety among individuals with ASD. They posited, based on extant research on typically developing individuals, that ER difficulties in ASD arise in part from ASD-associated symptomatology, such as challenges with emotion recognition and expression, difficulty with attentional processes such as shifting one's attention, neural hyper- and hypoconnectivity, physiological overarousal, and avoidance (White et al., 2014). Further empirical research is needed to better elucidate the relationship of maladaptive ER and ASD.

In terms of intervention, targeting maladaptive ER has also been posited as a means to address the underlying factors that contribute to anxiety disorders (Weiss, 2014). As transdiagnostic treatments, such as Barlow and colleagues' Unified Protocol (Barlow et al., 2004), have been used for the treatment of emotional disorders in individuals without ASD, such an approach has been suggested for ER difficulties, as they may underlie not only anxiety, but other common co-occurring difficulties in ASD such as irritability and depressive symptoms (Weiss, 2014).

MINDFULNESS AND ACCEPTANCE

Another potential mechanism for anxiety treatment is mindfulness and acceptance. As previously mentioned, adults with ASD often seem to demonstrate lack of insight into their and others' emotional states (Lombardo et al., 2007). Mindful awareness practices often ask individuals to attend to their thoughts, bodily sensations, and breathing, which can serve to improve one's ability to notice their own emotions (Segal et al., 2002). Similarly, cognitive inflexibility, which is often observed among adults with ASD (Eack et al., 2013), can also be facilitated by mindfulness/acceptance-based treatments, as the focus upon accepting negative thoughts and emotions when they occur can be applied towards rigidity, or the difficulties that arise from routines being broken (Lee and Orsillo, 2014).

A treatment study of adapted mindfulness-based cognitive therapy (MBCT) for adults with ASD looked at rumination as a potential mechanism of treatment for anxiety and depressive symptoms (Spek et al., 2013), and found that the treatment did decrease affective symptoms partially *via* reduction of rumination. Given the chronicity of ASD and the proposed relationship between ASD and anxiety (White et al., 2014), utilizing mindfulness- and acceptance-based interventions (MABIs) may be especially useful to target anxiety in this population. MABIs focus upon redirecting one's attention and one's relationship to negative or maladaptive thoughts and emotions such as worries and anxiety, rather than the traditional cognitive-behavioral therapy (CBT) focus upon identifying and changing maladaptive cognitions.

BEHAVIORAL TREATMENTS
Evidence Base in Adults Without ASD

CBT is well-investigated and widely regarded as the first-line psychological intervention for adults without ASD who struggle with anxiety (Butler et al., 2006). CBT includes graduated exposure to feared stimuli and cognitive restructuring (i.e., modifying dysfunctional cognitions). In addition to the already well-established CBT approaches, there has been increasing interest in "third wave" or "new wave" behavioral and cognitive-behavioral therapies, such as acceptance and commitment therapy (ACT) and mindfulness-based interventions for the treatment of anxiety disorders (Newby et al., 2015). Acceptance- and mindfulness-based treatments aim to increase a person's psychological flexibility through mindfulness, nonjudgmental awareness, and acceptance (Hayes et al., 2006). These newer approaches are beginning to demonstrate efficacy in treating anxiety (particularly GAD, SAD, and OCD) in adults without ASD (Bluett et al., 2014). For example, in a randomized controlled trial (RCT) comparing CBT, ACT, and a waitlist control for 87 adults with SAD, both treatment groups outperformed the control group, with no significant differences between the CBT and ACT groups on self-report, clinician-rated, or public-speaking outcomes (Craske et al., 2014).

EXTANT RESEARCH IN ADULTS WITH ASD

Although the majority of work in this field has focused on children and adolescents with ASD (see Chapter 8: Group Cognitive Behavior Therapy for Children and Adolescents with Anxiety and Autism Spectrum Disorders and this chapter), an emerging body of research suggests that cognitive-behavioral interventions—including CBT and mindfulness-based techniques—can effectively reduce anxiety in adults on the autism spectrum (Kiep et al., 2015; Spain et al., 2015). Cardaciotto and Herbert (2004) reported a case study of treating anxiety in an adult with ASD. A 23-year-old male with Asperger's Disorder and SAD demonstrated a consistent decrease in symptoms of social anxiety and comorbid depression, as determined by self-report measures, throughout the 14-week individual CBT program. At the 2-month follow-up assessment, the young man no longer met diagnostic criteria for SAD.

Weiss and Lunsky (2010) conducted a case series of group-based, manualized CBT for three adults with Asperger's and co-occurring anxiety or mood disorders. One male participant in his mid-50s had a diagnosis of panic disorder with agoraphobia, along with impairing symptoms of SAD. Although his self-report of anxiety symptoms did not significantly decrease across the 12 weekly sessions, he showed notable gains behaviorally in the group setting (e.g., less flushed while speaking, reduced tremble in his voice, increased eye contact with others). The other two group members (one male with depression and one female with depression and post-traumatic stress disorder) showed a decrease in self-reported anxiety symptoms over the course of treatment. Another study of a group-based CBT program with 32 older adolescents and young adults with ASD (23 males; age 15−25; mean age = 20.6 years) found significant reductions in self-reported depression and stress, but not anxiety, for the treatment group, relative to the waitlist control group (McGillivray and Evert, 2014). The improvements were maintained at 3- and 9-month follow-up assessments.

Promising results have also been reported regarding the treatment of adults with ASD and co-occurring OCD (Russell et al., 2009, 2013). The first published study (Russell et al., 2009) was a nonrandomized trial comparing CBT for OCD to treatment as usual (TAU) in 24 adults with ASD and co-occurring OCD (21 males; mean age = 28 years). All participants had average cognitive abilities. OCD symptoms, as measured by the Y-BOCS (Goodman et al., 1989) total severity score, significantly decreased pre- to post-treatment for the CBT group ($d = 1.01$), but not the TAU group. However, in 50% of the CBT cases, the Y-BOCS was completed by the treating therapist, which is a potential confound. In addition, the CBT group had more severe OCD symptoms at baseline, relative to the TAU group. To improve upon this initial pilot study, Russell and colleagues (2013) conducted a RCT of CBT for OCD with 46 cognitively unimpaired adolescents and adults with ASD (35 males; mean age = 27 years). The control group received an equivalent number of sessions of anxiety management (AM), which included psychoeducation about anxiety and general anxiety reduction techniques (e.g., diaphragmatic breathing, progressive muscle relaxation, problem solving training). The AM manual did not include any of the active ingredients of CBT (e.g., exposure–response prevention) for OCD or any cognitive techniques addressing OCD-related beliefs. Study assessors were blind to treatment assignment. Both groups demonstrated a significant reduction in OCD symptoms, based on Y-BOCS total severity score (within-group effect sizes of 1.01 for the CBT group and 0.6 for the AM group). The groups did not significantly differ in OCD symptoms at post-treatment, although the CBT group had more responders (45% *versus* 20%, with treatment response defined as >25% reduction in Y-BOCS total severity score). In addition, the CBT group (but not the AM group) completed a one-year follow-up assessment, and the treatment gains were sustained over this period (Russell et al., 2013).

In a RCT conducted by Spek et al. (2013), the results demonstrated that adults with ASD and co-occurring anxiety can benefit from modified mindfulness-based therapy (MBT). Their treatment was based on MBCT for depression in adults without ASD (Segal et al., 2002), with the cognitive elements (e.g., examining the content of one's thoughts) omitted, given the difficulties with information processing that are characteristic of ASD. Primary program content included mindful meditation exercises (e.g., eating, walking, breathing), along with psychoeducation about physical reactions to stress and ruminative thoughts. Forty-two cognitively unimpaired participants with ASD (27 males; mean age = 42 years) were randomized to the 9-week group-based MBT program (with each session lasting 2.5 hours) or a waitlist control group. At post-treatment, the intervention group demonstrated a significant decrease in self-reported anxiety and a significant increase in self-reported positive effect, whereas the control group did not. Kiep and colleagues (2015) examined the same MBT protocol in 50 cognitively unimpaired adults with ASD (34 males; mean age = 40 years) and found similar results. The reduction in anxiety symptoms remained stable at a 9-week follow-up.

In addition to preliminary evidence for treatment efficacy for traditional CBT and MBT approaches, these studies document treatment feasibility and acceptability with adults who have ASD (e.g., high attendance rate, high homework completion rate). The rule-bound, analytical style of thinking that is characteristic of people with ASD may be particularly well-suited to a CBT approach (Gaus, 2011). Case reports of adults receiving CBT suggest that the clients liked the structure and predictability of the treatment sessions, along with the scientific aspects of the CBT model (Weiss and Lunsky, 2010). However, clinicians can also face significant challenges when conducting CBT with adults who have ASD (Kerns et al., 2016). For example, parental involvement is a key component of effective CBT for children with ASD and anxiety, but including parents in treatment of adults may interfere with the adult client's independence or may not be possible due to practical considerations. Without a parent or other support person to help with treatment engagement and the generalization of skills, some adult clients may struggle to complete in-session or between-session therapeutic activities due to limited inherent motivation or executive functioning difficulties.

More research on behavioral treatments for anxiety in adults with ASD is clearly needed. As highlighted here, only a handful of fairly small *n* studies have addressed this common comorbidity, with most lacking a rigorous design. In addition, these studies have focused exclusively on cognitively unimpaired adults with ASD, leaving important questions about the appropriateness of cognitive-behavioral approaches for adults with intellectual disability and anxiety unaddressed.

PRIMARY MODIFICATIONS TO BEHAVIORAL TREATMENTS FOR ADULTS WITH ASD AND ANXIETY

Research suggests that behavioral treatments demonstrated to be effective with clients who do not have ASD are applicable to people with ASD, with some adjustments. Adapting the structure, content, and process of cognitive-behavioral approaches may be important due to differences in learning styles between adults with and without ASD, core ASD symptoms such as social communication impairments that affect therapeutic rapport, and common difficulties with emotion recognition and executive function (Gaus, 2007, 2011). These modifications to improve engagement, acceptability, and utility of CBT have mostly been evaluated in anxiety treatment studies for youth with ASD (Lang et al., 2010).

Several studies for adults with ASD have described adaptations to CBT or mindfulness techniques, and these adaptations often include an increased number of sessions with more frequent practice of cognitive restructuring and exposure exercises, emphasis on social skills training, additional information using concrete examples to enhance the client's understanding of emotions, inclusion of visual aids and written materials, avoidance of colloquialisms or metaphors, reliance on a more directive (rather than Socratic) therapeutic style, and incorporation of the client's circumscribed interests (Ekman and Hiltunen, 2015; Spain et al., 2015). In the two published studies of MBT for anxiety in adults with ASD (Kiep et al., 2015; Spek et al., 2013), the cognitive elements (e.g., exercises examining the content of one's thoughts) were omitted, the original program length was increased from 8 weekly sessions to 9 weekly sessions, and the original three-minute breathing exercise was extended to five minutes.

MEDICAL/PHARMACOLOGICAL TREATMENTS

Evidence Base in Adults With ASD

Research into pharmacological treatment for anxiety among typically developing adults has yielded promising results. Across the anxiety disorders and OCD, pharmacological and cognitive-behavioral treatments have been found to be equally effective in meta-analyses, although debate over relative efficacy, in the context of side-effects and gain longevity, continues (American Psychiatric Association [APA], 2007). In the APA's existing treatment guidelines, individual factors such as symptom severity, comorbid mental health conditions, and previous treatment history should be considered.

In contrast, relatively little research has been conducted at this point on pharmacological treatment of anxiety disorders among adults with ASD (see Table 9.1). An epidemiological study of adults with ASD, first diagnosed with ASD in childhood approximately 30 years prior, observed that 71% of the sample were taking at least one prescription medication, and 58.9% were taking one or more psychotropic medications, with antipsychotics used by over 1/3 of the sample despite an anxiety disorder listed as the most frequent comorbid psychiatric diagnosis (Buck et al., 2014). However, only two medications (risperidone and

Table 9.1 Adult ASD medication trials for anxiety and repetitive behaviors

	Medication	Methodology	Target	Symptom assessment
McDougle et al. (1992)	Clomipramine	Case series of 5 Age: 13–33 years old	OCD symptoms and impulsivity	Clinician observation of OCD symptoms and Aberrant Behavior Checklist
McDougle et al. (1996)	Fluvoxamine	Double-blind, placebo controlled trial 30 adults age 18–60 years old	Repetitive thoughts and behaviors	Y-BOCS and Ritvo-Freeman Real-Life Rating Scale (including Sensory Motor Behaviors and Sensory Responses)
Hollander et al. (2012)	Fluoxetine	Double-blind, placebo controlled trial 37 adults age 18–60 years old	Repetitive thoughts	Y-BOCS compulsions score
Brodkin et al. (1997)	Clomipramine	Open-label 33 adults 18–44 years old	Repetitive thoughts and behaviors	Y-BOCS and Ritvo-Freeman Real-Life Rating Scale (including Sensory Motor Behaviors and Sensory Responses)
Cook et al. (1992)	Fluoxetine	Open-label 23 individuals 7–28 years old	Repetitive behaviors	Via clinical judgment

aripiprazole) are currently FDA-approved specifically for individuals with ASD (Handen et al., 2011).

In light of the common usage of selective serotonin reuptake inhibitors (SSRIs), several studies have looked at the frequency of usage of antianxiety and antidepressant medications in ASD, and these medications' efficacy in treating repetitive behaviors and anxiety (although these studies did not specifically require individuals to have a comorbid anxiety disorder diagnosis). Among adolescents and adults with ASD who have had one or more prior psychiatric emergencies (defined as an acute behavior or mood episode requiring immediate attention and care by family and community), approximately 30% were taking an anxiolytic medication (Lake et al., 2012), while in a study of adolescents and adults with ASD without such an event in their history, 19% of the sample was prescribed either anxiolytic or sedative/hypnotic medications (Esbensen et al., 2009). In a meta-analysis reviewing SSRI usage among individuals with ASD, small positive effects were observed for adults in mostly small-sample studies, and adults with ASD experienced fewer side effects from the medications compared to children with ASD (Williams et al., 2010). However, it has been posited that publication bias may partially account for the generally positive, though small, effect when considering the extant research in composite (Carrasco et al., 2012).

In a review of pharmacotherapy for anxiety and repetitive behaviors in ASD, Propper and Orlik (2014) found evidence for efficacy of fluoxetine, fluvoxamine, and clomipramine among adults with ASD, although they cited limitations in the size and methodology of the studies. In addition to these medications, one open-label study among 42 adults aged 18–39 years with ASD found that sertraline was associated with improvement in repetitive and aggressive behaviors (McDougle et al., 1998). Again, it should be noted that individuals in these studies were not diagnosed with anxiety disorders or OCD, but rather displayed some level of such symptoms. Given that common anxiety symptoms such as repetitive behaviors or thoughts are also ASD core symptoms, focus upon these symptoms as representative of anxiety may not be ideal. Many of these studies, however, have focused specifically upon repetitive behaviors as indicative of anxiety, especially when the adults were cognitively impaired.

PRIMARY MODIFICATIONS TO MEDICAL TREATMENTS OF ANXIETY IN ASD

No guidelines for medication usage exist for treating anxiety in adults with ASD, although clinical case studies and reviews of extant literature provide some instruction. Handen and colleagues (2011) recommend using lower doses than typically given, as adults with ASD often seem to have stronger negative reactions to medications. In addition, they suggest slower dosage titration due to these difficulties (Handen et al., 2011). Propper and Orlik (2014) recommend combined treatments (both psychological and pharmacological) for anxiety or repetitive behaviors in this population. Similar to typically developing individuals with anxiety disorders, pharmacological treatment of anxiety is recommended when comorbid conditions are present, in cases of treatment resistant symptoms, or when treating severe psychopathology that prevents psychological interventions (Soorya et al., 2008). Furthermore, careful monitoring of the medication's effectiveness in treating anxiety symptoms and potential side effects is vital (Propper and Orlik, 2014).

LOOKING FORWARD: NEXT STEPS IN RESEARCH AND PRACTICE

The extant research suggests that anxiety is endemic in ASD. Anxiety is a common experience for adults who have ASD, and often the impetus for treatment referral. Within-person factors such as sex, cognitive/verbal ability, and insight may moderate the experience and severity of anxiety, though more research on factors that affect risk is needed. The adverse impact of anxiety disorders on psychosocial functioning and quality of life in adult samples without ASD has been well-documented (Mendlowicz and Stein, 2000; Olatunji et al., 2007). Although anxiety has not yet been explored as a mechanism that is predictive of, or causally related to, the adverse outcomes often documented among even cognitively more able adults with ASD (Howlin et al., 2004; Taylor and Seltzer, 2011), it is reasonable to expect that untreated anxiety adversely affects quality of life and other outcomes. For instance, anxiety can diminish social relationships, limit willingness to take on new challenges or risks, and decrease enjoyment in daily activities.

Our empirical understanding of the experience of anxiety in adults with ASD has been informed by correlational and cross-sectional research. To move the field forward, longitudinal research is needed, as well as treatment research that is sufficiently powered to detect moderators and identify mechanisms of action that underlie change in observed symptoms.

REFERENCES

Aldao, A., Nolen-Hoeksema, S., 2012. The influence of context on the implementation of adaptive emotion regulation strategies. Behav. Res. Ther. 50 (7), 493–501.

Aldao, A., Nolen-Hoeksema, S., Schweizer, S., 2010. Emotion-regulation strategies across psychopathology: a meta-analytic review. Clin. Psychol. Rev. 30 (2), 217–237.

American Psychiatric Association, 2007. Practice Guideline for the Treatment of Patients with Panic Disorder, second ed. Author, Arlington, VA.

American Psychiatric Association, 2013. Diagnostic and Statistical Manual of Mental Disorders, fifth ed. Author, Washington, DC.

Barlow, D.H., Allen, L.B., Choate, M.L., 2004. Toward a unified treatment for emotional disorders. Behav. Ther. 35 (2), 205–230.

Baron-Cohen, S., Wheelwright, S., Skinner, R., Martin, J., Clubley, E., 2001. The Autism Spectrum Quotient (AQ): evidence from Asperger syndrome/high-functioning autism, males and females, scientists and mathematicians. J. Autism Dev. Disord. 31, 5–17.

Beck, A.T., Steer, R.A., 1990. Beck Anxiety Inventory (BAI). Psychological Corporation, San Antonio, TX.

Bejerot, S., Eriksson, J.M., Möortberg, E., 2014. Social anxiety in adult autism spectrum disorder. Psychiatry Res. 220, 705–707.

Bluett, E.J., Homan, K.J., Morrison, K.L., Levin, M.E., Twohig, M.P., 2014. Acceptance and commitment therapy for anxiety and OCD spectrum disorders: an empirical review. J. Anxiety Disord. 28, 612–624.

Brodkin, E.S., McDougle, C.J., Naylor, S.T., Cohen, D.J., Price, L.H., 1997. Clomipramine in adults with pervasive developmental disorders: a prospective open label investigation. J. Child Adolesc. Psychopharmacol. 7 (2), 109–121.

Brown, T.A., Di Nardo, P.A., Barlow, D.H., 1994. Anxiety Disorders Interview Schedule for DSM-IV (ADIS-IV). Psychological Corporation. Graywind Publications Incorporated, San Antonio, TX.

Bruggink, A., Huisman, S., Vuijk, R., Kraaij, V., Garnefksi, N., 2016. Cognitive emotion regulation, anxiety and depression in adults with autism spectrum disorder. Res. Autism Spectrum Disord. 22, 34–44.

Buck, T.R., Viskochil, J., Farley, M., Coon, H., McMahon, W.M., Morgan, J., et al., 2014. Psychiatric comorbidity and medication use in adults with autism spectrum disorder. J. Autism Dev. Disord. 44, 3063–3071.

Butler, A.C., Chapman, J.E., Forman, E.M., Beck, A.T., 2006. The empirical status of cognitive-behavioral therapy: a review of meta-analyses. Clin. Psychol. Rev. 26, 17–31.

Cardaciotto, L., Herbert, J.D., 2004. Cognitive behavior therapy for social anxiety disorder in the context of Asperger's syndrome: a single-subject report. Cogn. Behav. Pract. 11, 75–81.

Carrasco, M., Volkmar, F.R., Bloch, M.H., 2012. Pharmacologic treatment of repetitive behaviors in autism spectrum disorders: evidence of publication bias. Pediatrics 129 (5), e1301–e1310.

Cervantes, P.E., Matson, J.L., 2015. Comorbid symptomology in adults with autism spectrum disorder and intellectual disability. J. Autism Dev. Disord. 45, 3961–3970.

Cook, E.H., Rowlett, R., Jaselskis, C., Leventhal, B.L., 1992. Fluoxetine treatment of children and adults with autistic disorder and mental retardation. J. Am. Acad. Child Adolesc. Psychiatry 31 (4), 739–745.

Craske, M.G., Niles, A.N., Burklund, L.J., Wolitzky-Taylor, K.B., Vilardaga, J.C.P., Arch, J.J., et al., 2014. Randomized controlled trial of cognitive behavioral therapy and acceptance and commitment therapy for social phobia: outcomes and moderators. J. Consult. Clin. Psychol. 82, 1034–1048.

Croen, L.A., Zerbo, O., Qian, Y., Massolo, M.L., Rich, S., Sidney, S., et al., 2015. The health status of adults on the autism spectrum. Autism 19 (7), 814–823.

Derogatis, L.R., 1977. SCL-90: Administration, scoring, and procedures manual-I for the revised version. Johns Hopkins University School of Medicine, Clinical Psychometrics Research Unit, Baltimore, MD.

Eack, S.M., Bahorik, A.L., Hogarty, S.S., Greenwald, D.P., Litschge, M.Y., Mazefsky, C.A., et al., 2013. Brief report: is cognitive rehabilitation needed in verbal adults with autism? Insights from initial enrollment in a trial of cognitive enhancement therapy. J. Autism Dev. Disord. 43 (9), 2233–2237.

Eack, S.M., Mazefsky, C.A., Minshew, N.J., 2015. Misinterpretation of facial expressions of emotion in verbal adults with autism spectrum disorder. Autism 19, 308–315.

Ekman, E., Hiltunen, A.J., 2015. Modified CBT using visualization for autism spectrum disorder, anxiety and avoidance behavior—a quasi-experimental open pilot study. Scand. J. Psychol 56, 641–648.

Esbensen, A.J., Greenberg, J.S., Seltzer, M.M., Aman, M.G., 2009. A longitudinal investigation of psychotropic and non-psychotropic medication use among adolescents and adults with autism spectrum disorders. J. Autism Dev. Disord. 39 (9), 1339–1349.

Gaus, V.L., 2007. Cognitive-behavioral therapy for adult Asperger syndrome. Guilford Press, New York, NY.

Gaus, V.L., 2011. Adult Asperger syndrome and the utility of cognitive-behavioral therapy. J. Contemp. Psychother. 41, 47–56.

Gillott, A., Standen, P.J., 2007. Levels of anxiety and sources of stress in adults with autism. J. Intellect. Disabil. 11 (4), 359–370.

Goodman, W.K., Price, L.H., Rasmussen, S.A., Mazure, C., Fleischmann, R.L., Hill, C.L., et al., 1989. The Yale-Brown Obsessive Compulsive Scale: I. Development, use, and reliability. Arch. Gen. Psychiatry 46, 1006–1011.

Gotham, K., Brunwasser, S.M., Lord, C., 2015. Depressive and anxiety symptom trajectories from school age through young adulthood in samples with autism spectrum disorder and developmental delay. J. Am. Acad. Child Adolesc. Psychiatry 54 (5), 369–376.

Gross, J.J., 2002. Emotion regulation: affective, cognitive, and social consequences. Psychophysiology 39 (3), 281–291.

Gross, J.J., Thompson, R.A., 2007. Emotion Regulation: Conceptual Foundations. Handbook of Emotion Regulation. Guilford Press, New York, NY, pp. 3–24.

Handen, B.L., Bodea, T., Tumuluru, R.V., Lubetsky, M.J., 2011. Pharmacological interventions. In: Lubetsky, M.J., Handen, B.L., McGonigle, J.J. (Eds.), Autism Spectrum Disorder. Oxford University Press, pp. 295–323.

Hayes, S.C., Luoma, J.B., Bond, F.W., Masuda, A., Lillis, J., 2006. Acceptance and commitment therapy: model, processes and outcomes. Behav. Res. Ther. 44, 1–25.

Hofvander, B., Delorme, R., Chaste, P., Nyden, A., Wentz, E., Stahlberg, O., et al., 2009. Psychiatric and psychosocial problems in adults with normal-intelligence autism spectrum disorders. BMC Psychiatry 9.

Hollander, E., Soorya, L., Chaplin, W., Anagnostou, E., Taylor, B.P., Ferretti, C.J., et al., 2012. A double-blind placebo-controlled trial of fluoxetine for repetitive behaviors and global severity in adult autism spectrum. Am. J. Psychiatry 169 (3), 292–299.

Howlin, P., 2000. Outcome in adult life for more able individuals with autism or asperger syndrome. Autism 4 (1), 63–83.

Howlin, P., Goode, S., Hutton, J., Rutter, M., 2004. Adult outcome for children with autism. J. Child Psychol. Psychiatry 45, 212–229.

Kazdin, A.E., 2007. Mediators and mechanisms of change in psychotherapy research. Ann. Rev. Clin. Psychol. 3, 1–27.

Keehn, B., Müller, R.-A., Townsend, J., 2013. Atypical attentional networks and the emergence of autism. Neurosci. Biobehav. Rev. 37 (2), 164–183.

Kendall, P.C., Compton, S., Walkup, J., Birmaher, B., Albano, A.M., Sherrill, J., et al., 2010. Clinical characteristics of anxiety disordered youth. J. Anxiety Disord. 24, 360–365.

Kerns, C.M., Kendall, P.C., 2012. The presentation and classification of anxiety in autism spectrum disorder. Clin. Psychol. Sci. Pract. 19, 323–346.

Kerns, C.M., Roux, A., Connell, J.E., Shattuck, P.T., et al., 2016. Adapting cognitive behavioral techniques to address anxiety and depression in cognitively-able emerging adults on the autism spectrum. Cogn. Behav Pract 23 (3), 329–340.

Kiep, M., Spek, A.A., Hoeben, L., 2015. Mindfulness-based therapy in adults with an autism spectrum disorder: do treatment effects last? Mindfulness 6, 637–644.

Kreiser, N.L., White, S.W. (2011). Measuring social anxiety in adolescents and adults with high functioning autism: the development of a screening instrument. In: Kreiser, N.L., Pugliese, C. (Chairs), Co-occurring Psychological and Behavioral Problems in Adolescents and Adults with Features of Autism Spectrum Disorder: Assessment and Characteristics. Symposium Presented at the Meeting of the Association for Behavioral and Cognitive Therapies, Toronto, Canada.

Kuusikko, S., Pollock-Wurman, R., Jussila, K., Carter, A.S., Mattila, M., Ebeling, H., et al., 2008. Social anxiety in high-functioning children and adolescents with autism and asperger syndrome. J. Autism Dev. Disord. 38, 1697–1709.

La Greca, A.M., Lopez, N., 1998. Social anxiety among adolescents: linkages with peer relations and friendships. J. Abnorm. Child Psychol. 26 (2), 83–94.

Lai, M.C., Baron-Cohen, S., 2015. Identifying the lost generation of adults with autism spectrum conditions. Lancet Psychiatry 2, 1013–1027.

Lake, J.K., Balogh, R., Lunsky, Y., 2012. Polypharmacy profiles and predictors among adults with autism spectrum disorders. Res. Autism Spectr. Disord. 6 (3), 1142–1149.

Lang, R., Regester, A., Lauderdale, S., Ashbaugh, K., Haring, A., 2010. Treatment of anxiety in autism spectrum disorders using cognitive behaviour therapy: a systematic review. Dev. Neurorehabil. 13, 53–63.

Lee, J.K., Orsillo, S.M., 2014. Investigating cognitive flexibility as a potential mechanism of mindfulness in generalized anxiety disorder. J. Behav. Ther. Exp. Psychiatry 45 (1), 208–216.

Lombardo, M.V., Barnes, J.L., Wheelwright, S.J., Baron-Cohen, S., 2007. Self-referential cognition and empathy in autism. PloS One 2 (9), e883.

Louwerse, A., Eussen, M.L.J., Van der Ende, J., de Nijs, A., Van Gool, A.R., Dekker, L.P., et al., 2015. ASD symptom severity in adolescence of individuals diagnosed with PDD-NOS in childhood: stability and the relation with psychiatry comorbidity and societal participation. J. Autism Dev. Disord. 45, 3908–3918.

Lugnegård, T., Hallerbäck, M.U., Gillberg, C., 2011. Psychiatric comorbidity in young adults with a clinical diagnosis of Asperger syndrome. Res. Dev. Disabil. 32, 1910–1917.

Maddox, B.B., White, S.W., 2015. Comorbid social anxiety disorder in adults with autism spectrum disorder. J. Autism Dev. Disord. 45, 3949–3960.

May, T., Cornish, K., Rinehart, N., 2013. Does gender matter? A one year follow-up of autistic, attention and anxiety symptoms in high-functioning children with autism spectrum disorder. J. Autism Dev. Disord. 44, 1077–1086.

Mazefsky, C.A., Herrington, J.D., 2014. Autism and anxiety: etiologic factors and trans-diagnostic processes. In: Davis III, T.E., White, S.W., Ollendick, T.H. (Eds.), Handbook of Autism and Anxiety. Heidelburg. Springer.

Mazefsky, C.A., White, S.W., 2014. Emotion regulation. Child Adolesc. Psychiatr. Clin. N. Am. 23 (1), 15–24.

Mazefsky, C.A., Herrington, J., Siegel, M., Scarpa, A., Maddox, B.B., Scahill, L., et al., 2013. The role of emotion regulation in autism spectrum disorder. J. Am. Acad. Child Adolesc. Psychiatry 52 (7), 679–688.

McDougle, C., Brodkin, E., Naylor, S., Carlson, D., Cohen, D., Price, L., 1998. Sertraline in adults with pervasive developmental disorders: a prospective open-label investigation. J. Clin. Psychopharmacol. 39 (18), 62−66.

McDougle, C.J., Price, L.H., Volkmar, F.R., Goodman, W.K., Ward-O'Brien, D., Nielsen, J., et al., 1992. Clomipramine in autism: preliminary evidence of efficacy. J. Am. Acad. Child Adolesc. Psychiatry 31 (4), 746−750.

McDougle, C.J., Naylor, S.T., Cohen, D.J., Volkmar, F.R., Heninger, G.R., Price, L.H., 1996. A double-blind, placebo-controlled study of fluvoxamine in adults with autistic disorder. Arch. Gen. Psychiatry 53 (11), 1001−1008.

Mendlowicz, M.V., Stein, M.B., 2000. Quality of life in individuals with anxiety disorders. Am. J. Psychiatry 157, 669−682.

McGillivray, J.A., Evert, H.T., 2014. Group cognitive behavioural therapy program shows potential in reducing symptoms of depression and stress among young people with ASD. J. Autism Dev. Disord. 44, 2041−2051.

Moss, P., Howlin, P., Savage, S., Bolton, P., Rutter, M., 2015. Self and informant reports of mental health difficulties among adults with autism: findings from a long-term follow-up study. Autism 19 (7), 832−841.

Newby, J.M., McKinnon, A., Kuyken, W., Gilbody, S., Dalgleish, T., 2015. Systematic review and meta-analysis of transdiagnostic psychological treatments for anxiety and depressive disorders in adulthood. Clin. Psychol. Rev. 40, 91−110.

Norcross, J.C., Wampold, B.E., 2011. What works for whom: tailoring psychotherapy to the person. J. Clin. Psychol. 67 (2), 127−132.

Olatunji, B.O., Cisler, J.M., Tolin, D.F., 2007. Quality of life in the anxiety disorders: a meta-analytic review. Clin. Psychol. Rev. 27, 572−581.

Paul, G.L., 1967. Strategy of outcome research in psychotherapy. J. Consult. Psychol. 31 (2), 109−118.

Propper, L., Orlik, H., 2014. Pharmacotherapy of anxiety and repetitive behaviors in autism spectrum disorders. Child Adolesc. Psychopharmacol. News 19 (1), 5−14.

Russell, A.J., Mataix-Cols, D., Anson, M.A.W., Murphy, D.G.M., 2009. Psychological treatment for obsessive-compulsive disorder in people with autism spectrum disorders: a pilot study. Psychother. Psychosom. 78, 59−61.

Russell, A.J., Jassi, A., Fullana, M.A., Mack, H., Johnston, K., Heyman, I., et al., 2013. Cognitive behavior therapy for comorbid obsessive-compulsive disorder in high-functioning autism spectrum disorders: a randomized controlled trial. Depress. Anxiety 30, 697−708.

Samson, A.C., Hardan, A.Y., Lee, I.A., Phillips, J.M., Gross, J.J., 2015. Maladaptive behavior in autism spectrum disorder: the role of emotion experience and emotion regulation. J. Autism Dev. Disord.3424−3432.

Scahill, L., McDougle, C.J., Williams, S.K., Dimitropoulos, A., Aman, M.G., McCracken, J.T., et al., 2006. Children's Yale-Brown Obsessive Compulsive Scale modified for pervasive developmental disorders. J. Am. Acad. Child Adolesc. Psychiatry 45, 1114−1123.

Segal, Z.V., Williams, J.M.G., Teasdale, J.D., 2002. Mindfulness-based Cognitive Therapy for Depression: A New Approach to Preventing Relapse. Guilford Press, New York, NY.

Solomon, M., Miller, M., Taylor, S.L., Hinshaw, S.P., Carter, C.S., 2012. Autism symptoms and internalizing psychopathology in girls and boys with autism spectrum disorders. J. Autism Dev. Disord. 42, 48−59.

Soorya, L., Kiarashi, J., Hollander, E., 2008. Psychopharmacologic interventions for repetitive behaviors in autism spectrum disorders. Child Adolesc. Psychiatr. Clin. N. Am. 17 (4), 753−771.

Spain, D., Sin, J., Chalder, T., Murphy, D., Happé, F., 2015. Cognitive behaviour therapy for adults with autism spectrum disorders and psychiatric co-morbidity: a review. Res. Autism Spectrum Disord. 9, 151–162.

Spek, A.A., van Ham, N.C., Nyklíček, I., 2013. Mindfulness-based therapy in adults with an autism spectrum disorder: a randomized controlled trial. Res. Dev. Disabil. 34, 246–253.

Swain, D., Scarpa, A., White, S., Laugeson, E., 2015. Emotion dysregulation and anxiety in adults with ASD: does social motivation play a role? J. Autism Dev. Disord. 45, 3971–3977.

Taylor, J., Seltzer, M., 2011. Employment and post-secondary educational activities for young adults with autism spectrum disorder during transition to adulthood. J. Autism Dev. Disord. 41, 566–574.

Trembath, D., Germano, C., Johanson, G., Dissanayake, C., 2012. The experience of anxiety in young adults with autism spectrum disorders. Focus Autism Other Dev. Disabil. 27, 213–224.

Trubanova, A., 2015. Eye-gaze analysis of facial emotion expression in adolescents with ASD. Unpublished Masters thesis: Virginia Tech.

Uljarevic, M., Hamilton, A., 2012. Recognition of emotions in autism: a formal meta-analysis. J. Autism Dev. Disord.1517–1526.

Weiss, J.A., 2014. Transdiagnostic case conceptualization of emotional problems in youth with ASD: an emotion regulation approach. Clin. Psychol. Sci. Pract. 21, 331–350.

Weiss, J.A., Lunsky, Y., 2010. Group cognitive behaviour therapy for adults with Asperger syndrome and anxiety or mood disorder: a case series. Clin. Psychol. Psychother. 17, 438–446.

White, S.W., Mazefsky, C.A., Dichter, G.S., Chiu, P.H., Richey, J.A., Ollendick, T.H., 2014. Social-cognitive, physiological, and neural mechanisms underlying emotion regulation impairments: understanding anxiety in autism spectrum disorder. Int. J. Dev. Neurosci.1–15.

Williams, K., Wheeler, D.M., Silove, N., Hazell, P., 2010. Selective serotonin reuptake inhibitors (SSRIs) for autism spectrum disorders (ASD). J. Evid. Based Med. 3 (4), 231.

Woolfenden, S., Sarkozy, V., Ridley, G., Williams, K., 2012. A systematic review of the diagnostic stability of autism spectrum disorder. Res. Autism Spectrum Disord. 6, 345–354.

CHAPTER 10

Behavioral Treatments for Anxiety in Minimally Verbal Children With ASD

Louis P. Hagopian[1,2], Megan Lilly[3] and
Thompson E. Davis[3]
[1]Kennedy Krieger Institute, Baltimore, MD, United States
[2]Johns Hopkins University School of Medicine, Baltimore, MD, United States
[3]Louisiana State University, Baton Rouge, LA, United States

Individuals with Autism Spectrum Disorder (ASD) represent an extremely heterogeneous group in terms of intellectual functioning, communication skills, repetitive behavior, and psychiatric comorbidities (Myers and Johnson, 2007). Even minimally verbal children with ASD can show a range of skills and deficits. Determining the presence of anxiety in minimally verbal children with ASD can be especially challenging given their limited ability (or complete inability) to self-report coupled with the overlapping features of anxiety and ASD. Anxiety has been defined as a response to an actual or perceived threat that occurs across multiple response domains: behavioral, physiological, verbal/cognitive, and subjective (Davis and Ollendick, 2005). For minimally verbal individuals with ASD, the verbal/cognitive and subjective response domains can be particularly difficult, if not impossible to examine. Although the physiological domain can be measured using monitoring devices (e.g., Moskowitz et al., 2013), the use of such devices in clinical practice and research is limited because they can be impractical (due to noncompliance, tactile sensitivities, etc.) and there is limited knowledge of how such measures can be used clinically. Although the behavioral response domain is the most readily observable, the shared features of ASD and anxiety make it difficult to ascertain the extent to which avoidance and escape-related behaviors or agitated states reflect the presence of anxiety or are secondary to ASD.

In contrast to adaptive anxiety, wherein potentially harmful situations are avoided to the benefit of the individual, clinically problematic anxiety is present either: (a) when the avoided stimulus poses little actual risk or

Anxiety in Children and Adolescents with Autism Spectrum Disorder.
DOI: http://dx.doi.org/10.1016/B978-0-12-805122-1.00010-7

© 2017 Elsevier Inc.
All rights reserved.

(b) when the response is out of proportion to the actual threat. Another issue specific to ASD is that it can be difficult to know whether events or stimuli that appear benign to typically developing individuals may actually be aversive to the child with ASD. For example, some individuals with ASD react to certain sensory stimuli that are neutral or mildly unpleasant to most typically developing individuals (e.g., shirt tags, sounds of crying babies) in a manner that would suggest they are highly aversive unconditioned stimuli (APA, 2013).

As noted, a major challenge to determining the presence of anxiety in a person with ASD arises from the fact that clinically problematic anxiety (and avoidant behavior) and ASD share some common features, making it difficult to determine if behaviors typically thought of as indicative of anxiety (e.g., avoidance of certain situations) are secondary to ASD itself or indicative of the presence of anxiety. For example, problem behavior such as aggression and self-injury is more common in individuals with ASD, particularly those who are lower functioning and minimally verbal (Jang et al., 2010; Lecavalier, 2014). Negative emotional states and behaviors (including agitation and crying) frequently cooccur with escape or avoidant problem behavior. Such behaviors could reflect anxiety or are could simply be related to the avoidance of nonpreferred situations (such as academic tasks), which is common in this population (Hanley et al., 2003).

We have proposed the use of the term *anxious avoidance* to refer to avoidant behavior associated with overt indicators of anxiety (e.g., fearful affect); and *simple avoidance* to refer to avoidance of nonpreferred situations not associated with apparent anxiety (Hagopian and Jennett, 2008). Thus, for minimally verbal children, the distinction between simple and anxious avoidant behavior is based on the presence or absence of some indicator of emotional distress and subjective states thought to be characteristic of anxiety. When anxious avoidance markedly interferes with functioning, then this would constitute an *anxiety disorder.* Which particular diagnosis obviously depends on the nature of the feared stimulus and the response (see Diagnosis below). The extent to which avoidant behaviors interfere with functioning is often determined by variables such as the ubiquity of the avoided stimulus and the cost of avoiding it. For example, anxious avoidance of breaking waves at the beach might not significantly impair functioning and quality of life, whereas anxious avoidance of riding in a car would likely impair functioning, and therefore necessitate treatment. In short, not all avoidant behavior in minimally verbal children with ASD is associated with negative emotional states we might characterize as anxiety, and not all anxiety in ASD would constitute an anxiety disorder that requires treatment. Failing to identify and treat anxiety could lead to prolonged distress and establishment of other problem behavior aimed at escaping or avoiding anxiety inducing situations, while erroneously concluding a child is anxious could lead to unnecessary interventions and misallocation of therapy time that would be better directed elsewhere. Behavioral assessment is critical to make these discriminations, and guide appropriate intervention.

DIAGNOSIS

Anxiety disorders have been found to cooccur at highly variable rates, 11–84%, with ASD individuals (White et al., 2009). This variability may be due in part to the highly heterogeneous presentation of ASD as well as the complexity of the manifestations of anxiety in the ASD population, not to mention the biases which may be present for or against diagnosis in those with comorbid ASD. We continue to recommend use of the terms *simple and anxious avoidance* to help differentiate between stimuli and situations that may constitute an *anxiety disorder* in individuals with and without ASD. However, the current *Diagnostic and Statistical Manual of Mental Disorders, 5th edition* (*DSM-5*; American Psychiatric Association, 2013) classifies *anxiety* as the "anticipation of future threat" and furthermore, various anxiety disorders can be differentiated by the "specific content of the thoughts and beliefs that may induce the fear or anxiety." Given this definition, how can the current diagnostic classifications of anxiety disorders be applied to those individuals with limited cognitive and/or verbal abilities? Early studies conducted on ASD suggested approximately half of those individuals diagnosed were incapable of speech acquisition (Rutter, 1978). Recent estimates have shown a marked decrease in these estimates due in part to earlier assessment and detection techniques (Klingler et al., 2003); however, the fact remains that some individuals with ASD never develop functional speech.

These deficits in verbal communication in a subpopulation of individuals with ASD may account for some of the variability in comorbidity rates. Researchers have shown higher levels of anxiety to be associated with functional language in individuals with ASD (Gadow and Sprafkin, 1998, 2002). Researchers have also argued these findings may be complicated by diagnostic overshadowing (Mason and Scior, 2004), while data from other studies suggests that individuals with ASD simply do not meet cooccurring criteria for other psychiatric conditions (Leyfer et al., 2006; Witmer and Lecavalier, 2010, Kaat et al., 2013). Differential diagnosis of ASD and anxiety, then, requires a careful evaluation of those symptoms unique to each disorder as well as common presentations of symptom patterns for individuals evincing comorbidity. Additionally, findings from a number of studies have shown that fears and behavioral responses common among the typically developing population, are not necessarily replicated in individuals with ASD (e.g., Evans et al., 2005; Kanner, 1943; Matson and Love, 1990).

Due to the overlap of symptomology between ASD and anxiety disorders a number of studies have attempted to differentiate those factors which are inextricably shared from those that may be conceptually differentiable. For example, social avoidance and a preference to be alone are shared qualities between both anxiety and ASD (Baron-Cohen et al., 2001; Roberson-Nay et al., 2007; White et al., 2012). However, ASD individuals may be less aware or have less concern for the social rejection component found in social anxiety disorder (Leyfer et al., 2006; Muris et al., 1998). Also, excessive worries around environmental changes or deviations from a schedule can be common in both groups of disorders (generalized anxiety disorder and ASD), as can be highly rigid behaviors, verbal rituals, and compulsions (OCD and ASD). The difficulty comes from determining whether these behaviors occur to reduce distress in the case of OCD or are generalized worry and broad anxious avoidance in the case of GAD. Differential diagnosis would also require the clinician to assess those behaviors seen less typically in non-ASD populations such as strict adherence to routine, circumscribed interests, and repetitive behaviors.

Attempts to distinguish between the similarities between anxiety and ASD symptoms have typically supported distinctiveness within areas which do not necessarily lend themselves to application in those who are minimally verbal or lower functioning. For example, Farrugia and Hudson (2006) found the only difference between anxiety presentation in typically developing and nontypically developing groups was reported thought patterns of social threat and physical injury, areas which would be difficult if not impossible to assess in a minimally verbal population. Atypical presentations of anxiety are also common in those with ASD and can include social fear without a negative evaluative component, nontraditional specific phobias, and fear of change and novelty (Kerns et al., 2014). Leyfer et al. (2006) found typical phobias were rarely endorsed in the ASD population; however, fears of loud noises, crowds, and shots/needles were much more common. Additionally, idiosyncratic fears (e.g., flushing toilets, beards, mechanical objects) have also been found in ASD individuals (Richman et al., 2012). Many of these problematic or avoided stimuli raise additional questions as to whether the problem is fear or anxiety versus altered sensory function. For example, repetitive and ritualistic behaviors seen in obsessive-compulsive disorder (OCD) are also commonly observed in many persons with ASD (McDougle et al., 1995), including those individuals that are not suspected of experiencing any anxiety. In such cases, repetitive behaviors may be a preferred self-stimulatory activity, in contrast to ritualistic behavior triggered by obsessional thoughts that is the hallmark of OCD. Caution should be taken to not immediately characterize these ritualistic or stereotypic behaviors as "OCD" based on their repetitive nature. Avoidance is another area which may present itself differentially as younger children and those with verbal deficits have been shown to express fear and avoidance in conjunction with other behaviors such as aggression, destruction of property, and self-injurious behavior (Hagopian et al., 2001; Ricciardi et al., 2006).

Finally, of particular concern with the diagnosis of anxiety in minimally verbal ASD populations is that strict adherence to the *DSM-5* diagnostic criteria may miss a significant proportion of these individuals in need of clinical services due to verbal requirements of the diagnostic criteria. For example, Criterion A for separation anxiety disorder requires endorsement of 3 out of 8 symptoms; however, 4 of the 8 symptoms require the expression of "worry, thematic explanations of nightmares, or complaints" (APA, 2013). Additionally, some disorders such as selective mutism and GAD may inherently be unavailable to the minimally verbal ASD population when adhering to strict diagnostic classification. Given the host of challenges associated with differential diagnosis, thorough assessment procedures are considered to be vitally important.

BEHAVIORAL ASSESSMENT

Fundamental goals of behavioral assessment are to identify treatment targets and their controlling antecedents and consequences (i.e., a functional assessment of behavior). Minimally verbal children with ASD may be referred for treatment of "anxiety" that is later determined to not be anxiety; or they may be referred for other problem behavior, that is later determined to be related to anxiety. Because of the inherent challenges noted above related to overlap of ASD and anxiety, great caution should be taken not to make assumptions based on another's labeled presentation of the presenting problem(s).

Traditional assessments of individuals with ASD who possess verbal or communication deficits typically involve multimodal, multi–informant assessments including interviews and self-report measures of behavior (King et al., 1997; Velting et al., 2004). However, as previously described, those individuals with communication problems are in some cases inherently incapable of describing their own cognitive and affective states (Ollendick et al., 1993) which may further complicate the already challenging process of assessment within the ASD population. Despite the inherent problems with a lack of self-report data, there exist a number of caregiver assessments as well as behavioral methods that can be utilized to help determine the presence of anxiety in the minimally verbal ASD population. Behavioral methods with minimally verbal populations specifically face a set of unique challenges when assessing anxiety in ASD.

BEHAVIORAL INTERVIEWS

When interviewing parents or other primary care providers it is especially important to include assessment questions related to the individual's family history. Because the individual may not be able to self-report, a detailed family history of mental health concerns (and a working knowledge of what conditions have high heritability) will assist the clinician to disentangle anxiety from ASD when assessing individuals with communication deficits (Ghaziuddin and Greden 1998; Hollander et al., 2003). Thorough interview procedures should also include information on the nature of the anxiety, associated behavioral symptoms, known antecedents to anxious response patterns, the individual's observed affective states, and atypical behavioral responses such as aggressive or self-injurious behavior. Specific care should be taken to limit the reporter's interpretations of *why* the individual may be experiencing certain behaviors. Certain behavior patterns may have led to a care provider developing their own hypotheses as to the purpose of the behaviors; however, it is important to limit the initial interview to purely descriptive information. Identification of emotional states in individuals unable to verbally express their own fears may present in the form of crying, trembling, and certain facial expressions. Avoidance behaviors may present as dropping or running off and have been found to cooccur at times with self-injurious or aggressive behaviors and property destruction (Hagopian et al., 2001; Ricciardi et al., 2006).

STANDARDIZED RATING FORMS

Assessment of anxiety symptomology among ASD individuals without associated communication deficits has typically included self-report measures (White and Roberson-Nay, 2009). However, to date no measure currently exists which was specifically designed for assessing anxiety in the minimally verbal population. Amongst those measures used for individuals with ASD without associated verbal problems, the majority were created for typically developing youth and adults (Davis, 2012). Previous analyses utilizing differential item functioning have attempted to construct a clearer picture as to whether items are endorsed at the same rates across ASD and non-ASD children allowing for greater sensitivity for discrimination (Douglas et al., 1998; Holland and Wainer, 1993; Roussos and Stout, 2004). However, the result of these procedures has been the creation of specifically modified rating scales which tend to simply eliminate overlapping items. Those anxiety triggers which have been identified as commonly occurring within the ASD population are also not found on these modified rating scales (Ozsivadjian et al., 2012).

Therefore, the psychometric problems associated with this downward extension of theoretical constructs is further exacerbated by the struggle minimally verbal individuals may have with communicating emotional states. Whereas attempts have been made to reanalyze the factor structure and measure validity in the ASD population, these analyses were still performed on measures which include a number of items requiring language. For example, the Child and Adolescent Symptom Inventory-4R (CASI-4R; Gadow and Sprafkin, 1998, 2002; Sprafkin et al., 2002) asks parents whether their child "complains about feeling sick" as well as a number of other questions about whether the child, "worries, describes, complains" all of which require verbal communication for endorsement and would lead to lower overall anxiety levels on the measure. In fact, studies analyzing anxiety measures designed and normed for children without associated communication difficulties have been shown to be rarely endorsed in the minimally verbal population (Hallett et al., 2010; Witwer and Lecavalier, 2010). Instead, more behaviorally oriented items are commonly endorsed in this population and while these items may be less specific to anxiety disorders, they may represent a more accurate picture of symptomology in the minimally verbal population (Witmer and Lecavalier, 2010). Additionally, items which assess sleep difficulties and over-arousal are more consistently endorsed as manifestations of anxiety by parents in the minimally verbal ASD population (Hallett et al., 2010). Therefore, assessment measures which place a high demand on the individual's level of communication may result in lowered endorsement and the potential for a loss of measurement validity and should be utilized only with extreme caution when assessing minimally verbal individuals with ASD.

DIRECT OBSERVATION

Naturalistic observations

One form of behavioral assessment involves a descriptive analysis of the behavior in the natural setting through direct observation by the professional. This method allows for identification of common situations under which the anxious or avoidant behavior occurs, development of operational definitions of the behavior, and possible identification of idiosyncratic antecedent and/or behavioral consequences (Vollmer et al., 2009). This form of descriptive data collection also may identify patterns of reinforcement that may occur in the naturalistic setting that can be subsequently compared to data collected in the clinical setting (Borrero et al., 2005). In certain cases, specific stimuli may be difficult to control or present in the clinical setting and therefore behavioral monitoring by a parent or caregiver may serve as a primary source of data for assessment and treatment evaluation purposes.

Behavior monitoring

Behavioral monitoring entails recording observations made by parents or care providers in the natural context in which the behavior is concern occurs. A simple behavioral monitoring form records the antecedents and consequences associated with the observed behavior (i.e., ABC record forms). These forms can be tailored to the individual client and contain columns for a formal definition of the behavior to be observed and space for recording open-ended antecedents and consequences. Besides simplicity of use, these forms also benefit from the possibility of data collection on low-rate behaviors that may not always present themselves during formal clinical assessment procedures (Vollmer et al., 2009).

Behavioral avoidance test (BAT)

For certain specific stimuli, conditions can be arranged for direct in vivo behavioral observations. This process could involve the use of a BAT (Dadds et al., 1994; Ollendick and Davis, 2012) which generally involves progressive exposure to the feared stimulus in gradually more (presumed) fear-evoking steps using a predetermined hierarchy. BATs benefit from the potential for high levels of personalization and direct measurement, but should also be implemented with caution in this population to minimize possible to harm to the individual and possibly the stimulus (e.g., considering physical limitations and unsteadiness when stairs are used to assess heights or considering how to care for a dog until needed and if the dog itself is put at risk in the assessment). Safeguards should also be put in place for possible instances of elopement, self-injury, aggression, or other challenging behavior. Finally, since behavioral exposure (discussed in the following section) during treatment will likely involve a similar framework, these procedures have been thoroughly examined in a number of well-validated studies (e.g., Davis, Kurtz et al., 2007; Erfanian and Miltenberger, 1990; Rudy and Davis, 2012).

Functional behavioral assessment of problem behavior

Functional behavioral assessment of problem behavior can help differentiate between simple and anxious avoidance, and identify relationships between avoidance and problem behavior, which may become a larger issue during the course of treatment. In cases where more externalizing problem behaviors are part of the presentation (e.g., self-injury, aggression, property destruction) a functional behavioral assessment should be conducted. When less intensive functional behavioral methods fail to yield conclusive findings about the function of problem behaviors co-occuring with anxiety (or fail to inform the development of an effective intervention), an analog functional analysis may be indicated. Functional analysis is the most rigorous type of functional behavioral assessment and involves testing hypotheses through the manipulation of antecedent and consequent events (Iwata et al., 1994; Lovaas and Simmons, 1969).

CAREGIVER ANXIETY AND ITS ROLE IN CHILD ANXIETY

A thorough understanding of the role parents and caregivers may be playing in the maintenance of certain avoidant behaviors should be a focus during assessment. The increased dependence on parents or other care providers within the minimally verbal ASD population (Shattuck et al., 2012) may increase the possibility that parents might actively avoid situations that occasion anxiety in their children, or inadvertently reinforce avoidant or anxious behavior with excessive attention aimed at quelling anxiety in the child. Identifying these interaction patterns is critical to understanding the controlling variables of child anxiety, but also has implications for the assessment and treatment process. For instance, it is important to determine whether parents are anxious themselves and avoid situations where their child may encounter the feared stimulus because exposure is a necessary part of the assessment and treatment process.

BEHAVIORAL TREATMENT

Behavioral treatments demonstrated to be effective with typically developing children (and adults) appear applicable to individuals with ASD—though minimally verbal children are likely to not be able to participate in intervention that requires verbal interchange, such as cognitive-behavioral therapy (CBT). A review by Jennett and Hagopian (2008) identified behavioral treatment as an evidence-based treatment for "phobic avoidance" in individuals with intellectual disabilities (ID). The authors identified 38 studies, 12 of which were well-designed, single-case, experimental studies. Four of these studies reported on five participants who were reported to have an ASD diagnosis, and ranged from having mild to profound intellectual disability (Love et al., 1990; Rapp et al., 2005; Ricciardi et al., 2006; Shabani and Fisher, 2006). Among these, two (Rapp et al., 2005; Shabani and Fisher, 2006) could be characterized as minimally verbal.

Subsequently, three additional studies have been published that used single-case experimental designs to evaluate treatments for avoidance of a particular stimulus (i.e., "phobic avoidance") in individuals with ASD (Ames and Weiss, 2013; Chok et al., 2010; Schmidt et al., 2013; only Chok et al., 2010 reported a diagnosis of Specific Phobia). Based on APA Division 12 and 16 criteria for empirically supported treatments, graduated exposure with reinforcement can be considered "well-established" for individuals with ID (Chambless et al., 1998; Chambless and Hollon, 1998; Krotochwill and Stoiber, 2002). To date, seven good single case design studies exist for individuals with ASD showing an effect of graduated exposure plus reinforcement (see Table 10.1). Thus, this treatment can also be characterized as a "probably efficacious" treatment for individuals with autism according to the same guidelines. When specifically reviewing those studies which reported analyses within the minimally verbal population, three good single case design studies have been conducted, suggesting further research is needed before it can be considered efficacious.

Table 10.1 Behavioral treatments for anxious avoidance in individuals with autism spectrum disorders

Author (year)	N	Participant characteristics	Stimulus avoided	Anxiety characteristics	Treatment components	Treatment outcomes
Ames and Weiss (2013)	1	9 y.o. male with ASD, low average IQ, verbal reasoning skills in the 2nd percentile	Social	Aggressive behaviors (hitting, punching, kicking)	Modified Coping Cat program (12-week CBT protocol)	Improved overall functioning in group settings and at home
Chok et al. (2010)	1	15 y.o. male with ASD, mod ID, Specific phobia	Dogs	Running away (including into running into street or woods), screaming, self-injury, elevated heart rate	Graduated exposure, positive reinforcement, prompting	Participant approached and touched 4 different dogs without elevated heart rate; results maintained at 6 mo follow-up
Love et al. (1990)	2	4.5 y.o. and 6 y.o. males with ASD	Going outside alone, Water	Shaking, wide eyes, grimacing, crying, physical resistance, running away	Graduated exposure, positive reinforcement, participant modeling, prompting	Both participants showed increase in approach, decrease in fear verbalizations, and decrease in ratings of appearance of fear
Rapp et al. (2005)	1	14 y.o. female with ASD, severe ID	Swimming pools	Screaming, running away, flopping, self-injury, and choking	Graduated exposure, positive reinforcement, extinction (response prevention)	Participant entered pool without problem behavior and remained in 4ft water

(Continued)

Table 10.1 (Continued)

Author (year)	N	Participant characteristics	Stimulus avoided	Anxiety characteristics	Treatment components	Treatment outcomes
Ricciardi et al. (2006)	1	8 y.o. male with ASD, Specific phobia	Animatronic objects	Screaming, attempts to run away, aggression when blocked from leaving area	Graduated exposure, positive reinforcement	Participant approached animatronic objects and remained within a meter distance without negative behavior
Schmidt et al. (2012)	1	16 y.o. male with ASD, severe ID	Particular school settings	Appearance of distress, agitation, physical resistance, running away, self-aggression, self-injury, destructive behavior	Graduated exposure, positive reinforcement	Participant attended activities with classmates in these settings without problem behavior for at least 5 min at a time
Shabani and Fisher (2006)	1	18 y.o. male with ASD, ID, Diabetes	Blood draws/ needles	Crying, screaming, running away, self-injury, aggression, pulling hand away; this resulted in no blood draws for 2 years	Graduated exposure, positive reinforcement	Participant remained still for blood draws; results maintained over 2 mo on daily glucose measures

GRADUATED EXPOSURE AND REINFORCEMENT

The main components of behavioral treatment for anxiety included graduated exposure to the feared stimulus coupled with reinforcement for approach behavior. Graduated exposure is most appropriate when the avoided stimulus is identifiable and controllable—as with specific phobia and social anxiety disorder. Graduated exposure involves presenting the avoided stimulus in increasing intensity along some physical dimensions—such as duration of presentation, proximity, size, mode of presentation (pictorial to actual)—while maintaining low levels of anxiety and avoidant behavior. In the case of minimally verbal children with ASD, determining the tolerance level can be difficult because of their limited abilities to self-report.

The goals of the graduated exposure are to: (a) extinguish any associations between the avoided stimulus and aversive events (such as intense physiological arousal) by presenting the avoided stimulus in the absence of those aversive events (i.e., Pavlovian extinction); and (b) extinguish negative reinforcement associated with escape or avoidance (i.e., operant extinction). Ideally, the stimulus should be encountered with little subjective distress and no avoidance, and so that approach responses can contact reinforcement (e.g., receiving a preferred edible or tangible object for successful steps along the exposure continuum). It is imperative that the procedure not result in anxious escape/avoidance from the stimulus in a manner that could further strengthen the avoidance response. Because minimally verbal children with ASD are limited in their ability to guide the development of an exposure hierarchy and inform the clinician when they are becoming anxious, the pace of graduated exposure should be very slow.

In addition to graduated exposure, which should decrease the likelihood of avoidant behavior, reinforcement procedures aimed at increasing approach responses should involve potent reinforcers. In contrast to verbal children who can simply name their reinforcers, a systematic preference assessment will likely be needed to identify reinforcers for minimally verbal children with ASD (see Hagopian et al., 2004, for a comprehensive summary of preference assessment procedures). Because many minimally verbal children will also have difficulties understanding the purpose and nature of graduated exposure sessions, beginning therapy sessions with more preferred activities might help establish the therapy context as reinforcing, and thus increase compliance (nevertheless, attempts should be made to inform the child about the procedures). Therefore, we have recommended that before initiating graduated exposure, initial sessions should be arranged in a way that maximizes the chances that the individual will contact the programmed reinforcement contingencies for cooperation.

ADDITIONAL TREATMENT COMPONENTS

For those that are unable to comprehend instructions, the use of prompting strategies commonly used with individuals with ASD may be needed to assist the individual with graduated exposure and other procedures. Following verbal prompts, it may be helpful to prompt the individual how to approach the avoided stimulus (e.g., touch the shoe)—and how to appropriately request pausing at the current hierarchy step (Runyan et al., 1985). However, prompting should be used to teach approach responses, not "force" them, as this could likely lead to adverse responses including increased negative emotional states and problem behavior. Modeling can also be used to facilitate learning (Erfanian and Miltenberger, 1990; Love et al., 1990); and for those who prefer watching videos over observing live models, video modeling can be used. Finally, use of distracting stimuli or alterative activities can also be helpful during graduated exposure (particularly free access to preferred activities; Luscre and Center, 1996). Distracting stimuli can divert attention away from the stimulus, and increase the overall level of reinforcement in the context of exposure. The combination of the specific treatment components listed above can be highly individualized based the functioning level and needs of the individual.

CAREGIVER INVOLVEMENT

Parents of minimally verbal children with ASD struggle with identifying the presence of anxiety in their children, for the same reasons that professionals do: shared features of anxiety and ASD, and the child's limited ability to report thoughts and subjective states. As noted, behavioral assessment must include an analysis of parent–child interactions that may reinforce anxiety and avoidant behavior, as well as evaluate parental anxiety, which is common in parents of children with anxiety (e.g., Beidel and Turner, 2005; Nebel-Schwalm and Davis, 2013). It important to educate parents about what behavior is actually anxiety (versus other emotional states), the uncertainties inherent to identifying anxiety in minimally verbal children with ASD, and how their interactions may inadvertently reinforce anxious and avoidant behavior. Because minimally verbal children with ASD are particularly vulnerable and highly dependent upon their caregivers, caregivers can be highly protective, and sensitive about their child being in distress. Clinicians must be aware of these possibilities, and take care to ensure parents that graduated exposure will be designed to be minimally aversive to the child. Furthermore, efforts aimed at enlisting parents to participate in treatment is necessary to ensure success in therapy sessions and to establish them as change agents in the home setting. As a result, care should be taken to plan for how to generalize treatment to other settings as necessary (e.g., to the home, school, doctor's office) and empower parents to be effective change agents in these settings. In some cases, it may be necessary to focus additional attention on parental anxiety related to treatment recommendations to ensure adherence with recommendations.

REFERENCES

American Psychiatric Association, 2013. Diagnostic and Statistical Manual of Mental Disorders, *fifth ed.* Author, Washington D.C.

Ames, M., Weiss, J., 2013. Cognitive behaviour therapy for a child with autism spectrum disorder and verbal impairment: a case study.

Baron-Cohen, S., Wheelwright, S., Skinner, R., Martin, J., Clubley, E., 2001. The Autism-Spectrum Quotient (AQ): evidence from asperger syndrome/High-functioning autism, males and females, scientists and mathematicians. J. Autism Dev. Disord. 31 (1), 5—17. Available from: http://dx.doi.org/10.1023/ A:1005653411471.

Beidel, D.C., Turner, S.M., 2005. Childhood Anxiety Disorders: A Guide to Research and Treatment. Routledge, New York, NY.

Borrero, C.S., Vollmer, T.R., Borrero, J.C., Bourret, J., 2005. A method for evaluating parameters of reinforcement during parent—child interactions. Res. Dev. Disabil. 26 (6), 577—592.

Chambless, D.L., Hollon, S.D., 1998. Defining empirically supported therapies. J. Consult. Clin. Psychol. 66, 7—18.

Chambless, D.L., Baker, M.J., Baucom, D.H., Beutler, L.E., Calhoun, K.S., Crits-Christoph, P., et al., 1998. Update on empirically validated therapies, II. Clin. Psychol. 51, 3—16.

Chok, J.T., Demanche, J., Kennedy, A., Studer, L., 2010. Utilizing physiological measures to facilitate phobia treatment with individuals with autism and intellectual disability: a case study. Behav. Intervent. 11, 325—337.

Dadds, M., Rapee, R., Barrett, P., 1994. Behavioral observation. In: Ollendick, T., King, N., Yule, W. (Eds.), International Handbook of Phobic and Anxiety Disorders in Children and Adolescents. Plenum Press, New York, NY, pp. 349—364.

Davis III, T.E., 2012. Where to from here for ASD and anxiety? Lessons learned from child anxiety and the issue of DSM-5. Clin. Psychol. 19, 358—363. Available from: http://dx.doi.org/10.1111/cpsp.12014.

Davis III, T.E., Ollendick, T.H., 2005. Empirically supported treatments for specific phobia in children: do efficacious treatments address the components of a phobic response? Clin. Psychol. 12, 144–160.

Davis III, T.E., Kurtz, P., Gardner, A., Carman, N., 2007. Cognitive-behavioral treatment for specific phobias with a child demonstrating severe problem behavior and developmental delays. Res. Dev. Disabil., 28, 546-558. Available from: http://dx.doi.org/10.1016/j.r.

Douglas, J.A., Stout, W., DiBello, L.V., 1998. A Kernel-Smoothed version of SIBTEST with applications to local DIF inference and function estimation. J of Educational and Behavioral Statistics 21, 333–363.

Erfanian, N., Miltenberger, R.G., 1990. Contact desensitization in the treatment of dog phobias in persons who have mental retardation. Behavioral Interventions 5, 55–60.

Evans, D.W., Canavera, K., Kleinpeter, F.L., Maccubbin, E., Taga, K., 2005. The fears, phobias and anxieties of children with autism spectrum disorders and Down syndrome: Comparisons with developmentally and chronologically age matched children. Child Psychiatry and Human Development 36, 3–26. Available from: http://dx.doi.org/10.1007/s10578-004-3619-x.

Farrugia, S., Hudson, J., 2006. Anxiety in adolescents with Asperger Syndrome: Negative thoughts, behavioral problems, and life interference. Focus on Autism and Other Developmental Disabilities 21, 25–35.

Gadow, K.D., Sprafkin, J., 1998. Adolescent symptom inventory-4 norms manual (Vol. Stony Brook, NY: Checkmate Plus). Checkmate Plus, Stony Brook, NY.

Gadow, K.D., Sprafkin, J., 2002. Child symptom inventory-4 screening and norms manual. Checkmate Plus, Stony Brook, NY.

Ghaziuddin, M., Greden, J., 1998. Depression in children with autism/pervasive developmental disorders: a case-control family history study. J. Autism Dev. Disord. 28 (2), 111–115.

Hagopian, L.P., Crockett, J.L., Keeney, K.M., 2001. Multicomponent treatment for blood-injury-injection phobia in a young man with mental retardation. Res. Dev. Disabil. 22, 141–149.

Hagopian, L.P., Jennett, H.K., 2008. Behavioral assessment and treatment of anxiety in individuals with intellectual disabilities and autism. Journal of Developmental and Physical Disabilities 20 (5), 467–483.

Hagopian, L.P., Long, E.S., Rush, K.S., 2004. Preference assessment procedures for individuals with developmental disabilities. Behav. Modif. 28, 668–677.

Hallett, V., Ronald, A., Rijsdijk, F., Happé, F., 2010. Association of autistic-like and internalizing traits during childhood: a longitudinal twin study. Am. J. Psychiatry.

Hanley, G.P., Iwata, B.A., McCord, B.E., 2003. Functional analysis of problem behavior: a review. J. Appl. Behav. Anal. 36, 147–185.

Holland, P.W., Wainer, H., 1993. Differential item functioning. Hillsdale, NJ, 137-166.

Hollander, E., King, A., Delaney, K., Smith, C.J., Silverman, J.M., 2003. Obsessive–compulsive behaviors in parents of multiplex autism families. Psychiatry Res. 117 (1), 11–16.

Iwata, B., Dorsey, M., Slifer, K., Bauman, K., Richman, G., 1994. Toward a functional analysis of self-injury. J. Appl. Behav. Anal. 27, 197–209.

Jang, J., Dixon, D., Tarbox, J., Granpeesheh, D., 2010. Symptom severity and challenging behavior in children with ASD. Res. Autism Spectr. Disord. 5, 1028–1032.

Jennett, H.K., Hagopian, L.P., 2008. Identifying empirically supported treatments for phobic avoidance in individuals with intellectual disabilities. Behav. Therapy 39, 151–161.

Kaat, A.J., Gadow, K.D., Lecavalier, L., 2013. Psychiatric symptom impairment in children with autism spectrum disorders. J. Abnormal Child Psychol. 41 (6), 959–969.

Kanner, L., 1943. Autistic disturbances of affective contact. Nervous Child 2, 217–250.

Kerns, C.M., Kendall, P.C., Berry, L., Souders, M.C., Franklin, M.E., Schultz, R.T., et al., 2014. Traditional and atypical presentations of anxiety in youth with autism spectrum disorder. J. Autism Dev. Disord. 44 (11), 2851–2861.

Klinger, L.G., Dawson, G., Renner, P., 2003. Autistic disorder. In: Marsh, E., Barkley, R. (Eds.), Child Psychopathology, second ed Guilford press, New York.

Krotochwill, T.R., Stoiber, K.C., 2002. Evidence-based interventions in school psychology: conceptual foundations of the *Procedural and Coding Manual* of Division 16 and the Society for the Study of School Psychology Task Force. School Psychol. Q. 17, 341–389.

Lecavalier, L., 2014. Phenotypic variability in autism spectrum disorder: Clinical considerations. In: Davis III, T.E., White, S.W., Ollendick, T.H. (Eds.), Handbook of Autism and Anxiety. Springer Science and Business Media, LLC, New York, pp. 137–152. . Available from: http://dx.doi.org/10.1007/978-3-319-06796-4_10.

Leyfer, O.T., Folstein, S.E., Bacalman, S., Davis, N.O., Dinh, E., Morgan, J., et al., 2006. Comorbid psychiatric disorders in children with autism: Interview development and rates of disorders. J. Autism Dev. Disord. 36, 849–861.

Lovaas, O.I., Simmons, J.Q., 1969. Manipulation of self-destruction in three retarded children. J. Appl. Behav. Anal. 2 (3), 143–157.

Love, S.R., Matson, J.L., West, D., 1990. Mothers as effective therapists for autistic children's phobias. J. Appl. Behav. Anal. 23, 379–385.

Luscre, D.M., Center, D.B., 1996. Procedures for reducing dental fear in children with autism. J. Autism Dev. Disord. 26, 547–556.

Mason, J., Scior, K., 2004. "Diagnostic overshadowing" amongst clinicians working with people with intellectual disabilities in the UK. J. Appl. Res. Intellect. Disabil. 17 (2), 85–90.

Matson, J.L., Love, S.R., 1990. A comparison of parent-reported fear for autistic and nonhandicapped age-matched children and youth. Aust. NZ J. Dev. Disabil. 16 (4), 349–357.

McDougle, C.J., Kresch, L.E., Goodman, W.K., Naylor, S.T., Volkmar, F.R., Cohen, D.J., et al., 1995. A case-controlled study of repetitive thoughts and behavior in adults with autistic disorder and obsessive-compulsive disorder. Am. J. Psychiatry 152, 772–777.

Moskowitz, L., Mulder, E., Walsh, C., McLaughlin, D., Proudfit, G., Carr, E., 2013. A multimethod assessment of anxiety and problem behavior in children with autism spectrum disorders and intellectual disability. Am. J. Intellect. Dev. Disabil. 118, 419–434. Available from: http://dx.doi.org/10.1352/1944.7558.118.6.419.

Muris, P., Steerneman, P., Merckelbach, H., Holdrinet, I., Meesters, C., 1998. Comorbid anxiety symptoms in children with pervasive developmental disorders. J. Anxiety Disord. 12 (4), 387–393.

Myers, S.M., Johnson, C.P., 2007. American Academy of Pediatrics Council on children with disabilities. Management of children with autism spectrum disorders. Pediatrics 120, 1162–1182.

Nebel-Schwalm, M., Davis III, T.E., 2013. Nature and etiological models of anxiety disorders. In: Storch, E., McKay, D. (Eds.), Handbook of Treating Variants and Complications in Anxiety Disorders. Springer Science and Business Media, LLC, New York, pp. 3–21.

Ollendick, T.H., Davis III, T.E., 2012. Evidence-based assessment and treatment of specific phobias in children and adolescents. In T. E. In: Davis III, T.H., Ollendick, Öst, L.-G. (Eds.), Intensive One-Session Treatment of specific phobias. Springer Science and Business Media, LLC, New York, pp. 43–56. Available from: http://dx.doi.org/10.1007/978-1-4614-3253-1_3.

King, N.J., Ollendick, T.H., Murphy, G.C., 1997. Assessment of childhood phobias. Clin. Psychol. Rev. 17, 667–687.

Ollendick, T.H., Oswald, D.P., Ollendick, D.G., 1993. Anxiety disorders in mentally retarded persons. In: Matson, J.L., Barrett, R.P. (Eds.), Psychopathology in the Mentally Retarded. Allyn & Bacon, Needham Heights, MA, pp. 41–85.

Ozsivadjian, A., Knott, F., Magiati, I., 2012. Parent and child perspectives on the nature of anxiety in children and young people with autism spectrum disorders: a focus group study. Autism 16 (2), 107–121.

Rapp, J.T., Vollmer, T.R., Hovanetz, A.N., 2005. Evaluation and treatment of swimming pool avoidance exhibited by an adolescent girl with autism. Behav. Therapy 36, 101–105.

Ricciardi, J.N., Luiselli, J.K., Camare, M., 2006. Shaping approach responses as intervention for specific phobia in a child with autism. J. Appl. Behav. Anal. 39, 445–448.

Richman, D.M., Dotson, W.H., Rose, C.A., Thompson, S., Abby, L., 2012. Effects of age on the types and severity of excessive fear or the absence of fear in children and young adults with autism. J. Mental Health Res. Intellect. Disabil. 5 (3-4), 215–235.

Roberson-Nay, R., Strong, D.R., Nay, W.T., Beidel, D.C., Turner, S.M., 2007. Development of an abbreviated Social Phobia and Anxiety Inventory (SPAI) using item response theory: The SPAI-23. Psychol. Assess. 19 (1), 133.

Roussos, L.A., Stout, W.F., 2004. Differential item functioning analysis: Detecting DIF items and testing DIF hypotheses. In: Kaplan, D. (Ed.), The SAGE Handbook of Quantitative Methodology for the Social Sciences. Sage, Thousand Oaks, CA, pp. 107–115.

Rudy, B., Davis III, T.E., 2012. Interventions for specific phobia in special populations. In: Davis III, T.E., Ollendick, T.H., Öst, L.-G. (Eds.), Intensive One-Session Treatment of Specific Phobias. Springer Science and Business Media, LLC, New York, pp. 177–193. Available from: http://dx.doi.org/10.1007/978-1-4614-3253-1_9.

Runyan, M.C., Stevens, D.H., Reeves, R., 1985. Reduction of avoidance behavior of institutionalized mentally retarded adults through contact desensitization. Am. J. Mental Deficiency 90, 222–225.

Rutter, M., 1978. Diagnosis and definition of childhood autism. J. Autism Childh. Schizophr. 8 (2), 139–161.

Shabani, D.B., Fisher, W.W., 2006. Stimulus fading and differential reinforcement for the treatment of needle phobia in a youth with autism. J. Appl. Behav. Anal. 39, 449–452.

Schmidt, J.D., Luiselli, J.K., Rue, H., Whalley, K., 2013. Graduated exposure and positive reinforcement to overcome setting and activity avoidance in an adolescent with autism. Behav. Modif. 37, 128–142.

Shattuck, P.T., Roux, A.M., Hudson, L.E., Taylor, J.L., Maenner, M.J., Trani, J.F., 2012. Services for adults with an autism spectrum disorder. Can. J. Psychiatry 57, 284–291.

Sprafkin, J., Gadow, K.D., Salisbury, H., Schneider, J., Loney, J., 2002. Further evidence of reliability and validity of the Child Symptom Inventory-4: Parent checklist in clinically referred boys. J. Clin. Child Adolesc. Psychol. 31 (4), 513–524.

Velting, O.N., Setzer, N.J., Albano, A.M., 2004. Update on and advances in assessment and cognitive-behavioral treatment of anxiety disorders in children and adolescents. Profes. Psychol. 35, 42–54.

Vollmer, T.R., Sloman, K.N., Borrero, C.S., 2009. Behavioral assessment of self-injury. Assessing Childhood Psychopathology and Developmental Disabilities. Springer, New York, pp. 341–369.

White, S.W., Roberson-Nay, R., 2009. Anxiety, social deficits, and loneliness in youth with autism spectrum disorders. J. Autism Dev. Disord. 39, 1006–1013.

White, S.W., Oswald, D., Ollendick, T.H., Scahill, L., 2009. Anxiety in children and adolescents with autism spectrum disorders. Clin. Psychol. Rev. 29, 216–229.

White, S.W., Bray, B.C., Ollendick, T.H., 2012. Examining shared and unique aspects of social anxiety disorder and autism spectrum disorder using factor analysis. J Autism Dev. Disord. 42 (5), 874–884.

Witmer, A.N., Lecavalier, L., 2010. Validity of comorbid psychiatric disorders in youngsters with autism spectrum disorders. J. Dev. Phys. Disabil. 22, 367–380.

CHAPTER 11

Anxiety and ASD in Schools: School-Related Issues and Individualized Education Programs

Christopher Lopata, James P. Donnelly and Marcus L. Thomeer
Institute for Autism Research, Canisius College, Buffalo, NY, United States

OVERVIEW

Youth with autism spectrum disorder (ASD) spend a significant amount of their development in educational settings and education law mandates that they be provided an appropriate education. School staff are increasingly challenged to adequately evaluate and treat symptoms of ASD, as well as any number of secondary symptoms. Anxiety is one of the most common co-occurring difficulties of students with ASD. Anxiety-related problems are a significant concern in school settings as they can exacerbate core symptoms of ASD, disrupt learning, and interfere with other interventions (American Psychiatric Association [APA], 2013; White et al., 2014b). Although the large majority of studies involving anxiety and youth with ASD have been conducted in nonschool settings, many have yielded findings that are highly relevant and applicable to schools (Lopata & Thomeer, 2014). This chapter examines anxiety and ASD in school settings, with an emphasis on research studies conducted in school settings or with school-derived samples, when available. Where school-based evidence is limited or nonexistent, data from the broader evidence-base are presented to inform the considerations and practices of educational teams. The chapter begins with an overview of how ASD is defined in clinical and educational settings, followed by a review of anxiety-related problems in youth with ASD in school settings. This is followed by a discussion of school-based assessment of anxiety in students with ASD and finally intervention development, implementation, and monitoring of anxiety symptoms using the Individualized Education Program (IEP).

Anxiety in Children and Adolescents with Autism Spectrum Disorder.
DOI: http://dx.doi.org/10.1016/B978-0-12-805122-1.00011-9
© 2017 Elsevier Inc.
All rights reserved.
211

CLINICAL DIAGNOSIS AND EDUCATIONAL CLASSIFICATION OF ASD

Clinical diagnostic and special education frameworks constitute two important classification systems used to identify students with ASD. Although both identify and characterize ASD features with considerable overlap between them, some differences exist. This is of interest given the increasingly important role of educational professionals in the assessment and treatment of youth with ASD. The *Diagnostic and Statistical Manual of Mental Disorders, Fifth Edition* (*DSM-5*; APA, 2013) represents a significant alteration in the diagnostic framework that in one way moved closer to the special education parameters, but in other ways encompasses a broader range of clinical impact.

The *DSM-5* collapsed the prior diagnostic categories of autistic disorder, Asperger's disorder, and pervasive developmental disorder — not otherwise specified (PDD-NOS) into a single category (autism spectrum disorder; ASD). This reflects the perspective that ASD exists on a continuum (spectrum) with varying degrees of severity and functional impairments (APA, 2013). The diagnostic criteria for ASD also collapsed the triad of features that characterized the prior diagnostic category of autism (i.e., communication, socialization, and circumscribed and repetitive behaviors and interests) into two primary symptom dimensions (i.e., social–communication/interaction and circumscribed and repetitive behaviors and interests) but continues to require a specific number of indicators within each of the two dimensions. The shift to a single *DSM-5* category (ASD) is consistent with the special education classification system which has used and continues to use a single category (i.e., *autism*). Under the educational classification system, *autism* is characterized by impairments in social interaction and verbal and nonverbal communication, and associated features such as repetitive activities and motor movements, behavioral rigidity, and atypical sensory sensitivities/responses (IDEIA, 2004). In contrast to the *DSM-5*, the educational classification scheme does not have specific indicators (or a minimum number of indicators) under each of these features or requires severity indicators or specifiers (for the presence of intellectual and/or language impairment). Another distinction involves the stipulation in the educational classification scheme that eligibility is based on an adverse effect on the student's *educational performance*; this is narrower than the *DSM-5* which considers the impact on a broader range of functional areas (e.g., social, occupational). One additional difference, of importance to this chapter, is the expanded recognition of comorbid symptoms/disorders (including anxiety) in the *DSM-5* for individuals with ASD. The educational classification system does not address other disorders, whereas the *DSM-5* indicates that these should be diagnosed when present (see APA, 2013 and IDEIA, 2004).

Discrepancies also exist in the national ASD prevalence data. The most recent data from 2010 indicated a national clinical ASD diagnosis prevalence of 1.5% (1 in 68; CDC, 2014), in contrast to a 0.8% (1 in 125) *autism* special education classification rate for that year (National Center for Education Statistics, 2015). The discrepancy may reflect a difference in data collection methods (i.e., CDC surveyed ASD diagnosis among 8-year-olds across 11 sites nationally vs. all students ages 3 to 21 years in school settings); however, it appears more likely to be due to under-classification of *autism* in schools. For example, studies have found that a sizable minority of students diagnosed with ASD do not receive special education services (e.g., 25%, Kaat et al., 2013; 19%, White et al., 2007). Additionally, students with a clinical diagnosis of ASD sometimes receive a different special education classification other than *autism*. The CDC (2014) data indicated that among children with an ASD clinical diagnosis, only 30% to 69% had a special education classification of *autism*. Despite the potential underestimate in the educational classification of *autism*, data suggest significant increases in the prevalence of autism in both educational classification (0.2% in 2002 to 0.8% in 2010) and clinical diagnosis (0.6% in 2002 to 1.5% in 2010).

ANXIETY AND ASD IN SCHOOLS

As noted, the *DSM-5* recognizes the presence of co-occurring psychiatric conditions and symptoms in individuals with ASD. Estimates suggest that nearly 70% of those with ASD also have at least one comorbid psychiatric condition (APA, 2013), with anxiety being among the most common (White et al., 2009). It is important to consider that studies of youth with ASD have differed in their measurement of anxiety. The majority of studies have relied on symptom level or severity ratings to evaluate anxiety problems, with fewer studies using formal diagnoses of anxiety disorders. Consistent with Lopata and Thomeer (2014) in their review of anxiety in school settings for students with ASD, this chapter will use the term *anxiety* to refer to anxiety symptoms. Examining comorbid anxiety from the symptom and severity level perspective is also more consistent with school practices as school-based clinicians do not render psychiatric diagnoses, special education includes only 13 categories, and the staff focuses on treating symptoms. In addition, symptoms at the subclinical level can cause impairment that warrants intervention (Kaat et al., 2013).

Anxiety in school-based samples with ASD

Research on anxiety in ASD has increased substantially over the last decade (Reaven et al., 2014) and is largely based on parent-reports and nonschool based samples (Hebron & Humphrey, 2014; Lopata & Thomeer, 2014; van Steensel et al., 2011). Information from these studies provides a broader context for interpreting the available school-based and school-related studies of anxiety in students with ASD. Many nonschool based studies have also examined potential risk factors for anxiety symptoms in this population and yielded mixed findings (Vasa & Mazurek, 2015). A review by White et al. (2009) of 40 studies examining anxiety in youth with ASD yielded prevalence rates of anxiety-related impairment ranging from 11% to 84%. Additionally, although anxiety was common across age and IQ ranges, findings suggested that older age and higher IQ were associated with greater levels of anxiety. van Steensel et al. (2011) conducted a meta-analysis of 31 studies of anxiety in youth with ASD and reported a 40% prevalence rate across studies for a comorbid anxiety disorder or clinically elevated symptoms. Findings from this study indicated that older age and lower IQ were associated with higher rates of overall anxiety; however, the directionality of the trends differed based on the type of anxiety disorder. Higher rates of anxiety were also associated with the use of diagnostic interviews (vs. questionnaires) suggesting that the method for assessing anxiety may affect prevalence and severity estimates.

Anxiety is of interest to educational professionals for many reasons. Anxiety can negatively impact school performance, social relationships, and behaviors of students with ASD (Reaven, 2009). Although clinically-referred samples provide essential information on comorbidity, studies of anxiety in school samples with ASD are needed (Hebron & Humphrey, 2014; White et al., 2009). Teachers and school-based professionals may be especially suited to provide ratings of students' anxiety because they spend extensive time with their students, and they have backgrounds that include training in development, disabilities, and emotional/behavioral problems (Lopata & Thomeer, 2014). Such studies would inform our current estimates of anxiety symptom and comorbidity rates in ASD and provide novel information on the impact of factors such as informant (e.g., parent vs. teacher) and setting (clinic vs. school) on anxiety prevalence in ASD.

In a study that included teacher ratings of comorbid symptoms in children with ASD evaluated at a developmental disabilities or psychiatric clinic, Weisbrot et al. (2005) found significantly higher levels of teacher-rated anxiety for 6-12-year-olds with ASD compared to a non-ASD clinical group. In addition, the high anxiety children with ASD had a higher mean IQ than the low anxiety children with ASD. Kaat et al. (2013) also found high rates of anxiety when examining impairment, symptom, and diagnostic criteria for teacher ratings of 6-12-year-olds with ASD referred to a developmental disabilities clinic. These studies suggest that teachers also perceive significant anxiety problems in students with ASD being evaluated at specialized clinics.

A small number of studies have evaluated self-reported and teacher-rated anxiety symptoms of students with ASD in public school samples. In a recent study of self-reported anxiety, Hebron and Humphrey (2014) found high-functioning adolescents with ASD (HFASD) in mainstream classrooms reported significantly more anxiety symptoms than comparison adolescents with no disability or a learning disability, with 59% of the HFASD group falling in the clinical range. Teacher ratings of school samples with ASD also reveal significant problems with anxiety. For example, Ashburner et al. (2010) found teacher ratings of anxiety were significantly higher for students (ages 6 to 10 years) with HFASD in mainstream classrooms compared to matched typically-developing controls. Our research team is currently conducting a randomized trial of a comprehensive school-based intervention (i.e., schoolMAX) targeting the social-communication skills of elementary school students with HFASD attending public schools (Institute of Education Sciences Grant R324A130216). Baseline measures of 77 students with HFASD have been collected including a broad clinical rating scale that includes an anxiety symptom scale. Teacher ratings indicated significantly higher anxiety levels for students with HFASD compared to normative estimates ($t[76] = 4.56$; $p < .001$, $d = 1.05$), with 33% of the sample having ratings at or above the at-risk cutoff score.

Although these self-report and teacher rating studies of school samples are informative, the samples are small (*ns* from 22 to 77) and relatively high-functioning. In one of the only large-scale studies, Lecavalier (2006) assessed comorbid symptoms of 3-21-year-olds with ASD (of various ability levels) receiving special education services across 37 school districts.

Teacher ratings of 437 students with ASD indicated prevalence rates (based on items rated to be a moderate problem or a severe problem) of 18% for nervous/tense, 14% for worrying, and 11% for fearful/anxious. Results also indicated that younger age and lower adaptive skills were associated with less anxiety related problems. Together, these school-based studies suggest that anxiety is a common problem in school settings for students with ASD and that age and level of functioning may be implicated. The broader research base also suggests that core impairments of students with ASD can contribute to anxiety (e.g., Mayes et al., 2011). For example, higher parent ratings of restricted, repetitive, and ritualistic behaviors were related to higher levels of anxiety in students with ASD (Rodgers et al., 2012; Stratis & Lecavalier, 2013; Sukhodolsky et al., 2008) and lower levels of social skills/social relationships were associated with higher levels of anxiety (e.g., Chang et al., 2012; Eussen et al., 2012). Anxiety may also serve to exacerbate core ASD impairments (i.e., bidirectional relationship; Mazefsky & Herrington, 2014; White et al., 2009).

School environments, stress, and anxiety

A broad range of environmental factors and interpersonal demands within schools appear to run counter to the preferences, traits, and impairments of students with ASD. Few studies have specifically examined school-related factors associated with increased anxiety in students with ASD. In one of the few studies, Hebron and Humphrey (2014) interviewed five adolescents with HFASD about their school experiences and found that problems with understanding social situations, social isolation, bullying, disrupted routines, and chaotic and unstructured environments (e.g., lunchroom, playground) were common and highly anxiety-provoking.

A number of authors have proposed anxiety-inducing factors that are commonly encountered in school environments. These factors reflect three general areas including social demands and exposure, sensory sensitivities, and disruptions to routines. Social demands are pervasive in school settings, ranging from academic instruction (i.e., social-communication) to group projects to adult and peer interactions (Lopata & Thomeer, 2014). These social interactions throughout the school day are likely challenging to students with ASD as a result of social-communication deficits. Prior experiences involving social failures, rejection, teasing, and bullying, as well as self-awareness of their social deficits, may increase anxiety for some students (Chang et al., 2012; Eussen et al., 2012; Schroeder et al., 2014; Szatmari &

McConnell, 2011; White et al., 2014a). In addition, unexpected interactions with unfamiliar peers or adults can increase stress and anxiety (Ashburner et al., 2010). The high level of social exposure in schools may contribute to the development of anxiety or exacerbate anxiety in students with ASD (Mayes et al., 2011). Beyond social demands, sensory-related features of school environments may also be anxiety producing. For example, students with ASD often exhibit hypersensitivity to sensory input (i.e., auditory and visual stimuli; Groden et al., 2006) and many school environments are characterized by loud noise and high activity levels (e.g., cafeteria, hallways, gymnasium; Mazefsky & Herrington, 2014). Loud and unpredictable environments may challenge the sensory tolerances of some students with ASD. The third feature of schools that may be anxiety-provoking involves disruptions to routines. Schools regularly impose changes to students' schedules, environments, and teaching staff (Ashburner et al., 2010). Schools also require multiple transitions across the school day and between years that can be challenging for students with ASD. The beginning of an academic year and the transition to secondary schools constitute significant transition points for students with ASD (Mazefsky & Herrington, 2014; Tsai, 2006; White et al., 2009). These changes and transitions can be difficult owing to the students' preference for structure, consistency, and predictability (APA, 2013; Mazefsky & Herrington, 2014). An inability to manage these stressors and self-regulate (i.e., down–regulate) can cause or exacerbate anxiety in students with ASD (White et al., 2014a; White et al., 2014b).

Anxiety may manifest in several ways including disclosures of negative cognitions, behaviors, and/or physical symptoms (Mazefsky & Herrington, 2014; White et al., 2014a). For students with ASD and higher cognitive and language abilities, symptoms of anxiety may be accurately reported in self-reports (Hagopian & Jennett, 2014). Still some caution is warranted, as these students often have difficulty labeling and reporting internalized states despite their higher cognitive and language abilities (Rotheram–Fuller & MacMullen, 2011). Anxiety can also manifest in behavioral excesses. The emergence of or increase in problem behaviors such as self-injury, self-stimulation, aggression, tantrums, yelling, crying, or general irritability may be indicators of anxiety in students with ASD (Groden et al., 2006; Mayes et al., 2011; Romanczyk & Gillis, 2006; White et al., 2014a). Increases in the frequency and/or intensity of ASD symptoms such as repetitive behaviors or circumscribed interests (Sukhodolsky et al., 2008; Stratis & Lecavalier, 2013;

White et al., 2014a), or avoidance of settings or individuals (isolation) may also signal anxiety (APA, 2013; White et al., 2014a). Gastrointestinal, sleep, and eating problems, and declines in academic performance have also been linked to anxiety in students with ASD (APA, 2013; Mazurek et al., 2013; Reaven, 2009; Williams et al., 2015). Lastly, anxiety may manifest in other elevated arousal states (e.g., shaking, rapid breathing) or nonverbal behaviors such as facial expressions of distress or fear (Hagopian & Jennett, 2014). While not comprehensive, these noted behaviors reflect a range of possible indicators of anxiety in students with ASD in school settings.

SCHOOL-BASED ASSESSMENT OF ANXIETY

Assessing anxiety in students with ASD is challenging due to symptom overlap (Kerns & Kendall, 2014; Lecavalier et al., 2014). As such, it is important to consider anxiety symptoms relative to core ASD symptoms, with comorbid anxiety identified if the anxiety symptoms are independent of, and result in additional impairment beyond, the ASD diagnosis (Szatmari & McConnell, 2011). Another barrier to assessing anxiety in the school setting is related to the fact that anxiety disorders are not a distinct special education category and school clinicians generally do not provide *DSM-5* diagnoses. As a result, anxiety-related problems, if identified, would be described in the student's psychoeducational assessment reports and Individualized Education Program (IEP).

Assessment of anxiety is also complex as it is comprised of several interrelated elements including a perceived threat (stimuli), cognitive appraisal, physiological reaction, and behavioral response (White et al., 2014a). Considering how anxiety may manifest in each of these elements is important to detecting anxiety and differentiating it from core ASD features (Mazefsky & White, 2013). Based on the high prevalence of anxiety in ASD, screening for anxiety should be part of all initial and ongoing assessments for students suspected of, or having ASD (Rodgers et al., 2012; Vasa & Mazurek, 2015). Multidisciplinary school teams may be ideally suited to conduct such assessments as they are typically comprised of parents, teachers, and service providers with diverse areas of expertise (e.g., school psychology, speech/language pathology, physical therapy; Lopata & Thomeer, 2014). In addition, they are responsible for conducting comprehensive evaluations that include all areas related to the disability (cognitive, language/communication, academic, social-emotional, and health/physical; IDEIA, 2004), and they have access to and observe the student with ASD in a variety of natural and demanding settings.

It is important to note that assessing and treating anxiety in students with ASD in school settings follows the same general framework as in clinical settings, only adapted to the expertise and setting characteristics of schools. Assessments for anxiety in students with ASD should involve multiple informants and measures (Mazefsky & White, 2013; White et al., 2009). Initially, it is necessary to assess the student's IQ and language level as these will inform both assessment and intervention techniques (Rotheram-Fuller & MacMullen, 2011; White et al., 2014a). Significant intellectual or language deficits will render some measures and techniques less valid or inapplicable. A multimodal approach can include rating scales, formal clinical interviews, other interviews, and behavioral assessment (observations and physiological indicators; Groden et al., 2006; Mazurek et al., 2013; White et al., 2014a). Although there are a range of instruments available, there is a lack of anxiety measures that have been validated for students with ASD (Kerns & Kendall, 2014).

One type of measure, familiar in schools, for assessing anxiety is rating scales. These are frequently used because they are brief, efficient, and can be completed by individuals from the student's natural environments (e.g., teachers and parents; Norris & Lecavalier, 2010). Although not diagnostic, these scales are commonly used to screen for anxiety symptoms and can contribute to diagnostic decisions. Despite the fact that most anxiety rating scales have not been validated for use with students with ASD, several have been identified as appropriate for these students (see review by Lecavalier et al., 2014); these may represent preferred scales for school evaluators. As noted, parent and teacher rating scales have been used extensively to study and detect anxiety in students with ASD. Discrepancies in informant ratings of anxiety are common and should be expected as teachers and parents are characterizing the students' symptoms in different settings (Stratis & Lecavalier, 2015). School evaluators should examine cross-informant ratings as they may provide important insights into the pervasiveness of symptoms or setting-specific symptoms and contributors (Romanczyk & Gillis, 2006). Rating scales also offer an additional advantage. In contrast to measures based on symptom counts and dichotomous scoring (i.e., present vs. absent), rating scales assess the extent and severity of anxiety in students with ASD (Achenbach, 2011; Gotham et al., 2015). Because some students with ASD may not reach diagnostic criteria for an anxiety disorder but are still in need of anxiety-reducing intervention (Kaat et al., 2013), continuous-scaled measures such as rating scales can help identify and monitor symptom severity including subclinical symptoms (Lecavalier, 2006; Mazefsky & White, 2013). A focus on symptom severity is also consistent with school practices that regularly assess and treat comorbid symptoms, even in the absence of a diagnosis. When appropriate, self-report rating scales should also be completed. These may be most appropriate for students with HFASD (Mazefsky & White, 2013), but caution is still warranted due to characteristic impairments in identifying and labeling internalized states including anxiety (Rotheram-Fuller & MacMullen, 2011).

Diagnostic clinical interviews are another type of measure that may be employed in school settings to assess for anxiety. Interviews can be conducted with parents and/or teachers to determine whether the student meets criteria for a specific anxiety disorder. While determining a clinical diagnosis is not the focus of school evaluators, these interviews allow for probing that can help differentiate anxiety symptoms from ASD symptoms (Szatmari & McConnell, 2011). These measures are often not feasible in applied settings such as schools because they require a high level of training and expertise (Norris & Lecavalier, 2010) and typically take one to three hours to administer (Mazefsky & White, 2013). In addition, the information they yield is less useful in treatment planning and progress monitoring than other forms of assessment (e.g., observations; Bolton et al., 2012). As a result, school evaluators will most likely rely on other assessment techniques. Informal interviews may also yield useful information. For example, interviews with school staff and parents may help identify anxiety-related symptoms, behaviors, and contingencies that are useful in behavioral assessments. When possible, interviews should be conducted with the students in order to better understand the cognitive aspects of the anxiety problems including cognitive distortions and deficiencies (Bolton et al., 2012; Mazefsky & Herrington, 2014). Understanding the specific cognitions will help inform intervention targets and strategies.

Behavioral assessment plays a critical role in measuring anxiety in all students with ASD, and in particular those with intellectual and language deficits (APA, 2013). Given that assessment techniques for anxiety in typically-developing students (self-reports and interviews) have significant limitations for students with ASD, evaluators commonly rely on behavioral assessments to measure symptoms and circumstances surrounding them. These assessments can include observations of behaviors and/or physiological measures to operationalize and track anxiety symptoms in order to determine antecedent and consequent variables (Hagopian & Jennett, 2014). As noted, anxiety can manifest in the emergence of a new problem behavior/symptom and/or change in a behavior/symptom relative to baseline. Once the anxiety symptom is operationalized it can be tracked along with antecedents and consequences (Hagopian & Jennett, 2014). This process is familiar to school staff that frequently conduct and collect data as part of functional behavioral assessments (FBAs). The accuracy of behavioral assessments can increase when the student with ASD is observed and tracked across settings (e.g., lunchroom, classroom, playground); this can provide greater specificity in identifying triggers and reactions under different setting demands (Bolton et al., 2012).

Physiological measures can also be used to assess anxiety. These may be particularly useful given the cognitive, language, and/or self-report limitations of students with ASD (Hagopian & Jennett, 2014; Kerns & Kendall, 2014), as well as potential problems with operationalizing anxiety behaviors. Common indicators can include salivary cortisol, heart rate, blood pressure, and skin conductance (Mazurek et al., 2013; Romanczyk & Gillis, 2006). Given significant variability in physiological arousal and anxiety within and/or across individuals with ASD (Romanczyk & Gillis, 2006), and the fact that normative comparisons are often unavailable (Lopata & Thomeer, 2014), these measures may be most useful when comparing the student's physiological responses to baseline levels (Groden et al., 2006). As part of an FBA, school evaluators can measure the student's reactive arousal and the circumstances under which it occurs across a range of settings (Mazurek et al., 2013; White et al., 2014a). Because physiological devices may cause stress and anxiety for the student with ASD (Hagopian & Jennett, 2014) evaluators should select the one that is most tolerable (Lopata & Thomeer, 2014). Many devices may not be feasible in schools due to practical limitations (e.g., cost, time, expertise), however, advances in technology (e.g., online applications) may make measuring physiological reactions increasingly available, affordable, and easy to do.

Findings from the comprehensive assessment may be delineated in several different educational reports (psychoeducational report, FBA, etc.), but the specific assessment results (scores, frequency counts, etc.) are reported on the student's IEP (IDEIA, 2004). For more details on the assessment of anxiety in children with ASD, please see Chapter 5 in this book.

INTERVENTION DEVELOPMENT, IMPLEMENTATION, AND MONITORING USING THE IEP

Special education programming is guided by an IEP which serves as the official record of the student's assessment results, present levels of performance (PLEP), measurable goals and objectives, and special education supports and services (IDEIA, 2004). Of relevance to this chapter, the IEP includes results of the anxiety (and IQ and language) assessment, including the student's associated performance levels which serve as the entry point for the intervention and baseline for measuring progress. It also includes the goals of the school intervention and a description of the program supports (i.e., anxiety-targeted intervention).

Although the student's IEP addresses academic, and developmental and functional needs (e.g., social, management, physical), anxiety will most likely be addressed using techniques that fall under the social (skills development) and management (structure/rules, exposures, and reinforcement) domains. The diverse expertise of school intervention teams, coupled with the range of authentic environments appear to make schools ideal for treating anxiety in students with ASD, yet there is a dearth of school-based models (Lopata & Thomeer, 2014). In the only identified school study, Reaven et al. (2014) described results of a pilot feasibility trial of a school adaptation of the Face Your Fears program for children with HFASD. Multidisciplinary school teams of youth with ASD and their parents reported positive views of the training and curriculum (which included behavioral rehearsal, roleplay, and exposure hierarchies). The findings suggested that such a program is feasible in school settings but no studies were identified showing efficacy. As such, the following should be considered as guidelines, informed by the broader treatment research on anxiety in youth with ASD.

A multimodal intervention approach is warranted given the multiple and interrelated components that comprise anxiety and the features of ASD (Hagopian & Jennett, 2014; White et al., 2013b). These interventions should target anxiety symptoms, as well as social and adaptive skills (Green & Wood, 2013). Although these treatments follow the same progression as for non-ASD students (assessment, psychoeducation, cognitive restructuring, and exposure; Moree & Davis, 2010), some of the techniques are modified (based on the unique features of ASD and functional level of the student) and supplemental instruction is often provided (Sukhodolsky et al., 2013). Results of the comprehensive assessment yield a disorder-specific hierarchy that delineates the specific ASD-related deficits and anxiety features to be targeted in the intervention (Moree & Davis, 2010). The intervention procedures are developed by the student's IEP and intervention team including the parent(s)/caregiver(s) and then communicated to the student's broader educational team.

Initially, training is provided to the intervention team. Team members may consist of professionals (teachers, school psychologists, counselors, speech/language pathologists, etc.) and paraprofessionals (one-to-one aides, classroom assistants, etc.) that work directly with the student and it is likely that many do not have experience in anxiety treatments for students with ASD (Reaven et al., 2014). Beyond presenting the intervention procedures, trainings can be used to increase shared responsibility, coordination, and generalization (Wood et al., 2009). Given the multicomponent nature of the treatment, feasibility may be increased by having all members of the team trained in the full intervention but assigning an individual treatment element(s) to different members. This requires coordination but it may increase implementation fidelity by decreasing the burden on any individual member (Lopata & Thomeer, 2014). Regardless of the procedures or functional level of the student with ASD, all will benefit from high levels of structure and predictability during the intervention (White et al., 2013a).

To date, studies targeting anxiety in ASD have used cognitive behavioral treatments (CBT) for students with HFASD. These treatments target maladaptive cognitive processing and reactions (thoughts, emotions, and behaviors) by teaching adaptive coping skills that alter the students' cognitive distortions (appraisals) and lower arousal levels so that they can gradually and successfully confront the feared stimulus (Green & Wood, 2013). Results of several studies have supported the efficacy of CBT for reducing anxiety in youth with HFASD (e.g., Reaven et al., 2012; Wood et al., 2009). A recent meta-analysis evaluating the efficacy of CBT for anxiety in youth with HFASD indicated large reductions in anxiety for those receiving treatment (relative to control conditions) based on clinician ($d = 1.21$) and parent ratings ($d = 1.19$; Sukhodolsky et al., 2013). These treatments provide a framework and adaptations that can be applied to school interventions for anxiety in students with ASD.

One component of a school intervention should involve remediation of ASD-related impairments (social, perspective taking, emotion recognition, etc.); this can be done prior to addressing the anxiety or concurrently (Moree & Davis, 2010; White et al., 2013a; Wood et al., 2009).

School clinicians (e.g., school psychologists, counselors) are well-qualified and regularly conduct such skills groups. Developing these skills will help the students better understand their cognitive distortions, as well as assist with their coping responses during exposure exercises.

The second component consists of psychoeducation and cognitive restructuring in which the student is taught about anxiety, how cognitive distortions affect emotions and behavioral reactions (avoidance), and adaptive coping strategies to confront the feared stimulus (Moree & Davis, 2010; White et al., 2013a). School clinicians are also qualified to conduct this portion but should adapt the traditional approach to take into account features of students with ASD. Concrete and visual techniques, hands-on activities (e.g., cartoons, worksheets, stress thermometers), simplified instruction, and a focus on physiological sensations have been recommended to accommodate the students' concrete learning style and increase their understanding of the link between distorted cognitions, physiological reactions, and behaviors (Green & Wood, 2013; Moree & Davis, 2010). Cognitive restructuring is achieved by challenging distortions and replacing them with adaptive self-statements (Bolton et al., 2012). In addition, the student is taught practical problem-solving skills and arousal reduction techniques (relaxation; deep breathing, muscle relaxation) and when to apply them (Groden et al., 2006; Reaven et al., 2012).

Once the student has developed these coping strategies, graded exposures are used to confront the anxiety-provoking stimulus in order to achieve habituation (White et al., 2013a). To the extent possible, these exposures should be conducted daily *in vivo* with escape prevention (Wood et al., 2009; Reaven, 2009). Classroom teachers and/or aides may be ideally suited for these trials because they are with the student throughout the day. As such, they can conduct planned exposures, but also assist the student when unplanned exposures occur (Lopata & Thomeer, 2014). The assigned staff member can rehearse the coping strategy (cognitive and arousal reduction) with the student prior to the exposure, as well as provide prompts and model the strategy during the exposure (Hagopian & Jennett, 2014; Rotheram-Fuller & MacMullen, 2011). Relaxation strategies can be antecedent- (prior to the event) or response-targeted (in response to the exposure; White et al., 2014a), and/or practiced daily to reduce general stress (Groden et al., 2006). Another important technique to use is reinforcement. School staff should reinforce the student for making approach behaviors, using coping strategies, completing exposures (Hagopian & Jennett, 2014), and using other social and adaptive skills across the school day (Lopata & Thomeer, 2014; Rotheram-Fuller & MacMullen, 2011). Parents can also conduct exposure trials outside of school using the same coping and reinforcement strategies. This may help generalize skills across settings. It is important for school teams and parents to ensure that movement along the graded hierarchy is contingent upon successful completion of the prior trial (Hagopian & Jennett, 2014). Lastly, self-monitoring skills should be developed to increase the student's sense of control (Bolton et al., 2012).

Although evidence has supported the use of CBT with students with HFASD, little is known about how to treat anxiety in lower-functioning students with ASD (LFASD; White et al., 2009). Significant cognitive and/or language deficits will likely require a more behaviorally-based approach as these students may be confronting anxiety-inducing stimuli with less cognitive understanding and fewer cognitive strategies than students with HFASD (Lopata & Thomeer, 2014). Despite these barriers, school clinicians may attempt to teach strategies using pictures that depict adaptive coping techniques (approach behaviors, deep breathing, etc.) and positive outcomes (Groden et al., 2006). Arousal reduction strategies (deep breathing, relaxation) can also be taught and practiced daily to reduce general stress and anxiety, and used before and/or during an exposure (Groden et al., 2006; White et al., 2014a). Even in the absence of cognitive understanding of anxiety, students with LFASD can benefit from exposure to reduce anxious avoidance (Hagopian & Jennett, 2014). Given the impairments of students with LFASD, exposure and reinforcement will be critical and can be provided by teaching and support staff (due to their contact with the student across the school day). Prompting, modeling, and reinforcement are used during the gradual exposure exercises (Rotheram-Fuller & MacMullen, 2011; Vasa & Mazurek, 2015) and staff must ensure the student's anxiety levels are kept low to ensure habituation (Hagopian & Jennett, 2014). School staff should reinforce the student for confronting the feared stimulus and use highly desirable reinforcers to counter the negatively reinforced avoidant behavior (Hagopian & Jennett, 2014). Daily *in vivo* exposures with escape prevention should be attempted (Wood et al., 2009; Reaven, 2009). Lastly, parents should conduct exposure trials outside of school to increase generalization. For more details on CBT approaches for children with ASD, including common modifications, group and individual programs, see Chapters 6-8 in this book.

The students' IEPs should contain specific goals and objectives related to anxiety reduction. These goals will be derived from the comprehensive assessment and will serve as the basis for progress monitoring throughout the intervention (Hagopian & Jennett, 2014; Mazefsky & White, 2013). Progress monitoring indicators will vary across students but should involve multiple measures and methods (Moree & Davis, 2010; Rotheram-Fuller & MacMullen, 2011). Although progress monitoring efforts may be hindered by the previously noted lack of reliable and valid measures of anxiety for students with ASD (White et al., 2013a), the meta-analysis by Sukhodolsky et al. (2013) suggested that parent and clinician rating scales were sensitive to changes in anxiety levels for students with HFASD. The continuous-scaling of rating scales also makes them useful indicators of symptom severity (Achenbach, 2011) and allows for evaluation of change in anxiety levels over time. Despite these positive features and indications, the treatment sensitivity of these rating scales for students with LFASD is unknown. Behavioral observations are another progress monitoring option and may be especially applicable as they are often used in the assessment process and are familiar to school staff. If using behavioral observations, the target behaviors must be clearly operationalized and checks of reliability (interrater) should be conducted (Bolton et al., 2012). Physiological measures can also be used to measure reductions in stress and anxiety during exposure trials. These measures avoid many of the limitations of other types of measures and may be more valid; however, they require staff expertise with the measure(s) and tolerance on the part of the student with ASD. If using physiological measures, stress and anxiety responses to a feared stimulus should be compared to baseline levels away from the stimulus (Groden et al., 2006). These measures may be less accessible and feasible in school settings (Lopata & Thomeer, 2014) but may become increasingly applicable with improvements in technology and online applications. A final consideration involves the proximity of the outcome indicator to the skills/responses targeted by the intervention. Proximal measures (e.g., direct observations of approach behaviors without avoidance) may be more sensitive and effective in determining treatment effects compared to broadbased measures which may fail to detect improvements and clinically meaningful changes (Bolton et al., 2012; Wood et al., 2009).

CONCLUSION

Prevalence data indicate a substantial increase in the number of students with ASD, a significant portion of which also experience problems with anxiety. In contrast to clinical settings, schools have access to and are responsible for serving all students with ASD. As such, schools are a critical resource for identifying and treating anxiety in this population. School evaluators have professional training and experiences that allow them to conduct comprehensive assessments of anxiety, ASD symptoms, and intellectual and language functioning. In school settings, anxiety interventions for students with ASD are formalized in the students' IEPs. Along with assessment results, the IEP delineates the goals of the anxiety–reducing intervention and the support services to meet those goals. School intervention teams are uniquely suited to implement anxiety interventions for students with ASD as they are multidisciplinary and have access to the students across the school day and under real-world demands. Despite these advantages, no school-based anxiety treatment model for students with ASD has been validated and controlled trials are needed (White et al., 2009). Until then, school staff may be best served by adapting outpatient strategies that have been shown to be effective into comprehensive school-based models.

FUNDING ACKNOWLEDGMENT

Some of the data reported in this chapter was supported by Department of Education, Institute of Education Sciences Grant R324A130216. Findings and conclusions are those of the authors and do not necessarily reflect the views of the funding agency.

REFERENCES

Achenbach, T.M., 2011. Commentary: Definitely more than measurement error: But how should we understand and deal with informant discrepancies? Journal of Child and Adolescent Psychology 40 (1), 80—86. Available from: http://dx.doi.org/10.1080/15374416.2011.533416.
American Psychiatric Association, 2013. Diagnostic and statistical manual of mental disorders, 5th ed. American Psychiatric Association, Arlington, VA.
Ashburner, J., Ziviani, J., Rodger, S., 2010. Surviving in the mainstream: Capacity of children with autism spectrum disorders to perform academically and regulate their emotions and behavior at school. Research in Autism Spectrum Disorders 4, 18—27. Available from: http://dx.doi.org/10.1016/j.rasd.2009.07.002.
Bolton, J.B., McPoyle-Callahan, J.E., Christner, R.W., 2012. Autism: School-based cognitive-behavioral interventions. In: Mennuti, R.B., Christner, R.W., Freeman, A. (Eds.), Cognitive-behavioral interventions in educational settings: A handbook for practice, 2nd ed. Routledge, New York, pp. 469—501.
Center for Disease Control and Prevention (CDC), 2014. Prevalence of autism spectrum disorder among children aged 8 years - Autism and Developmental Disabilities Monitoring Network, 11 states, United States, 2010. MMWR 63 (SS-2), 1—21.

Chang, Y., Quan, J., Wood, J.J., 2012. Effects of anxiety disorder severity on social functioning in children with autism spectrum disorders. Journal of Developmental and Physical Disabilities 24, 235−245. Available from: http://dx.doi.org/10.1007/s10882-012-9268-2.

Eussen, L.J.M., Van Gool, A.R., Verheij, F., De Nijs, P.F.A., Verhulst, F.C., Greaves-Lord, K., 2012. The association of quality of social relations, symptom severity and intelligence with anxiety in children with autism spectrum disorders. Autism 17 (6), 723−735. Available from: http://dx.doi.org/10.1177/1362361312453882.

Gotham, K., Brunwasser, S.M., Lord, C., 2015. Depressive and anxiety symptom trajectories from school age through young adulthood in samples with autism spectrum disorder and developmental delay. Journal of the American Academy of Child and Adolescent Psychiatry 54 (5), 369−376. Available from: http://dx.doi.org/10.1016/j.jaac.2015.02.005.

Green, S.A., Wood, J.J., 2013. Cognitive-behavioral therapy for anxiety disorders in youth with ASD: Emotional, adaptive, and social outcomes. In: Scarpa, A., White, S.W., Attwood, T. (Eds.), CBT for children and adolescents with high-functioning autism spectrum disorders. Guilford, New York, NY, pp. 73−96.

Groden, J., Baron, M.G., Groden, G., 2006. Assessment and coping strategies. In: Baron, M.G., Groden, J., Groden, G., Lipsitt, L.P. (Eds.), Stress and coping in autism. Oxford University Press, New York, pp. 15−41.

Hagopian, L., Jennett, H., 2014. Behavioral assessment and treatment for anxiety for those with autism spectrum disorder. In: Davis, T.E., White, S.W., Ollendick, T.H. (Eds.), Handbook of autism and anxiety. Springer, New York, pp. 155−169.

Hebron, J., Humphrey, N., 2014. Mental health difficulties among popole on the autistic spectrum in mainstream secondary schools: A comparative study. Journal of Research in Special Educational Needs 14 (1), 22−32. Available from: http://dx.doi.org/10.1111/j.1471-3802.2012.01246.x.

Individuals with Disabilities Education Improvement Act (IDEIA) of 2004, P.L. 108-446 § 34 CFR Part 300 (2004).

Kaat, A.J., Gadow, K.D., Lecavalier, L., 2013. Psychiatric symptom impairment in children with autism spectrum disorders. Journal of Abnormal Child Psychology 41, 959−969. Available from: http://dx.doi.org/10.1007/s10802-013-9739-7.

Kerns, C.M., Kendall, P.C., 2014. Autism and anxiety: Overlap, similarities, and differences. In: Davis, T.E., White, S.W., Ollendick, T.H. (Eds.), Handbook of autism and anxiety. Springer, New York, pp. 75−89.

Lecavalier, L., 2006. Behavioral and emotional problems in young people with pervasive developmental disorders: Relative prevalence, effect of subject characteristics, and empirical classification. Journal of Autism and Developmental Disorders 36, 1101−1114. Available from: http://dx.doi.org/10.1007/s10803-006-0147-5.

Lecavalier, L., Wood, J.J., Halladay, A.K., Jones, N.E., Aman, M.G., Cook, E.H., et al., 2014. Measuring anxiety as a treatment endpoint in youth with autism spectrum disorder. Journal of Autism and Developmental Disorders 44, 1128−1143. Available from: http://dx.doi.org/10.1007/s10803-013-1974-9.

Lopata, C., Thomeer, M.L., 2014. Autism and anxiety in school. In: Davis, T.E., White, S.W., Ollendick, T.H. (Eds.), Handbook of autism and anxiety. Springer, New York, pp. 201−214.

Mayes, S.D., Calhoun, S.L., Murray, M.J., Zahid, J., 2011. Variables associated with anxiety and depression in children with autism. Journal of Developmental and Physical Disabilities 23, 325−337. Available from: http://dx.doi.org/10.1007/s10882-011-9231-7.

Mazefsky, C.A., Herrington, J.D., 2014. Autism and anxiety: Etiologic factors and transdiagnostic processes. In: Davis, T.E., White, S.W., Ollendick, T.H. (Eds.), Handbook of autism and anxiety. Springer, New York, pp. 91−103.

Mazefsky, C.A., White, S.W., 2013. The role of assessment in guiding treatment planning for youth with ASD. In: Scarpa, A., White, S.W., Attwood, T. (Eds.), CBT for children and adolescents with high-functioning autism spectrum disorders. Guilford, New York, NY, pp. 45–69.

Mazurek, M.O., Vasa, R.A., Kalb, L.G., Kanne, S.M., Rosenberg, D., Keefer, A., et al., 2013. Anxiety, sensory over-responsivity, and gastrointestinal problems in children with autism spectrum disorders. Journal of Abnormal Child Psychology 41, 165–176. Available from: http://dx.doi.org/10.1007/s10802-012-9668-x.

Moree, B.N., Davis, T.E., 2010. Cognitive-behavioral therapy for anxiety in children diagnosed with autism spectrum disorders: Modification trends. Research in Autism Spectrum Disorders 4, 346–354. Available from: http://dx.doi.org/10.1016/j.rasd.2009.10.015.

National Center for Education Statistics, U. S. Department of Education (2015). Digest of Education Statistics, 2013.

Norris, M., Lecavalier, L., 2010. Screening accuracy of level 2 autism spectrum disorder rating scales: A review of selected instruments. Autism 14 (4), 263–284. Available from: http://dx.doi.org/10.1177/1362361309348071.

Reaven, J., Blakely-Smith, A., Culhane-Shelburne, K., Hepburn, S., 2012. Group cognitive behavior therapy for children with high-functioning autism spectrum disorders and anxiety: A randomized trial. Journal of Child Psychology and Psychiatry 53 (4), 410–419. Available from: http://dx.doi.org/10.1111/j.1469-7610.2011.02486.x.

Reaven, J., Blakeley-Smith, A., Hepburn, S., 2014. Bridging the research to practice gap in autism research: Implementing group CBT interventions for youth with ASD and anxiety in clinical practice. In: Davis, T.E., White, S.W., Ollendick, T.H. (Eds.), Handbook of autism and anxiety. Springer, New York, pp. 185–200.

Reaven, J.A., 2009. Children with high-functioning autism spectrum disorders and co-occurring anxiety symptoms: Implications for assessment and treatment. Journal for Specialists in Pediatric Nursing 14, 192–199. Available from: http://dx.doi.org/10.1111/j.1744-6155.2009.00197.x.

Rodgers, J., Riby, D.M., Janes, E., Connolly, B., McConachie, H., 2012. Anxiety and repetitive behaviours in autism spectrum disorders and Williams syndrome: A cross-syndrome comparison. Journal of Autism and Developmental Disorders 42, 175–180. Available from: http://dx.doi.org/10.1007/s10803-011-1225-x.

Romanczyk, R.G., Gillis, J.M., 2006. Autism and the physiology of stress and anxiety. In: Baron, M.G., Groden, J., Groden, G., Lipsitt, L.P. (Eds.), Stress and coping in autism. Oxford University Press, New York, pp. 183–204.

Rotheram-Fuller, E., MacMullen, L., 2011. Cognitive-behavioral therapy for children with autism spectrum disorders. Psychology in the Schools 48 (3), 263–271. Available from: http://dx.doi.org/10.1002/pits.20552.

Schroeder, J.H., Cappadocia, M.C., Bebko, J.M., Pepler, D.J., Weiss, J.A., 2014. Shedding light on a pervasive problem: A review of research on bullying experiences among children with autism spectrum disorders. Journal of Autism and Developmental Disorders 44, 1520–1534. Available from: http://dx.doi.org/10.1007/s10803-013-2011-8.

Stratis, E.A., Lecavalier, L., 2013. Restricted and repetitive behaviors and psychiatric symptoms in youth with autism spectrum disorders. Research in Autism Spectrum Disorders 7, 757–766. Available from: http://dx.doi.org/10.1016/j.rasd.2013.02.017.

Stratis, E.A., Lecavalier, L., 2015. Informant agreement for youth with autism spectrum disorder or intellectual disability: A meta-analysis. Journal of Autism and Developmental Disorders 45, 1026–1041. Available from: http://dx.doi.org/10.1007/s10803-014-2258-8.

Sukhodolsky, D.G., Scahill, L., Gadow, K.D., Arnold, E., Aman, M.G., McDougle, C.J., et al., 2008. Parent-rated anxiety symptoms in children with pervasive developmental disorders: Frequency and association with core autism symptoms and cognitive functioning. Journal of Abnormal Child Psychology 36, 117–128. Available from: http://dx.doi.org/10.1007/s10802-007-9165-9.

Sukhodolsky, D.G., Bloch, M.H., Panza, K.E., Reichow, B., 2013. Cognitive-behavioral therapy for anxiety in children with high-functioning autism: A meta-analysis. Pediatrics 132 (5), 1341–1350. Available from: http://dx.doi.org/10.1542/peds.2013-1193.

Szatmari, P., McConnell, B., 2011. Anxiety and mood disorders in individuals with autism spectrum disorder. In: Amaral, D.G., Dawson, G., Geschwind, D.H. (Eds.), Autism spectrum disorders. Oxford University Press, New York, pp. 330–338.

Tsai, L.Y., 2006. Diagnosis and treatment of anxiety disorders in individuals with autism spectrum disorder. In: Baron, M.G., Groden, J., Groden, G., Lipsitt, L.P. (Eds.), Stress and coping in autism. Oxford University Press, New York, pp. 388–440.

van Steensel, F.J.A., Bogels, S.M., Perrin, S., 2011. Anxiety disorders in children and adolescents with autistic spectrum disorders: A meta-analysis. Clinical Child and Family Psychology Review 14, 302–317. Available from: http://dx.doi.org/10.1007/s10567-011-0097-0.

Vasa, R.A., Mazurek, M.O., 2015. An update on anxiety in youth with autism spectrum disorders. Current Opinion in Psychiatry 28 (2), 83–90.

Weisbrot, D.M., Gadow, K.D., DeVincent, C.J., Pomeroy, J., 2005. The presentation of anxiety in children with pervasive developmental disorders. Journal of Child and Adolescent Psychopharmacology 15 (3), 477–496. Available from: http://dx.doi.org/10.1089/cap.2005.15.477.

White, S.W., Scahill, L., Klin, A., Koenig, K., Volkmar, F.R., 2007. Educational placements and service use patterns of individuals with autism spectrum disorders. Journal of Autism and Developmental Disorders 37, 1403–1412. Available from: http://dx.doi.org/10.1007/s10803-006-0281-0.

White, S.W., Oswald, D., Ollendick, T., Scahill, L., 2009. Anxiety in children and adolescents with autism spectrum disorders. Clinical Psychology Review 29, 216–229. Available from: http://dx.doi.org/10.1016/j.cpr.2009.01.003.

White, S.W., Ollendick, T., Albano, A.M., Oswald, D., Johnson, C., Southam-Gerow, M.A., et al., 2013a. Randomized controlled trial: Multimodal anxiety and social skill intervention for adolescents with autism spectrum disorder. Journal of Autism and Developmental Disorders 43, 382–394. Available from: http://dx.doi.org/10.1007/s10803-012-1577-x.

White, S.W., Scahill, L., Ollendick, T.H., 2013b. Multimodal treatment for anxiety and social skills difficulties in adolescents on the autism spectrum. In: Scarpa, A., White, S.W., Attwood, T. (Eds.), CBT for children and adolescents with high-functioning autism spectrum disorders. Guilford, New York, NY, pp. 123–146.

White, S.W., Mazefsky, C.A., Dichter, G.S., Chiu, P.H., Richey, J.A., Ollendick, T.H., 2014a. Social-cognitive, physiological, and neural mechanisms underlying emotion regulation impairments: Understanding anxiety in autism spectrum disorder. International Journal of Developmental Neuroscience 39, 22–36. Available from: http://dx.doi.org/10.1016/j.ijdevneu.2014.05.012.

White, S.W., Schry, A.R., Kreiser, N.L., 2014b. Social worries and difficulties: Autism and/or social anxiety disorder? In: Davis, T.E., White, S.W., Ollendick, T.H. (Eds.), Handbook of autism and anxiety. Springer, New York, pp. 121–136.

Williams, S., Leader, G., Mannion, A., Chen, J., 2015. An investigation of anxiety in children and adolescents with autism spectrum disorder. Research in Autism Spectrum Disorders 10, 30–40. Available from: http://dx.doi.org/10.1016/j.rasd.2014.10.017.

Wood, J.J., Drahota, A., Sze, K., Har, K., Chiu, A., Langer, D.A., 2009. Cognitive behavioral therapy for anxiety in children with autism spectrum disorders: A randomized, controlled trial. Journal of Child Psychology and Psychiatry 50 (3), 224–234. Available from: http://dx.doi.org/10.1111/j.1469-7610.2008.01948.x.

CHAPTER 12

Dissemination and Implementation of Behavioral Treatments for Anxiety in ASD

Amy Drahota[1,2], Colby Chlebowski[2,3], Nicole Stadnick[2,3], Mary Baker-Ericzén[2,4] and Lauren Brookman-Frazee[2,3]
[1]Michigan State University, East Lansing, MI, United States
[2]Child & Adolescent Services Research Center, San Diego, CA, United States
[3]University of California, San Diego, CA, United States
[4]Rady Children's Hospital, San Diego, CA, United States

GAPS BETWEEN RESEARCH AND ROUTINE CARE FOR ANXIETY IN YOUTH WITH AUTISM

Anxiety is a common co-occurring condition in autism spectrum disorder (ASD), that contributes to the complexity of youth's clinical presentation, functioning, and service needs (Joshi et al., 2010). Although there is a rapidly growing body of evidence for the efficacy of cognitive behavioral therapy for anxiety in youth with ASD (Wood et al., 2015a), there is also a well-documented gap between research-based interventions and routine care. Evidence-based interventions (EBIs) for ASD have traditionally been difficult to transport from university laboratory settings to community settings (Garland et al., 2013; Dingfelder & Mandell, 2011), and recent small-scale studies have found that EBIs are not consistently implemented in routine, community settings (Brookman-Frazee et al., 2010). Contributing to this research-to-practice gap, youth with ASD and anxiety are often provided services simultaneously from multiple community service systems targeting core and associated symptoms of ASD (Brookman-Frazee et al., 2009; Goin-Kochel et al., 2007). For example, providers from multiple disciplines deliver services to youth with ASD including psychologists, behavioral therapists, educators, pediatricians, nurses, speech-language pathologists, occupational therapists, physical therapists, audiologists, neurologists, and social workers (McLennan et al., 2008), each with diverse and unique characteristics, such as education level and training and attitudes toward delivery of EBIs. In addition, each

Anxiety in Children and Adolescents with Autism Spectrum Disorder.
DOI: http://dx.doi.org/10.1016/B978-0-12-805122-1.00012-0
© 2017 Elsevier Inc.
All rights reserved.
231

provider may use different terminology or identify different needs for intervention, bringing their own perspectives on community care for youth with ASD (Volkmar et al., 2011). For instance, mental health clinicians may have less specialized diagnostic or ASD intervention-specific training, which poses challenges to treating youth with ASD who have co-occurring psychiatric conditions, while community providers who specifically serve populations with ASD or developmental disabilities are not often trained in providing mental health services.

Additionally, the service systems in which these providers work vary in their policies, organizational structure, intervention utilization, and funding support. As a result, youth with ASD and co-occurring anxiety are often provided services from systems operating in a balkanized fashion that all too frequently yield fragmented care (Christon et al., 2015; Cidav et al., 2013; Swiezy et al., 2008). A recent study found that clinicians across disciplines reported using or recommending intervention elements based on Applied Behavioral Analysis (ABA) principles (e.g., reinforcement, visual supports and task analysis) most frequently for youth with ASD and co-occurring anxiety, with cognitive-behavior therapy (CBT) used or recommended the least (Christon et al., 2015). Even more surprising, clinicians reported providing and recommending play therapy significantly more than CBT for youth with ASD despite the efficacy literature supporting CBT with youth with ASD and co-occurring symptoms (see Scarpa et al., 2013 and Wood et al., 2011 for efficacy data for CBT).

While it is unclear if clinicians do not provide or recommend CBT due to lack of provider knowledge and training or due to a lack of readily available treatment models within the community, these findings demonstrate the gap between research and practice that has been a prominent discussion within mental health literature for over a decade (Warren et al., 2010), and highlight the ongoing challenges in translating research knowledge into clinical practice (Chambers et al., 2013; Garland et al., 2013). Fortunately, recent paradigm shifts in the field of psychology have pushed researchers to look beyond the question of efficacy—the extent to which interventions achieve outcomes under ideal circumstances—to translational science, which focuses on testing the effectiveness of interventions, the success of community clinicians who use them, and implementation of EBIs within community agencies and systems (Dingfelder & Mandell, 2011; Feldman, 2008; Wood et al., 2015b). Two specific time points are particularly pivotal for the translation of EBI into community settings: 1. during intervention development and 2. when facilitating implementation of existing EBIs within community care settings.

DEVELOPING EFFECTIVE ANXIETY INTERVENTIONS FOR YOUTH WITH AUTISM

In an effort to accelerate the bidirectional translation between research and routine care delivery, care must be taken at the intervention development stage to ensure the fit between the intervention and community settings (Dingfelder & Mandell, 2011). In order to do so, we offer the following recommendations to intervention developers:

1. *Consider the potential end users of an intervention at the outset of intervention development and/or adaptation.* What are the characteristics and needs of youth/families, clinicians, organizations and systems that may impact intervention uptake, sustained delivery, and effectiveness? How can a given intervention address the needs of youth, clinicians, and organizations of systems? How might the intervention fit within the service context and are adaptations to the intervention necessary? How may the clinical specialty (ASD vs mental health disorders) of clinicians impact the delivery of the intervention? What existing funding mechanisms are available to cover the cost of the intervention? Partnering with community stakeholders early in the intervention development and implementation process and systematically collecting data on the service context should help facilitate understanding of the needs and constraints of the service system (Drahota et al., 2016).

2. *Assume adaptions are necessary and will occur.* Ascertainment of efficacy research samples may result in relatively homogenous samples that are not representative of the target population. Furthermore, the context of routine care is likely very different than tightly controlled research contexts. As such, assume that adaptations may be needed to facilitate fit and adoption. Which adaptations are fidelity-consistent versus fidelity-inconsistent (Wiltsey-Stirman et al., 2013)? Are there ways to simplify the intervention? Consider what the hypothesized core mechanisms of change for the intervention are and pare down the intervention to only include those components (e.g., exposure, behavioral rehearsal).

3. *Combine clinical interventions with implementation strategies.* Translation from research to practice does not simply involve providing a treatment manual or conducting workshops with clinicians.

Implementation strategies (Powell et al., 2012; Powell et al., 2015; Proctor et al., 2011; Drahota et al., 2014b) are used in combination with clinical interventions to systematically implement them in routine care. Consider dissemination and implementation frameworks and research-based implementation strategies at multiple levels to facilitate the adoption, initial uptake, and sustained use of EBIs in ASD community care settings.

IMPLEMENTING EXISTING ANXIETY INTERVENTIONS WITH YOUTH WITH AUTISM

Born out of the need to minimize the substantial delay (up to 17 years) in translating only 14% of research findings to practice to increase the public health impact of EBIs (Balas, 1998; Balas & Boren, 2000), dissemination and implementation (D&I) science (see Table 12.1) is an emerging field that provides theoretical and empirical infrastructure for the promotion of EBI transportation to community settings (Rabin & Brownson, 2012). Specifically, *dissemination* is defined as "the targeted distribution of information and intervention materials to a specific public health or clinical practice audience. The intent is to spread knowledge and the associated evidenced-based interventions" (National Institutes of Health Program Announcement, 2016). *Implementation science* "is the scientific study of methods to promote the systematic uptake of research findings and other evidence-based practices into routine practice, and thereby improve the quality and effectiveness of health services and care" (p.1; Eccles & Mittman, 2006). Recognizing the complex interplay of variables integral in transporting an EBI to community practice, dissemination and implementation (D&I) science necessitates consideration of multiple levels of influence including the youth and families accessing care, the clinicians delivering care, the agencies or organizations through which care is delivered, and healthcare policy that effects service delivery (Bauer et al., 2015).

Several comprehensive, phased, and multilevel implementation frameworks have been developed (e.g., Aarons et al., 2011; Damschroder et al., 2007; Greenhalgh et al., 2004) that denote specific "inner" (e.g., consumer, provider characteristics) and "outer" (e.g., policy, fiscal environment) context factors that may facilitate or hinder the adoption, implementation, and sustainment of EBIs in community care settings. An overarching goal of D&I frameworks is to maximize the "fit" between the EBI and the service context in which it is to be implemented. This is

Table 12.1 Glossary of implementation science terms

Term	Definition	Reference
Adaptation	Planned or purposeful changes to the design or delivery of an EBI, as opposed to modifications that may be unintentional deviations	Wiltsey-Stirman et al. (2013)
Clinician (or Provider)	Individuals providing a broad array of services in any usual care service section (therapists, clinicians, case managers, paraprofessional, educational staff)	
De-Implementation	To reduce the use of strategies and interventions that are not evidence-based, have been prematurely widely adopted, yield sub-optimal benefits for patients, or are harmful or wasteful	National Institutes of Health Program Announcement (2016)
Dissemination	Active, intentional efforts aimed to encourage specified groups to adopt an innovation, which can be a new clinical program or practice	Greenhalgh et al. (2004)
Implementation	Active, intentional efforts to embed a clinical program or practice (innovation) within an organization or service system	Greenhalgh et al. (2004)
Implementation Model (or D & I Framework)	A conceptual framework of distinct factors that are hypothesized to strongly influence the implementation of evidence-based practices in service systems	Aarons et al. (2011), Tabak et al. (2012)
Implementation Science	The scientific study of methods to promote the systematic uptake of EBIs into routine clinical care settings with the overarching aim of improving the quality and effectiveness of health services	Eccles and Mittman (2006)
Implementation Strategies	Methods or techniques used to enhance the adaptation, implementation, and sustainability of an evidence-based clinical program or practice	Powell et al. (2015), Proctor et al. (2013)
Implementation Team	Agency leaders, designated agency staff members (e.g., clinicians), and other stakeholders who work through the multiple phases of implementation often by meeting, completing activities, and conducting actions necessary for implementation and sustainment of an EBI	
Sustainment	The (a) capacity to deliver and/or (b) maintain core elements of an intervention (e.g., remain recognizable or delivered at a sufficient level of fidelity or intensity to yield desirable results) after initial implementation support has been withdrawn	Wiltsey-Stirman et al. (2012)

done through comprehensive study of routine care practices and service systems (Drahota et al., 2012), including characteristics specific to the healthcare policy and legislative landscape, service system (outer context), and the organization, providers, and individual with ASD (inner context). One promising method that is highlighted to facilitate "fit" between EBIs and organizational contexts is the inclusion of strong, well-defined community–academic partnerships with community stakeholders (e.g., caregivers, service providers, clinicians, clinical supervisors, agency leaders) (Garland & Brookman-Frazee, 2015; Drahota et al., 2016).

Comprehensive understanding and ongoing monitoring of the contextual landscape of a service system is essential to facilitate adoption, uptake, and sustained delivery of EBIs without compromised treatment adherence, and to facilitate the de-adoption of practices that are not evidence-based (Bauer et al., 2015). For example, Drahota and colleagues (2015) utilized a mixed methods design to evaluate hindering and facilitating factors to implementation of EBI in community settings for youth with ASD. Agency leaders reported that there is not an existing systematic implementation process that fits the ASD usual care setting resulting in a lack of structure and consistency in implementation efforts. Further, agency leaders reported uncertainty about which implementation strategies best facilitate EBI adoption, uptake, and sustained use.

Utilizing a theory-based implementation framework and an ASD-specific implementation toolkit that addresses the unique client, provider, and contextual factors of ASD community service systems is a promising method for building upon existing EBIs while also accelerating D&I efforts for this population. The following section describes a D&I framework and corresponding implementation toolkit—the ACT SMART Implementation Toolkit—used to improve the implementation of EBIs within ASD community agencies.

ADAPTED EPIS MODEL OF IMPLEMENTATION

The EPIS (Exploration, Preparation, Implementation, Sustainment) model of implementation (Aarons et al., 2011) is a multi-phased, multi-level framework of implementation processes that was used to guide the development of the ACT SMART Implementation Toolkit. Recent discussions with ASD community stakeholders yielded an adapted EPIS conceptual model to better fit the needs of ASD community agencies (Drahota et al., 2012). Taken together, the five phases of the adapted

EPIS (see Table 12.2) provide useful guidance for consideration of both inner and outer contextual factors that may influence the implementation of an EBI within a specific service setting and organizational context.

Outer Context. Outer contextual factors include sociopolitical context, policy, advocacy, funding, and inter-organizational networks. For example, recent healthcare legislation, namely the Patient Protection and Affordable Care Act (Patient Protection and Affordable Care Act, 2010), has a core goal of improving access to and quality of healthcare while lowering per capita costs. Moreover, mental health parity is highlighted within the Affordable Care Act and has significant potential to shape mental health service access, quality, and receipt for children with ASD. Policies such as these shape the outer context to facilitate greater mental health coverage for individuals, including youth with ASD, who also are experiencing co-occurring anxiety disorders. As a result, service systems have been pushed by policy to provide evidence-based interventions to intervene and ameliorate the symptoms of anxiety and related interference. A second example of important outer contextual factors for the ASD population includes parent networks. Parent networks have played an important role in advocating for greater intervention services to treat the challenging behaviors and anxiety disorders often comorbid with ASD. The strength of ASD advocacy networks can been seen by the increase in public and private funding through organizations such as Autism Speaks and the Interagency Autism Coordinating Committee, which offer guidance to the National Institutes of Health on funding and research priorities.

Inner Context. The inner context of the EPIS varies by phase, and commonly includes factors such as organizational-, leadership-, provider-, and client-level characteristics. For example, organizational culture—an organizational-level characteristic—has been defined as "the behavioral expectations that members of an organization are required to meet in their work environment" (Verbeke et al., 1998; Glisson et al., 2013), and is associated with receptivity of an organization to a new EBI. That is, if the organizational culture is receptive to identifying new EBI to benefit clinicians or clients, it is more likely that it will be implemented and sustained successfully, thereby increasing the quality of service delivery and positive patient outcomes (Aarons et al., 2012; Glisson & Green, 2006; Glisson & Hemmelgarn, 1998). The converse may be true as well; organizations with a culture of low receptivity to innovations are likely to experience greater barriers to adoption, uptake, and sustained use, despite the EBI meeting client needs or being advantageous for the agency.

Additional inner contextual factors important for implementation include staffing and staff characteristics, EBI fit with agency values and needs, and EBI adaptability and training availability (Aarons et al., 2012).

While the adapted EPIS provides guidance for the implementation of EBIs within ASD community settings by emphasizing the need to consider both outer and inner contextual factors prior to and throughout the implementation process (Aarons et al., 2011), it does not offer concrete tools to support agency leader's implementation of EBIs. As a result, the ACT SMART Implementation Toolkit was developed in collaboration with a community-academic partnership to provide a systematized approach for progressing through the multi-phased EPIS (Table 12.2).

THE ACT SMART IMPLEMENTATION TOOLKIT

The *Autism Community Toolkit: Systems to Measure and Adopt Research-Based Treatments* (ACT SMART Implementation Toolkit) (Drahota et al., 2014a) is an evidence-informed, comprehensive, implementation toolkit designed to assist ASD agency leaders and clinicians to efficiently and effectively implement EBIs and de-implement unsupported strategies. It is comprised of a web-based implementation interface that has steps and activities to guide clinicians through the adapted EPIS phases and is accompanied by monthly facilitation meetings with ACT SMART facilitators who provide consultation about the process of implementation, de-implementation and sustainment. Facilitation is a consultation method that emphasizes change through encouragement and action promotion (Kitson et al., 1998; Kitson & Harvey, 2015), and has been found to help staff change work practices and behaviors successfully (Rycroft-Malone et al., 2002; Stetler et al., 2006) and improve the capacity of community-based agencies to plan, implement, and evaluate new EBIs in previous implementation studies (Hunter et al., 2009).

Phase 1: Exploration. The aims of the first phase of the ACT SMART Implementation Toolkit are to 1. identify practice and service delivery gaps within organizations by conducting a comprehensive organizational needs assessment to determine areas of strength and possible growth for the agency, 2. identify recommendations for next steps, and 3. assist with prioritizing agency goals. Factors important to consider when assessing an organization include client needs, effectiveness of interventions being delivered within the agency, perceived competency in the delivery of current interventions, staff attitudes toward innovations, staff training and

Table 12.2 Adapted EPIS implementation framework (Adapted from Aarons, Hurlburt and Horwitz, 2011) with ACT SMART implementation toolkit steps and activities

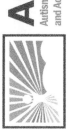

ACT SMART

Autism Community Toolkit: Systems to Measure and Adopt Research-Based Treatments

Adapted EPIS phases	ACT SMART implementation toolkit		Facilitation meetings
	Web-Based interface		
	Steps	Activities	
Phase 1: Exploration	Step 1: Conduct agency assessment Step 2: Evaluate receptivity to implementing new EBI	Activity 1: Encourage staff participation in the organizational needs assessment Activity 2: Form implementation team, if needed	• 12 monthly 30–60 minute meetings • Agency implementation team and ACT SMART facilitator collaborate to move through ACT SMART phases and activities • Structured facilitation meetings to review steps, phases and activities; troubleshoot previous action items; introduce next steps and phases; and plan for future steps
Phase 2: Adoption Decision	Step 1: Identify appropriate EBI(s) Step 2: Evaluate EBI and provider factors Step 3: Adoption decision	Activity 1: Identify EBI(s) to meet agency need Activity 1: EBI fit Activity 2: EBI feasibility Activity 3: Clinical value and research validity Activity 4: Training requirements Activity 5: Funding source Activity 6: Benefit-cost estimator Activity 1: Synthesize and weigh factors Activity 2: Formally make an adoption decision	
Phase 3: Preparation	Step 1: Develop prospective adaptation plan Step 2: Develop training plan Step 3: Develop implementation plan	Activity 1: Gather EBI materials Activity 2: Evaluate possible adaptations to EBI Activity 3: Adaptation planning worksheet Activity 1: Training plan worksheet Activity 1: Implementation plan worksheet	
Phase 4: Implementation	Step 1: Conduct adaptation plan Step 2: Conduct training plan Step 3: Conduct implementation plan Step 4: Task evaluation	Activity 1: Develop concrete tasks and establish due dates Activity 1: Evaluate tasks from Steps 1–3	
Phase 5: Sustainment	Step 1: Evaluate implementation success Step 2: Evaluate current sustainment Step 3: Develop sustainment plan	Activity 1: Synthesize task evaluations Activity 1: Identify current sustainment practices Activity 1: Sustainment planning	

attributes, agency resources, fidelity and performance measurements, organizational context, climate and culture, and previously used implementation and sustainment strategies. Using a structured and systematic method of conducting an organizational needs assessment allows for the most utility and ease. The ACT SMART Implementation Toolkit utilizes an assessment battery to achieve these goals. Numerous surveys are available for use and, fortunately with the continued development of implementation science as a discipline, measures and assessment tools are being placed in web-based repositories for use by researchers and clinicians (see the National Cancer Institute's Grid-Enabled Measures Database and the Society for Implementation Research Collaboration—Instrument Review Project).

The ultimate goal of Phase 1 is to determine an agency's receptivity to implementing a new EBI. This is an important consideration because if an agency is not receptive to implementing a new EBI, resources would be better spent improving the quality and organizational structure of the agency by recommending quality improvement literature and tools (c.f., Belson, 2014; Ovretveit, 2014). For agencies receptive to implementing new EBIs, an agency implementation team is formed and an ACT SMART facilitator is assigned to guide the implementation team through the continuation of the ACT SMART Implementation Toolkit.

Phase 2: Adoption Decision. The goals of Phase 2 is for the implementation team to identify an EBI that matches agency-identified needs and to make an informed decision about whether to adopt the EBI for use within the agency. Using the information identified in Phase 1, ACT SMART facilitators guide agency implementation teams through three steps: 1. identify an appropriate EBI to meet the needs derived from the organizational assessment; 2. evaluate EBI characteristics to determine whether it would be appropriate to meet client, clinician, and agency needs; and 3. synthesize this information to make a systematic decision whether or not to adopt the EBI. Specifically, during Step 1, the ACT SMART facilitator supports implementation team members' efforts to explore the literature and available EBI repositories to identify an intervention that will match the need identified through the organizational assessment. For example, if the organizational assessment indicates that the agency's clients with ASD are experiencing anxiety and the clinicians are not effectively treating anxiety symptoms, implementation teams may wish to explore current literature and available manuals to meet this agency-level need. By reading the literature and obtaining anxiety CBT manuals, the implementation team will be able to evaluate important factors of the intervention before making a formal intervention adoption decision (Step 3).

Once an EBI has been identified and intervention resources have been obtained, implementation team members evaluate treatment and provider factors (Step 2) that have been found to influence the EBI adoption decision. Adoption decision factors include EBI fit and feasibility with the agency's context and structure, the clinical value and research validity of the EBI, training requirements and availability, EBI funding sources, and the benefit of delivering a new EBI as compared with the cost. While these factors have been identified through interviews with agency leaders (Drahota et al., 2015), each factor may have variable influence over the final adoption decision for an implementation team. Thus, the ratings from each of these factors are synthesized and weighted by implementation teams to assist with making a systematic and informed adoption decision. Once an adoption decision is made, implementation teams either move onward to Phase 3 or return to evaluate a different EBI for possible adoption.

Phase 3: Preparation. The goals of the preparation phase are to 1. plan for EBI adaptation prior to staff training and implementation; 2. develop the staff training; and 3. select and plan for specific implementation strategy use. Especially with complex interventions developed in university settings, adaptations will be needed for the successful implementation of the EBI in community agencies. Literature suggests that clinicians often do not use EBIs due to disbelief in the research base, difficulty with implementation, requirement to change behaviors, manuals unable to meet complexity of usual care clinical population, and lack of infrastructure to support EBI implementation (Fixsen et al., 2005). Moreover, strict protocol adherence may be at odds with the implementation of EBIs in usual care settings (Aarons et al., 2012) by limiting the opportunity to tailor EBIs to client's needs and culture and the community in which the service is being delivered (Nock et al., 2003; Lyon et al., 2014; Lau, 2006; Berwick, 2003). The purpose of EBI adaptation is to promote a better fit between the context in which the EBI was tested and the service setting where it will be implemented, as well as the target population of the EBI (Aarons et al., 2011; Lundgren et al., 2011; McHugh et al., 2009). However, caution should be taken to ensure that adaptations do not interfere with core elements of the EBI (Aarons et al., 2012). Therefore, it is important to classify the types of EBI adaptations needed and examine how these changes may potentially impact key outcomes in a broad set of circumstances and a variety of settings (Wiltsey-Stirman et al., 2012, 2013).

Specifically, implementation teams are asked to consider whether adaptations to the EBI will be necessary for its use within their agency and to consider whether adaptations are necessary to the content of the EBI and/or to the delivery context. Examples of adaptations to the content include, for example, tailoring or refining the intervention (e.g., changing terms or language, modifying worksheets), shortening session duration, frequency or number, or adjusting the order of the intervention modules, topics, or segments. Adaptations to the context may include changing the setting (e.g., delivering the EBI in a school rather than a clinic) or changing the format by which the treatment is delivered (e.g., offering an individual treatment in a group or telephone format). Once implementation teams consider the possible adaptations needed to deliver the EBI within their agency, they are asked to consider the reasons for making the adaptation, identify any specific concerns about the adaptation, identify how the concern will be addressed, and then specify how the adaptation will be made and by whom.

That Preparation phase also includes developing a comprehensive staff training plan. Training the staff who will be involved in delivering the EBI is a crucial step in the implementation process. The quality of staff training can greatly impact the implementation, effectiveness, and ongoing fidelity of the EBI being delivered and is often a difficult task (Beidas et al., 2012; Drahota et al., 2014a). To this end, use of training planners, such as the ACT SMART Training Plan worksheet, can guide implementation teams through systematically planning each component of training.

The third step in the Preparation phase is to develop an implementation plan. Passive implementation efforts often lead to limited implementation or discontinuation of EBIs (Powell et al., 2015). Therefore, many evidence-based implementation strategies have been developed and researched to support the successful implementation of EBIs (Fixsen et al., 2005; Fixsen et al., 2009; Powell et al., 2012; Powell et al., 2015) (Table 12.3).

These strategies vary greatly in their level of involvement, time commitment, cost and feasibility. Yet, research suggests that when discrete and feasible implementation strategies are utilized, successful implementation outcomes are observed, such as knowledge and use of specific EBIs when appropriate, intervention fidelity, provider and client satisfaction with EBI, improved client outcomes, and improved organizational outcomes

Table 12.3 Implementation and sustainment strategies grouped by domain

Relationship-Based Strategies	The focus of relationship-based strategies is to identify agency leader characteristics, staff buy-in, and partnerships that encourage and support the use of the selected practice or strategy and implementation effort. • Build agency leader characteristics to support innovation acceptance and use • Build buy-in among agency clinicians and clients • Develop relationships to support the implementation process
Financial Strategies	These are financial strategies that help to incentivize the use of new practices or strategies and provide resources for training and ongoing support for clinical staff. • Modify incentives • Facilitate financial support
Restructuring Strategies	These strategies include altering staffing, professional roles, the physical structure of the agency or service setting, intervention equipment, materials and resources, and data systems. • Change staffing or professional roles • Change physical structure or service setting • Change or update data and reminder systems
Implementation Testing Strategies	These strategies focus on systems that rollout or scale up interventions within an agency. • Pilot test implementation effort on a small scale, gradually moving to system-wide roll out • Model or simulate changes that will be implemented prior to system-wide implementation • Implementation changes in a recursive, cyclical fashion
Quality Management Strategies	These strategies involve developing support networks or data systems that act to continually evaluate and enhance client's quality of care. These systems also ensure that new practices or strategies are delivered with fidelity. • Develop performance and fidelity monitoring systems for the intervention • Evaluate the implementation effort
Sustainment Strategies	The focus of these strategies are to facilitate the continued use of new practices or strategies. These are strategies that are distinctly different from implementation strategies but may fall in similar domains as the implementation strategies, such as: • Relationship-building sustainment strategies • Financial sustainment strategies • Quality management sustainment strategies.

Adapted from Powell et al. (2012) and Powell et al. (2015)

(Proctor et al., 2011). Therefore, it is critical for implementation teams to select and plan for use of 1–3 specific implementation strategies in order to facilitate the initial implementation of the EBI.

Phase 4: Implementation. The purpose of Phase 4 is for implementation teams to track progress toward completing the adaptation, training, and implementation plans as designed in the previous phase, and evaluate the progress and satisfaction of completing the action steps. For the ACT SMART Implementation Toolkit, implementation teams are asked to complete a brief evaluation survey after each action step has either been completed or when the scheduled due date for the action step has passed. The evaluation survey allows the implementation team to reflect on the progress being made. If the progress is considered satisfactory, the implementation team may wish to continue to follow the plans as previously designed. If the progress is considered to be neutral or challenging, the evaluation with facilitator assistance will guide the implementation team to consider making changes to the adaptation, training, and implementation plans. This is designed to fit the adaptive and dynamic process inherent in the implementation of an EBI within community-based agencies (Aarons et al., 2012).

Phase 5: Sustainment. The purpose of the sustainment phase is to transition efforts from initial EBI implementation to ongoing EBI sustainment within an agency. Sustainment is defined as the (a) capacity to deliver and/or (b) maintain core elements of an intervention (e.g., remain recognizable or delivered at a sufficient level of fidelity or intensity to yield desirable results) after initial implementation support has been withdrawn (Wiltsey-Stirman et al., 2012). For the ACT SMART Implementation Toolkit, once the majority of the implementation tasks have been completed, the ACT SMART facilitator works with the implementation team to identify specific sustainment strategies that will facilitate the continued use of the EBI. This may include continued training in the EBI to new staff hires and ongoing support or supervision of the use of the EBI with current staff and providers. In addition, structural changes to the organization may be necessary to support the sustained use of the EBI and implementation strategies. For example, if fidelity monitoring was the implementation strategy selected to facilitate the uptake of an anxiety CBT protocol within an agency, allowing providers to have time to self-monitor in a systematic manner will be necessary to continue to sustain both the use of the implementation strategy and the EBI. However, the period of sustainment is not entered into until active implementation has been completed and ACT SMART facilitators have concluded their meetings with the agency implementation team.

CONCLUSION

In conclusion, the ultimate goal for intervention developers, ASD and anxiety researchers, and community agency leaders and clinicians is to increase the quality of life for youth with ASD and co-occurring anxiety disorders and their families. There are a growing number of evidence-based interventions for anxiety and ASD. However, similar to other populations, there is a concerning gap between ASD interventions delivered in research studies and routine care. Traditional unidirectional models of research to practice translation have resulted in minimal public health impact; however, practice-based approaches rooted in implementation science have the potential to bridge this gap. This chapter highlighted the importance of explicit attention to the routine care context in which an intervention could be used and to the process through which evidence-based interventions are developed, selected, implemented, and sustained in routine care. Based on the ASD services and broader dissemination and implementation science research described in this chapter, we recommend that intervention developers consider implementation outcomes during development of innovative interventions for youth with ASD, and community agency leaders utilize a systematic process to facilitate the implementation and sustainment of EBI within their agencies.

REFERENCES

Aarons, G.A., Hurlburt, M., Horwitz, S.M., 2011. Advancing a conceptual model of evidence-based practice implementation in public service sectors. Administration and Policy in Mental Health and Mental Health Services Research 38 (1), 4–23.

Aarons, G.A., Green, A.E., Palinkas, L.A., Self-Brown, S., Whitaker, D.J., Lutzker, J.R., et al., 2012. Dynamic adaptation process to implement an evidence-based child maltreatment intervention. Implementation Science 7 (1), 32.

Balas, E.A., 1998. Appropriate care to evidence-based medicine. Pediatric Annual 27, 581–584.

Balas, E.A., Boren, S.A., 2000. Managing clinical knowledge for health care improvement. In: Bemmel, J., McCray, A.T. (Eds.), Yearbook of Medical Informatics 2000: Patient-Centered Systems. Schattauer Verlagsgesellschaft, Stuttgart, Germany.

Bauer, M.S., Damschroder, L., Hagedorn, H., Smith, J., Kilbourne, A.M., 2015. An introduction to implementation science for the non-specialist. BMC Psychology 3, 32.

Beidas, R.S., Edmunds, J.M., Marcus, S.C., Kendall, P.C., 2012. Training and consultation to promote implementation of an empirically supported treatment: A randomized trial. Psychiatric Services 63 (7), 660—665.

Belson, D., 2014. Quality improvement methods for use in QUERI research proposals and grant projects (2nd Ed).

Berwick, D.M., 2003. Disseminating innovations in health care. JAMA 289 (15), 1969.

Brookman-Frazee, L., Baker-Ericzen, M., Stahmer, A., Mandell, D., Haine, R.A., Hough, R.L., 2009. Journal of Mental Health Research Intellect Disability 2 (3), 201—219.

Brookman-Frazee, L., Taylor, R., Garland, A., 2010. Characterizing community-based mental health services for children with autism spectrum disorder and disruptive behavior problems. Journal of Autism and Developmental Disorders 40 (10), 118—1201.

Chambers, D., Glasgow, R., Stange, K., 2013. The dynamic sustainability framework: Addressing the paradox of sustainment amid ongoing change. Implementation Science. 8, 117.

Christon, L.M., Arnold, C.C., Myers, B.J., 2015. Professionals' reported provision and recommendation of psychosocial interventions for youth with autism spectrum disorder. Behavior Therapy 46 (1), 68—82.

Cidav, Z., Lawer, L., Marcus, S.C., Mandell, D.S., 2013. Age-related variation in health service use and associated expenditures among children with autism. Journal of Autism and Developmental Disorders 43 (4), 924—931.

Damschroder, L.J., Aron, D.C., Keith, R.E., Kirsh, S.R., Alexander, J.A., Lowery, J.C., 2007. Fostering implementation of health services research findings into practice: A consolidated framework for advancing implementation science. Implementation Science 4 (1), 50.

Dingfelder, H.E., Mandell, D.S., 2011. Bridging the research-to-practice gap in autism intervention: An application of diffusion of innovation theory. Journal of Autism and Developmental Disorders 41 (5), 597—609.

Drahota, A., Aarons, G.A., Stahmer, A.C., 2012. Developing the Autism Model of Implementation for autism spectrum disorder community providers: Study protocol. Implementation Science 7 (1), 85.

Drahota, A., Stadnick, N., Brookman-Frazee, L., 2014a. Therapist perspectives on training in a package of evidence-based practice strategies for children with autism spectrum disorders served in community mental health clinics. Administration and Policy in Mental Health and Mental Health Research 41 (1), 114—125.

Drahota, A., Meza, R., & Martinez, J.I. (2014b). The Autism-Community Toolkit: Systems to Measure and Adopt Research-Based Treatments. www.actsmarttoolkit.com

Drahota, A., Martinez, J.I., Meza, R., Brikho, B., Gomez, E., Stahmer, A.C., et al., 2015. ACT SMART Toolkit: Developing and pilot testing a comprehensive implementation strategy for ASD service providers. Paper presented at the 49th Annual Association for Behavioral and Cognitive Therapies Convention, Chicago, IL.

Drahota, A., Meza, R., Brikho, B., Naaf, M., Estabillo, J., Gomez, E., et al., 2016. Community-Academic Partnerships: A systematic review of the state of the literature and recommendations for future research. Milbank Quarterly 94 (1), 163—214.

Eccles, M., Mittman, B., 2006. Welcome to implementation science. Implementation Science 1 (1), 1.

Feldman, A.M., 2008. CTS: A new discipline to catalyze the transfer of information. Clinical and Translational Science 1 (1), 1—2.

Fixsen, D.L., Naoom, S.F., Blase, K.A., Friedman, R.M., Wallace, F., 2005. Implementation research: A synthesis of the literature. National Implementation Research Network, Tampa, FL.

Fixsen, D., Blase, K., Naoom, S., Wallace, F., 2009. Core implementation components. Research on Social Work Practice 19 (5), 531.

Garland, A.F., Brookman-Frazee, L., 2015. Therapists and reseachers: Advancing collaboration. Psychotherapy Research 25 (1), 95−107.

Garland, A.F., Haine-Schlagel, R., Brookman-Frazee, L., Baker-Ericzen, M., Trask, E., Fawley-King, K., 2013. Improving community-based mental health care for children: Translating knowledge into action. Administration and Policy In Mental Health And Mental Health Services Research 40 (1), 6−22.

Glisson, C., Green, P., 2006. The effects of organizational culture and climate on the access to mental health care in child welfare and juvenile justice systems. Administration and Policy in Mental Health and Mental Health Services Research 33 (4), 433−448.

Glisson, C., Hemmelgarn, A., 1998. The effects of organizational climate and inter-organizational coordination on the quality and outcomes of children's service systems. Child Abuse & Neglect 22 (5), 401−421.

Glisson, C., Hemmelgarn, A., Green, P., Williams, N.J., 2013. Randomized trial of the Availability, Responsiveness and Continuity (ARC) organizational intervention for improving youth outcomes in community mental health programs. Journal of the American Academy of Child & Adolescent Psychiatry 52 (5), 493−500.

Greenhalgh, T., Robert, G., Macfarlane, F., Bate, P., Kyriakidou, O., 2004. Diffusion of innovations in service organizations: Systematic review and recommendations. Milbank Quarterly 82 (4), 581−629.

Goin-Kochel, R.P., Mackintosh, V.H., Myers, B.J., 2007. Parental reports on the use of treatment and therapies for children with autism spectrum disorder. Research in Autism Spectrum Disorders 1 (3), 195−209.

Hunter, S.B., Chinman, M., Ebener, P., Imm, P., Wandersman, A., Ryan, G., 2009. Technical assistance as a prevention capacity-building tool: A demonstration using the Getting To Outcomes framework. Health Education and Behavior 36 (5), 810−828.

Joshi, G., Petty, C., Wozniak, J., Henin, A., Fried, R., Galdo, M., et al., 2010. The Heavy Burden of Psychiatric Comorbidity in Youth with Autism Spectrum Disorders: A Large Comparative Study of a Psychiatrically Referred Population. Journal of Autism and Developmental Disorders 40 (11), 1361−1370.

Kitson, A., Harvey, G., 2015. Translating evidence into healthcare policy and practice: Single versus multi-faceted implementation strategies—Is there a simple answer to a complex question?. International Journal of Health Policy and Management 4 (3), 123−126.

Kitson, A., Harvey, G., Mccormack, B., 1998. Enabling the implementation of evidence based practice: A conceptual framework. Quality and Safety in Health Care 7 (3), 149−158.

Lau, A., 2006. The why's, when's, what's, and how's of cultural adaptation of evidence-based treatments. PsycEXTRA Dataset.

Lundgren, L., Krull, I., Zerden, L.D., McCarty, D., 2011. Community-based addiction treatment staff attitudes about the usefulness of evidence-based addiction treatment and CBO organizational linkages to research institutions. Evaluation and Program Planning 34 (4), 356−365.

Lyon, A.R., Lau, A.S., McCauley, E., Vander Stoep, A., Chorpita, B.F., 2014. A case for modular design: Implications for implementing evidence-based interventions with culturally diverse youth. Professional Psychology: Research and Practice 45 (1), 57−66.

McHugh, R.K., Murray, H.W., Barlow, D.H., 2009. Balancing fidelity and adaptation in the dissemination of empirically-supported treatments: The promise of transdiagnostic interventions. Behaviour Research and Therapy 47 (11), 946−953.

McLennan, J.D., Huculak, S., Sheehan, D., 2008. Brief report: Pilot investigation of servicereceipt by young children with autistic spectrum disorders. Journal of Autism and Developmental Disorders 38 (6), 1192−1196.

National Institutes of Health Office of Behavioral and Social Science Research. Dissemination and implementation 2016; http://obssr.od.nih.gov/scientific_areas/translation/dissemination_and_implementation/index.aspx. Accessed September 21, 2016.

Nock, M.K., Goldman, J.L., Wang, Y., Albano, A.M., Jellinek, M.S., 2003. From science to practice: The flexible use of evidence-based treatments in clinical settings. Journal of the American Academy of Child & Adolescent Psychiatry 43 (6), 777−780.

Ovretveit, J., 2014. Evaluating Improvement and Implementation for Health. McGraw-Hill.

Powell, B.J., McMillen, J.C., Proctor, E.K., Carpenter, C.R., Griffey, R.T., Bunger, A.C., et al., 2012. A compilation of strategies for implementing clinical innovations in health and mental health. Medical Care Research and Review 69 (2), 123−157.

Powell, B.J., Waltz, T.J., Chinman, M.J., Damschroder, L.J., Smith, J.L., Matthieu, M.M., et al., 2015. A refined compilation of implementation strategies: Results from the Expert Recommendations for Implementing Change (ERIC) project. Implementation Science 10, 21.

Proctor, E.K., Silmere, H., Raghavan, R., Hovmand, P., Aarons, G., Bunger, A., et al., 2011. Outcomes for implementation research: Conceptual distinctions, measurement challenges, and research agenda. Administration and Policy in Mental Health and Mental Health Services Research 38 (2), 65−76.

Proctor, E.K., Powell, B.J., McMillen, J., 2013. Implementation strategies: Recommendations for specifying and reporting. Implementation Science 8 (1), 139.

Rabin, B.A., Brownson, R.C., 2012. Developing the terminology for dissemination and implementation research. Dissemination and Implementation Research in Health Translating Science to Practice 23−52, Section 1.

Rycroft-Malone, J., Kitson, A., Harvey, G., McCormack, B., Seers, K., Titchen, A., et al., 2002. Ingredients for change: Revisiting a conceptual framework. Quality and Safety in Health Care 11 (2), 174−180.

Scarpa, A., Wells, A., Attwood, T., 2013. Exploring feelings for young children with high-functioning autism or Asperger's disorder: The STAMP treatment manual. Jessica Kingsley Publishers.

Stetler, C.B., Legro, M.W., Wallace, C.M., Bowman, C., Guihan, M., Hagedorn, H., et al., 2006. The role of formative evaluation in implementation research and the QUERI experience. Journal of General Internal Medicine 21 (S2).

Swiezy, N., Stuart, M., Korzekwa, P., 2008. Bridging for success in autism: Training and collaboration across medical, educational, and community systems. Child and Adolescent Psychiatric Clinics of North America 17 (4), 907−922.

Tabak, R.G., Khoong, E.C., Chambers, D.A., Brownson, R.C., 2012. Bridging research and practice: Models for dissemination and implementation research. American Journal of Preventive Medicine 43 (3), 337−350.

Verbeke, W., Volgering, M., Hessels, M., 1998. Exploring the conceptual expansion within the field of organizational behaviour: Organizational climate and organizational culture. Journal of Management Studies 35 (3), 303−329.

Volkmar, F.R., Reichow, B., Doehring, P., 2011. Evidence-based practices and treatments for children with autism. Springer Science Business Media, LLC, New York.

Warren, J.S., Nelson, P.L., Mondragon, S.A., Baldwin, S.A., Burlingame, G.M., 2010. Youth psychotherapy change trajectories and outcomes in usual care: Community mental health versus managed care settings. Journal of Consulting and Clinical Psychology 78 (2), 144−155.

Wiltsey-Stirman, S., Kimberly, J., Cook, N., Calloway, A., Castro, F., Charns, M., 2012. The sustainability of new programs and innovations: A review of the empirical literature and recommendations for future research. Implementation Science 7 (1), 12.

Wiltsey-Stirman, S., Miller, C.J., Toder, K., Calloway, A., 2013. Development of a framework and coding system for modifications and adaptations of evidence-based interventions. Implementation Science 8 (1), 65.

Wood, J.J., Fujii, C., Renno, P., 2011. Autism symptom severity during school recess: A preliminary randomized, controlled trial. Journal of Autism and Developmental Disorders 44 (9), 2264—2276.

Wood, J.J., Ehrenreich-May, J., Alessandri, M., Fujii, C., Renno, P., Laugeson, E., et al., 2015a. Cognitive behavioral therapy for early adolescents with autism spectrum disorders and clinical anxiety: A randomized, controlled trial. Behavior therapy 46 (1), 7—19.

Wood, J.J., McLeod, B.D., Klebanoff, S., Brookman-Frazee, L., 2015b. Toward the implementation of evidence-based interventions for youth with autism spectrum disorders in schools and community agencies. Behavior Therapy 46 (1), 83—95.

INDEX

Note: Page numbers followed by "*t*" refer to tables.

Printed and bound by CPI Group (UK) Ltd, Croydon, CR0 4YY

08/06/2025

01896873-0001